Psychiatric Management for Medical Practitioners

Psychiatric Management for Medical Practitioners

Edited by

Donald S. Kornfeld, M.D.
Professor of Clinical Psychiatry
Columbia University College of Physicians and Surgeons
Chief, Psychiatric Consultation-Liaison Service
Presbyterian Hospital
New York, New York

Jerry B. Finkel, M.D.
Assistant Professor of Clinical Psychiatry
Columbia University College of Physicians and Surgeons
Chief, Psychiatry Liaison Service, Internal Medicine
Presbyterian Hospital
New York, New York

GRUNE & STRATTON
A Subsidiary of Harcourt Brace Jovanovich, Publishers
New York London
Paris San Diego San Francisco São Paulo
Sydney Tokyo Toronto

Library of Congress Cataloging in Publication Data
Main entry under title:

Psychiatric management for medical practitioners.

Bibliography: p.
Includes index.
1. Psychiatry. 2. Family medicine. I. Kornfeld, Donald S. II. Finkel, Jerry B. [DNLM: 1. Mental disorders. 2. Family practice. WM 100 P97752]
RC454.4.P76 616.89 81-7101
ISBN 0-8089-1420-0 AACR2

Grune & Stratton, Inc.
111 Fifth Avenue
New York, New York 10003

Distributed in the United Kingdom by
Academic Press Inc. (London) Ltd.
24/28 Oval Road, London NW 1

Library of Congress Catalog Number 81-7101
International Standard Book Number 0-8089-1420-0
Printed in the United States of America

To my parents, Rebecca and the late Benjamin Kornfeld, my wife Edythe, and our daughters, Anne, Deborah, and Harriet.

DSK

To my mother, Gertrude, and my father, the late Samuel Finkel, and my dear son, Benjamin.

JBF

Contents

Preface

Experienced clinicians do not need to be told that a large percentage of their patients come to them with emotional problems. However, these clinicians often feel inadequately equipped to deal with these matters; they usually attribute their failure to provide these patients with adequate treatment to two factors: insufficient training and lack of time.

Unfortunately, the typical medical school curriculum in psychiatry emphasizes diagnosis and neglects treatment. Most often, the medical student learns to do a work-up of a patient, make a diagnosis, speculate on etiology, and "refer the patient for psychiatric treatment." Such training offers little help to the average practitioner in those situations where it is necessary to manage a patient without a referral. It also fails to prepare the student to deal with those kinds of patients who do not present at the psychiatric clinic or hospital of the typical medical school but who appear significantly often in the doctor's office. A partial list of these would include patients with marital and family problems, hypochondriasis, terminal illness, presurgical anxiety, chronic pain, sleep disorders, and alcoholism. We believe that this book can do a great deal to help by focusing on practical issues such as these and by teaching practicing physicians, house officers, and medical students efficient methods of dealing with them.

Clinicians will learn that they can do effective psychiatric evaluation and psychotherapy, and that this need not clog their waiting rooms nor demand a major financial sacrifice on the part of the patient or the physician. Indeed, practitioners use psychotherapeutic techniques all the time. Like the man who was shocked to learn that he had been speaking "prose" all his life, physicians should be made aware that they have psychotherapeutic skills. What they need to learn, however, is how to apply these skills in a more sophisticated and, therefore, more effective manner. Once properly trained, practitioners will find that this can become one of the most gratifying areas of medical practice.

Nonpsychiatrists probably write the majority of the prescriptions for psychopharmaclogical agents in this country; they should be better equipped to do so. We believe that these practitioners can be confused by the plethora of agents available and that as a result the wrong drug or the wrong dosage is too often prescribed. Psychopharmacology need not be so complicated. We believe that a physician can practice good office psychiatry with a few select drugs if these agents are properly used. Our chapters on the management of anxiety, depression, and psychosis explain how this can be done.

This book, therefore, is designed to be a supplement to standard textbooks of psychiatry. The table of contents reflects our basic orientation: each chapter discusses a specific and common type of problem and then outlines practical diagnostic and treatment approaches. Chapters that deal with topics not usually covered in medical school curricula also include some necessary background material.

The contributors are all clinician–teachers who have spent much of their professional careers working with physicians in a general hospital and its clinics. Thus they are aware of the problems with which medical practitioners must deal and of the limitations placed on them by time and training. However, to be certain that the problems and potential solutions presented would be useful to practicing physicians, we submitted individual chapters to our medical and surgical colleagues, who were asked to comment specifically on their completeness and practicality. Chapters were then revised to incorporate their suggestions. This book, then, is the product of an active collaboration with a group of physicians experienced in the day-to-day practice of medicine. It is hoped that this collaboration has produced a volume that will contribute to better patient care and greater physician satisfaction.

Acknowledgments

We are pleased that we were able to elicit the help of a group of experts in areas where we believed special knowledge was needed to make a chapter more helpful. Dr. Glenda Garvey, Chief of the Medical Intensive Care Unit, and Dr. Thomas Bigger, Chief of the Coronary Care Unit at the Presbyterian Hospital, provided considerable help in the preparation of the material dealing with the management of drug overdose. Dr. Joseph Tenenbaum of the Cardiology Department reviewed the material dealing with the management of sexual activity in cardiac patients. Dr. Lawrence Kolb reviewed the material on the management of pain, and Dr. Herbert Spiegel helped in the preparation of the section dealing with the use of hypnosis in pain management. Dr. Wilma Harrison made a major contribution to the material dealing with dysmenorrhea and the premenstrual syndrome. We are grateful for the benefits of their special expertise.

We are also very grateful to Drs. Harvey Schneier, Samuel Teichman, Carmen Neu, Arnold Lisio, Ramon Murphy, Anne Moore, Jeffrey Redmond, Bernard Edelstein, Gail Williams, Edward Bowe, and Mildred Bowen, who took time out from their busy professional lives to review individual chapters and to help make this volume as useful a work as we hope it can be. For advice and support, our thanks to Dr. John Schimel.

We are also particularly grateful to Ms. Sandra Bligen and her associate Ms. Elissa Pyatt for their many hours at the typewriter converting our illegible scrawlings into a workable manuscript.

D. S. K.
J. B. F.

Contributors

Kenneth Altschuler, M.D.	Professor and Chairman, Department of Psychiatry Southwestern Medical School Dallas, Texas
Paul Califano, M.D.	Assistant Clinical Professor of Psychiatry Columbia University College of Physicians and Surgeons and Assistant Attending Psychiatrist Presbyterian Hospital New York, New York
Richard Gardner, M.D.	Associate Clinical Professor of Psychiatry Columbia University College of Physicians and Surgeons and Associate Attending Psychiatrist Presbyterian Hospital New York, New York
Richard Glavin, M.D.	Assistant Clinical Professor of Psychiatry Columbia University College of Physicians and Surgeons and Assistant Attending Psychiatrist Presbyterian Hospital New York, New York
Elizabeth Hegeman, Ph.D.	Assistant Professor of Anthropology City University of New York New York, New York
Arthur Jacobs, M.D.	Assistant Clinical Professor of Psychiatry Columbia University College of Physicians and Surgeons and Liaison Psychiatrist, Renal Dialysis and Transplant Unit Presbyterian Hospital New York, New York

Lila Kalinich, M.D.
Assistant Clinical Professor of Psychiatry
Columbia University College of Physicians and Surgeons and
Liaison Psychiatrist, Obstetrics and Gynecology Service
Presbyterian Hospital
New York, New York

Neil Kavey, M.D.
Assistant Clinical Professor of Psychiatry
Columbia University College of Physicians and Surgeons and
Director, Sleep Disorders Center
Presbyterian Hospital
New York, New York

Samuel Klagsbrun, M.D.
Associate Clinical Professor of Psychiatry
Columbia University College of Physicians and Surgeons and
Associate Visiting Professor of Pastoral Psychiatry
Jewish Theological Seminary
New York, New York and
Medical Director, Four Winds Hospital
Katona, New York

Alexander Levay, M.D.
Associate Clinical Professor of Psychiatry
Columbia University College of Physicians and Surgeons and
Associate Attending Psychiatrist
Presbyterian Hospital
New York, New York

Michael R. Milano, M.D.
Assistant Clinical Professor of Psychiatry
Columbia University College of Physicians and Surgeons and
Liaison Psychiatrist, Surgery Service
Presbyterian Hospital
New York, New York

Philip Muskin, M.D.
Assistant Clinical Professor of Psychiatry
Columbia University College of Physicians and Surgeons and
Assistant Attending Psychiatrist
Presbyterian Hospital
New York, New York

Irene Seeland, M.D.
Assistant Clinical Professor of Psychiatry
Columbia University College of Physicians and Surgeons and
Liaison Psychiatrist, Oncology Service
Presbyterian Hospital
New York, New York

Lawrence Sharpe, M.D.
Assistant Professor of Clinical Psychiatry
Columbia University College of Physicians and Surgeons and
Research Psychiatrist
New York State Psychiatric Institute
New York, New York

Ralph N. Wharton, M.D.
Associate Clinical Professor of Psychiatry
Columbia University College of Physicians and Surgeons and
Associate Attending Psychiatrist
Presbyterian Hospital
New York, New York

Richard Wortman, M.D.
Assistant Professor of Psychiatry
Mt. Sinai School of Medicine and
Clinical Director, Mental Health Division
Adolescent Health Center
Mt. Sinai Hospital
New York, New York

Stuart Yudofsky, M.D.
Associate Professor of Clinical Psychiatry
Columbia University College of Physicians and Surgeons and
Assistant Attending Psychiatrist
Presbyterian Hospital
New York, New York

Sheldon Zimberg, M.D.
Associate Professor of Psychiatry
Mt. Sinai School of Medicine and
Director of Psychiatry Service
North General Hospital
New York, New York

Jerry B. Finkel, M.D.

1

The Medical Interview and the Therapeutic Alliance

I. THE MEDICAL INTERVIEW

The most powerful tool a physician has is the relationship that develops between physician and patient. Without your patient's trust you may not obtain the data necessary to make a complete and accurate diagnosis. Without an adequate understanding of your patient's personality you will not be able to develop or make optimal therapeutic use of the relationship. Therefore, you must acquire the data that will help you to know your patient as an individual.[1, 2]

The medical interview that should provide these data is not the usual "psychiatric interview" taught in medical school. The information you need can be acquired in a less formal manner in the course of each medical interview, and throughout your ongoing relationship with your patient. You can train yourself to organize the data in meaningful categories that will help you diagnostically and therapeutically. This chapter describes the best ways of obtaining and organizing needed data and reviews some basic principles of developing and maintaining the therapeutic alliance. Both the collection of data and the development of an alliance proceed simultaneously from the moment patient and doctor first meet.

When a physician and patient first meet, anxiety is often aroused in both. For the patient, a visit to the physician is a reminder of a basic fact of life: the vulnerability of all people to illness. A visit to the doctor, no matter how minor the complaint or how routine the visit, brings this fact closer to consciousness, and this can arouse considerable anxiety.

To some extent, all patients are wary and distrustful of a stranger who asks for carte blanche. In a psychologically healthy patient, this initial anxiety is tempered by good reality testing, which leads to reduced anxiety and increased trust. Thus during their early meetings with patients, physicians need to keep in mind that they are dealing with anxious strangers. Moreover, people who are under stress are more likely than others to distort what transpires in an interaction. Until physicians learn with whom they are dealing, they must maintain appropriate neutrality, avoiding either too much intimacy or too much reserve. Throughout the course of the relationship the physician will have to gauge the emotional distance each individual requires.

OBTAINING MEDICAL AND PSYCHOSOCIAL INFORMATION

The history and the physicial and mental status examinations should provide sufficient information to establish a medical and psychiatric diagnosis. However, the physician also needs to obtain information that will provide:

- An overview of the patient's personal history and development with some knowledge of the cultural background and of the important people and events in the patient's life
- An evaluation of the patient's emotional maturity as measured by the capacity to function in marriage, family, work, and other relationships
- An appraisal of the patient's family's ability and willingness to offer support during illness.
- An understanding of the conscious and unconscious meanings of illness to the patient[3]
- An understanding of the patient's capacity to adapt to stress and illness[4]
- Some assessment of how stress might influence illness, pain, and other symptoms[5–7]

Data collection proceeds as we move along through the "flow-sheet" of history-taking and physical exam. There may never be a single point in an interview where we feel we are collecting only psychosocial data. There is a weaving in and out as we "converse," noting such things as a reaction to a question, a tone of voice, or a facial expression. The sections that follow will point out how to obtain and organize the necessary information.

General Principles of Interviewing

Opening the Initial Review

During the initial conversation, the usual rules of courtesy between two strangers need to be observed. Proper names should be used at the outset of every initial interview, and the doctor should be mindful of the patient's anxiety. Since no health examination is routine for the person experiencing it, the physician must not be fooled by superficial calm. Within a short period after the interview begins, the physician must determine just how anxious the patient is and what coping mechanisms he or she is using. Occasionally, early intervention is needed to reduce anxiety and prevent regressive and inappropriate behavior; such intervention is discussed in the following chapters. The physician's primary concern must be to recognize and accommodate to the psychological needs and limitations of the patient.

Language and Jargon: Designing Questions to Suit Patients

Learning to use plain English, after medical school and residency training, is not an easy task. The use of medical jargon or of English that is beyond the educational level of the patient will impede a physician's ability to collect relevant data. It is often difficult to determine whether questions are appropriate for a particular patient. Patients may be too embarrassed to communicate their difficulties in understanding to the physician. The simplest language remains the most effective technique for communicating with patients. For example:

Doctor: "Have you a history of peptic ulcers or gall bladder disease?
Patient: "No."

but

Doctor: "Mr. Jones, have you ever had any pains in the stomach?
Patient: "Yes, for two years, right up here (pointing to his abdomen). The pain goes all the way through to my back. My family doctor told me I had a sore in my stomach.

Directive and Nondirective History Taking

The two major approaches to history taking, the directive and nondirective, employ closed-end and open-ended questions, respectively.[8] Both approaches are necessary for any medical evaluation. The directive, closed-end technique is recommended when the physician requires specific responses regarding aspects of the patient's history. It is important not to force negatives. Hurried physicians who rush through a past medical history or review of systems by prefacing their questions with, "There is no history of ——— is there?" will miss data.

Here is an example of a structured sequence in a directive interview.

Doctor: Mr. Jones, have you had any pain in your chest?
Patient: Yes, I've had some pain in my chest that would come and go mainly while I was walking.
Doctor: What did the pain feel like?
Patient: What do you mean?
Doctor: Did the pain feel as if it were coming from outside or inside your chest?
Patient: Outside.
Doctor: Did it ever feel as if someone were sitting on your chest?
Patient: Yes, that's exactly how it felt.
Doctor: Did you ever have any pain in your left arm or in your right arm, or on your chin or in your teeth?
Patient: Yes, last night I felt a pain in my fingers and along the left side of my jaw.
Doctor: How long did the pain last?
Patient: It lasted about three minutes, then slowly went away.

Note how each question in this sequence is designed to elicit a specific, short answer.

Although an interview like the preceding one is helpful in obtaining concrete medical information, it will usually not allow certain pathological thinking disorders to appear. For example, tangential or loosened associations are not likely to become apparent until open-ended questions are asked. In a less structured interview, you will get a more precise picture of how your patient's thought processes operate. The more structured questions should be used early in the interview, but always after the patient has been allowed to tell you about the chief complaint in his or her own words. The directive technique will provide much needed information and will help put the patient at ease. Later in the interview open-ended questions can be introduced.

The nondirective approach using open-ended questions is preferable for eliciting psychosocial information. This technique is more likely to allow the patient to express emotional and unconscious material. A question such as "Is your marriage okay?" answered "Yes" or "No," does not give us much information. Open-ended questions that may begin with "Tell me about—" such as "Tell me about your spouse," or "What sort of person is your spouse?" or "Describe your relationship with your spouse," are more likely to allow patients to express their feelings.

Open-ended questions help elicit emotional responses and facilitate a deeper understanding of the nature of a relationship. The interviewer should follow the patient's lead in developing the interview. If the patient provides hints of areas that are emotionally important, these should be explored by means of nondirective, open-ended questions. In this technique, the physician follows the lead in the flow of the patient's responses rather than staying within a preconceived format. This technique allows associative processes to facilitate a freer production of information. It is important to remember that patients unconsciously try to keep painful or conflictual material out of awareness. Direct confrontation will only produce defensive responses. The physician should use open-ended questions and pay attention to the developing themes as they emerge. Here is an example of a sequence in an open-ended interview:

Patient: The back pain I was telling you about began in the morning about two weeks ago.

Doctor: What were you doing at that time?

Patient: My wife and I were going over the bills, and I must say we were quite upset.

Doctor: What was the problem?

Patient: There doesn't seem to be enough money to go around, and I cannot seem to convince my wife that we need to cut down on our spending.

Doctor: Tell me more about it.

Patient: Well, the money issue has been a tough one for us on the salary that I make.

Doctor: Can you tell me more about your wife and the problems?

Patient: Basically, she is a decent person. We get along well in other matters. I feel that she just doesn't understand me or the financial realities of life.

Doctor: How does this make you feel?

Patient: Very unhappy and angry with her. There are times when I feel like exploding and walking out, but I don't because I care about her.

Parallel History Taking

It is often difficult, if not impossible, for some patients to associate their physical complaints with stressful events in their personal lives. Therefore, a direct inquiry regarding such an association—for example, asking a patient who complains of physical pain, "Do you think your pain can be related to any stress in your life?"—may not get you the information you need for an accurate appraisal. On the other hand, if you take two histories, a history of the physical complaint and a history of the patient's recent personal life, and place them in parallel, striking associations can become apparent. In addition to the obvious common sources of stresses such as job or marital problems, anniversaries are often stressful events, in particular the anniversaries of the deaths of close friends or relatives.

A 20-year-old single male was admitted to the hospital with an eleven-month history of ulcerative colitis. The patient understood that the consultant was inquiring into his personal life because it was thought that emotional factors might play a role in triggering an episode of ulcerative colitis. The patient was not aware of any connection between his illness and personal problems.

Following a careful medical evaluation, the doctor proceeded to take a history of the patient's life. He learned that the patient was the oldest son of a successful businessman. The patient had considerable academic difficulty in school, and on completion of high school he had taken a job working as an office boy for a local firm. He experienced increasing conflict with his parents living at home, so he moved out, took his own apartment, and shortly thereafter began living with his girlfriend. He was given increasing responsibility on his job but very little additional pay. Because of the financial pressures of maintaining the household, he left the office job and took a job in a local factory, where the pay was considerably better. However, he found that the working conditions were very bad. He was surrounded by toxic fumes and great heat; it was generally a very uncomfortable place in which to work. However, he felt that he could not leave the job, because he very much needed the money to maintain his independence, and that was his overriding concern. It was in this setting of conflict that the first episode of ulcerative colitis took place.

Having this information, the physician suggested to the patient that perhaps the episode of colitis was related to the stress of that situation. The patient was then able to make the connection between the conflict with which he was living at the time of the initial episode and the onset of the illness.

Listening with the Third Ear

Sometimes patients' communications are understood only by listening for themes in the seemingly unconnected thoughts of an interview. Eliciting such themes is a skill that calls for listening with what psychiatrists call "the third ear." Identifying such themes can help the physician understand what the patient is in conflict about but cannot communicate directly. For example, suppose a patient tells her physician that she has been suffering abdominal pains. She also mentions her husband's frequent business trips. She discusses some problems with one of her children. The physician may sense that the patient is angry about the frequent separations which leave her alone to deal with family problems, even though the patient does not express that thought or emotion directly. He may infer some connection between the physical pain, the separations, and the patient's conflict regarding her husband's career and her own needs. These communications are very important in understanding a patient's illness and in developing a treatment plan. The parallel history-taking technique already described helps in obtaining these kinds of data.

The process of the interview—that is, the developing relationship—must be monitored at all times. Defensive responses, anger, silence, or other nonverbal communications should alert you to the fact that a patient is in conflict. You must then decide if you wish to pursue the matter further or switch to another topic. In most situations, after reassuring the patient you can explore a topic further, but you must always give the patient the right not to answer your questions. Inappropriate and ill-timed interpretations concerning these areas may lead to denial and defensive responses and may weaken the therapeutic alliance. The reader is referred to Chapter 3 for advice regarding the exploration of anxiety-laden areas.

Using The Family

The physician must try to develop a working relationship with significant people in the patient's life, as they are an invaluable source of information and can help in influencing a patient to comply with a treatment plan. Often, for the patient who is acutely ill, anxiety may preclude any real comprehension of what a physician is asking. Therefore, the family should be utilized to help provide the information needed. This is easily accomplished when a patient is hospitalized and the family is readily available. For the office patient, such interviews are more difficult to arrange. In some situations, however, they are worth the special effort. Where both husband and wife are your patients, obvious opportunities for such background information-gathering are present.

The patient's spouse may provide the best information about compliance with a medication regimen, a diet, or the like and may also provide insight regarding recent life stresses that the patient himself or herself may not be able to identify or acknowledge. Be wary of patients who respond to questions with one-word answers: "How are things going at home, Mr. Jones?" "Fine." "How are things at work?" "Fine." Chances are that this patient's wife will give you a much better history.

It is important to begin to gather data regarding how family members relate to each other as early as possible in your relationship with the patient. Such information regarding the reliability of family support will prove invaluable should one member of the family become seriously ill.

Specific Areas of Inquiry

Each section of the medical history allows the physician to obtain some of the data needed. Questions can be designed which fit into the framework of the medical evaluation. Some examples are explored in the next several sections.

Chief Complaint and Present Illness

Patients are preoccupied with the distress of their illness and need to communicate this to the physician. This need takes precedence over everything else. Patients need to feel that they have been given enough time to tell the story their way. Specific questions asked too early may be misinterpreted as a lack of concern or as a sign of an impatient doctor. Therefore, during the "Chief Complaint" portion of the inquiry, the physician does best to listen to the story as the patient presents it. During the "Present Illness" inquiry, closed-ended questions may be used to obtain more specific information. This type of questioning is reassuring to patients, but only if they are convinced that their view of the trouble has been communicated. If it is possible to reassure patients about their concerns, do it as soon as possible. Do not wait until the end of the consultation.

Past Health

The physician should explore patients' reactions to previous illness and hospitalizations, including the effect of such experience on their lives and families. How did the patients respond psychologically to these stresses?

Most people tend to respond to specific kinds of stresses in a similar way each time they occur. Therefore, your patient's previous response to the enforced dependency of illness will probably serve as a reasonably good predictor of a future response. However, certain illnesses and their treatment have very particular meaning for individual patients and thus will arouse special responses. For example, malignancies, problems and/or procedures involving sexual organs, and myocardial infarction are likely to elicit such responses. Later chapters will deal with these issues in detail.

For some patients the emotional and psychiatric aftermath of a previous illness can be a particularly painful memory. For example, the patient who has experienced a post-operative delirium may fear a repetition of that experience more than the pain of future surgery. The physician who knows this can reassure the patient that should some type of surgery be required in the future, steps will be taken to prevent a recurrence of such an earlier experience. Some patients will focus on the terrible pain they experienced, pain that did not respond to the medicine they were given. These patients can be reassured that they were probably undermedicated and that no patient need suffer as they apparently did. By thus encouraging patients to share their experiences with you, you will acquire information that will be useful should they become ill in the future.

The physician should explore how well the patient has complied with treatment plans in the past. If the patient is found to have been a poor complier, the first thing to examine is the previous working alliance. What role did the physician's personality play? Exploration is then required to define whether the problem was denial of illness; oppositional, negativistic, or self-destructive behavior; educational or cultural problems; or a poorly informed patient. We will consider this problem again later.

Personal and Family History

Information regarding the patient's development, including significant events in his or her life, marriage, family, and other relationships should be obtained in some detail. Try to obtain data that gives you some sense of the personality style of individual family members and how they relate to each other. Are there family stresses? Begin with general open-ended questions such as "Tell me something about each of your children." Most patients will be pleased that you are interested in them as individuals and will discuss these matters. An occasional patient will not want to discuss these things and will tell you so. You have lost nothing by asking the questions. Perhaps, at a later date, such a patient will remember your expression of interest and communicate a personal problem to you.

Work History

It is essential to have some understanding of your patients' work experience. Are they steadily employed? Do they get a sense of satisfaction from their work? How do they get along with fellow workers and subordinates? Do they feel competent in their work? Get some sense of the way the patient approaches work and co-workers. Also, explore patients' sense of their areas of strength and limitation in their work.

With a woman who is a full-time homemaker and mother, be sure to discuss the stresses of these occupations. How long is the patient's day? Does she have any free time for herself? Does her husband understand the problems? Does he provide support? What kind? Homemakers and mothers resent our taking their role for granted, by not acknowledging the problems that accompany it. Further, it is especially important for women who also work outside the home to tell you about how their lives are organized and about the great pressure of this double role.

Excessive Drinking, Smoking, Eating

Managing these problems requires information regarding the patient's behavior, educating the patient regarding the medical consequences of that behavior, and acquiring an understanding of the patient's unconscious motivation for persisting in a self-destructive course.

How much does your patient drink and under what circumstances? Try to understand what function alcohol serves in their lives. For example, is it a tranquilizer for an anxious person? An antidepressant for a person who is depressed? A social disinhibitor for someone who is shy? Only by understanding the reasons for their use of this drug can you hope to help patients with an alcohol problem to deal with it. These patients probably do not need a lecture on the dangers of excessive drinking. You can be sure they have heard such a lecture. Patients expect you to understand that if you ask them to give up alcohol, they will suffer and, therefore, will require something in its place. If you establish that supportive base your treatment plan is more likely to succeed. Chapter 11 deals in more detail with the management of alcohol-related problems.

Similar information is needed about their smoking. You need to know the number of cigarettes smoked and under what circumstances. You should be knowledgeable regarding the various techniques used to help patients who want to stop smoking. Knowledge of the amount of tobacco used will help you determine whether the patient is physically addicted to nicotine, and will need a withdrawal regimen.

The obese patient requires a careful history. Information regarding personal and family nutrition and eating patterns is essential. It is important to understand the patient's personality structure, family dynamics, and methods of dealing with stress since overeating can be related to these factors. Your understanding of the complex nature of the patient's motivation to eat will prove valuable in developing a workable diet program.[9, 10]

Living Arrangements

The physician should explore the circumstances of the patient's living situation. What is the home like? What are the sleeping arrangements? How much privacy is there? The patient should be asked how he or she feels about the present situation and what stresses on the family the living arrangements may cause.

Financial Situation

The physician should explore the patient's financial situation. Although patients need not reveal specific details of their income, general questions such as "How are you managing financially?" can determine whether the patient wishes to discuss this further. Obviously, financial problems cause a great deal of stress, but they can also be used to obscure other family problems. The impact of illness on a patient's finances should also be explored. Knowledge acquired earlier can be helpful in your planning when illness occurs.

Emotional History

The initial interviews with a new patient should be directed toward obtaining, in addition to past psychiatric history, information helpful in appraising his or her emotional maturity and capacity to function in relationships, work, and leisure. The patient's strengths as well as maladaptive character traits should be evaluated. Try to determine the patient's sense of himself as an independent, stable person and his or her capacity for a relatively unambivalent, empathic caring relationship. How much do entitlement, dependency, or transference distortions interfere?

Establish a climate in which patients feel you care about their emotional state. Questions should be asked in a way that communicates an interested, nonjudgmental attitude. For example: "Do you consider yourself to be a nervous person?" "Do you consider yourself to be a sensitive person?" "Are you hard-driving?" "Are you able to relax?" "Are you emotional or do you keep your feelings under tight control?" "Does your mood tend to fluctuate?" "Are you impatient or easygoing?"

General inquiries such as, "How is your mood?" "Are there any tensions or worries in your life these days?" or "Any major changes in your family or career since you were here last?" are useful. However, personalized questions are even more likely to get a meaningful reply: for example, "How are things going for you at the office? "How do you feel about moving?" "How do you like your new job?" "How does it feel to be retired?" "How are your kids?" "Mary is due to graduate from high school, isn't she? What are her plans?" "What is it like for you now that John's a teenager?" "How is it going now that your mother is living with you?" Such questions tell patients you know them as individuals and consider data regarding their emotional lives to be an important part of their medical history.

Systems Review

Some parts of the routine systems review provide additional opportunities for obtaining important data. For example, the genitourinary section can be used to explore questions relating to the patient's sex life. You can begin with a general question such as, "Do you have a satisfactory and pleasurable sex life?" You can ask, "What birth control method do you use?" Most patients will accept these questions as an understandable part of the history dealing with an important part of their lives. Many will be grateful for your giving them the opportunity to discuss these issues. For those who do not wish to talk about their sexual activity, no further inquiries should be made during the initial history. However, by including such an inquiry in the routine review of systems, you have let your patient know that you consider this to be an important area of medical concern. When ready, he or she may return to this topic. Our patients expect us to be knowledgeable about sex. A feeling that this is too personal a matter to be discussed is usually a projection of our own feelings, and reflects our anxiety about dealing with these issues. Chapter 9 deals with the management of sexual problems.

The Psychiatric Diagnosis and Mental Status Examination

The mental status examination assesses a patient's state of mental functioning at a given time and is part of the psychiatric examination. Most of the information required can be obtained during the course of the regular history. For example, you can judge a patient's recent and remote memory reasonably well in the course of taking a detailed medical history. If any organic or psychiatric syndrome is suspected, a formal mental status examination should be conducted. Such an examination is designed to elicit signs of organic and psychiatric disorders. Standard textbooks of psychiatry contain detailed descriptions of how to do a mental status examination, and later chapters of this book discuss the mental status in specific disorders. Figure 1-1 presents a short mental status examination that can be used as a quick screening device.[11]

Figure 1–1. Mental status examination.[11]

Examiner ______________________________ Date __________

Instructions for Examiner: Check items answered correctly. Write incorrect or unusual answers in space provided. If necessary, urge patient, once only, to complete task.

Introduction to Patient: "I would like to ask you a few questions. Some you will find very easy and others may be very hard. Just do your best."

1. What day of the week is this? __________
2. What month? __________
3. What day of the month? __________
4. What year? __________
5. What place is this? __________
6. Repeat the numbers: 8 7 2. __________
7. Say them backwards. __________
8. Repeat these numbers: 6 3 7 1. __________
9. Listen to these numbers: 6 9 4. Count from 1 through 10 out loud. Then repeat 6 9 4. (Help, if needed; then use numbers 5 7 3). __________
10. Listen to these numbers: 8 1 4 3. Count from 1 through 10 out loud; then repeat 8 1 4 3. __________
11. Beginning with Sunday, say the days of the week backwards. __________
12. 9 + 3 equals __________
13. Add 6 (*to the previous answer, or to 12*) __________
14. Take away 5 (*from 18*). Repeat these words *after me* and *remember them.* I will ask for them later: *hat, car, tree, twenty-six.* __________
15. The opposite of *fast* is *slow*. The opposite of *up* is __________
16. The opposite of *large* is __________

17. The opposite of *hard* is ______
18. An orange and a banana are both fruits. Red and blue are both ______
19. A penny and a dime are both ______
20. What were those words I asked you to remember (*hat*) ______
21. (*Car*) ______
22. (*Tree*) ______
23. (*Twenty-six*) ______
24. Take away 7 from 100; then take away 7 from what is left and keep going: 100 − 7 equals ______
25. Minus 7 (*Write down answers; check correct subtraction of 7*) ______
26. Minus 7 ______
27. Minus 7 ______
28. Minus 7 ______
29. Minus 7 ______
30. Minus 7 ______

Total Correct (maximum score = 30) ______

Patient's occupation (previous, if not employed) ______
Education ______ Age ______.
Estimated intelligence (based on education, occupation, and history, not on a test score):

______

(Below average, average, above average)

Patient was: Cooperative ______ Uncooperative ______
Depressed ______ Lethargic ______ Other ______

Medical Diagnosis:

A score of less than 20, indicates diminished cognitive capacity. In this case, an organic mental syndrome should be suspected and the following information obtained.

Temp. ______
BP ______
Hct ______
Na ______
K ______
Cl ______
CO_2 ______
EEG ______
ECG ______

BUN ______
Glu ______
PO_2 ______
PCO_2 ______

Endocrine dysfunction? ______
T_3 T_4 Ca, P, etc.
History of previous psychiatric difficulty ______

______

Use of drugs, including steroids? L-Dopa? amphetamines? tranquilizers? digitalis? ______

______

Focal neurological signs: ______
DIAGNOSIS: ______

______

The Physical Examination

Do not deceive yourself that you can forget about communication during the physical exam. The average patient becomes closely attuned to nonverbal cues at this time. For example, a patient may think, why did the doctor spend so much time listening in that one spot? What did that change in the doctor's facial expression mean? You must, therefore, avoid sending messages in this way. You must also be sensitive to the possibility that your patient may easily misinterpret what transpires. Give patients a chance to express these concerns by asking them, at the conclusion of the physical exam, if they have any questions about your findings.

You can also do a great deal to reduce anxiety as you go along by communicating some significant findings that are negative. For example, "Your blood pressure is just fine," or "That rectal exam was normal." This procedure tells patients that you are aware of their unspoken anxiety and will do what you can to make them more comfortable, whenever you can.

THE PHYSICIAN-PATIENT ALLIANCE

In the working alliance between physician and patient there is an unsigned, unspoken treatment contract. Both understand what behavior is expected and the limitations of the relationship. This is the real relationship between the two, and it requires a nondistorted appraisal of each other. This developing alliance, however, can be complicated by social, cultural, and unconscious processes. The most common unconscious mechanisms are referred to as transference and countertransference reactions.

Transference

Transference is an unconscious phenomenon, potentially ubiquitous in all relationships. It refers to an unconscious tendency to assign feelings and attitudes originally linked to significant figures of the patient's early life to someone in the present. When it is intense, it interferes with the capacity to relate to others without distortions. In the medical setting, it may interfere with the working alliance between patient and physician. For example, patients may reactivate an infantile need for an omnipotent, nondemanding, gratifying parent in the relationship with their physician. When we fail to meet unrealistic expectations, the relationship suffers. The age and sex of the physician is immaterial, as patients can make mothers and sisters from middle-aged male physicians. Some patients develop a transference reaction to a hospital or institution. This allows them to be indifferent to the changing personnel as long as the setting remains the same.

Transference, like our early relationships with our parents, always contains positive and negative feelings. Usually trusting, cooperative feelings prevail, but negative reactions including mistrust, anger, and even hatred may occur. Often both exist with one or the other repressed and emerging, without awareness, through action, e.g., noncompliant behavior.

Some positive, and most negative, transference reactions are difficult for physicians because they evoke strong counterresponses which interfere with their ability to work with patients. Patients who exhibit demanding, hostile, suspicious, or competitive transferences can evoke angry, hateful responses from physicians. The management of such patients is discussed in detail in Chapter 2. Some patients will sexualize the transference. For example, the seductive female patient may be expressing her need for care in the only way she knows how. The management of this problem is discussed in detail in Chapter 4.

Unconscious Conflict and Countertransference in Physicians

Physicians are as vulnerable to transference and other unconsciously determined emotional responses and behavior as their patients. Their reactions to their patients will also be affected by their own life experience, expectations, cultural background, and psychologic maturity. All of these may lead to misperceptions and inappropriate behavior, which will be referred to here as countertransference. For example, the physician who suspects every patient is potentially litiginous may be unconsciously reliving an important mistrustful relationship in childhood. The doctor who "forgets" to visit a dying patient may be expressing an unconscious fear of death; guilt over not providing adequate care; or unacceptable wishes for the patient's death. Here is a clinical example:

> A young female medical resident was treating an elderly, confused woman suffering from a pneumoccocal pneumonia. During the workup, the physician was aware of an increasing sense of involvement, sympathy, and affection for the patient. When the diagnosis was established and treatment instituted, small doses of haloperidol (Haldol) were also begun to control the patient's aggressive and confused organic mental syndrome. Although the nursing and medical care were adequate on the ward where the patient was being treated the physician began to feel that this patient required transfer to the Intensive Care Unit. When the case was reviewed by the ICU staff, they recommended that the patient remain on the ward, where she was receiving proper attention. Angered, the medical resident accused the attending staff of being insensitive to the needs of this sick woman. Again, the ICU staff reassured her, and by the following morning, it was clear that the patient was making significant improvement.
>
> In discussing her feelings with the liaison psychiatrist, the medical resident became aware that the requested transfer reflected a variety of conscious and unconscious motives. She was afraid that this patient, who was critically ill, might die. She feared she was too inexperienced to deal with this problem. She hoped the "gifted" physicians in the ICU could save her. This confused, aggressive, elderly woman was also not allowing

the resident to provide optimal care. She felt helpless, then angry. This anger was unacceptable to her and initially repressed. Later, it evoked a guilty response.

In the course of the discussion with the psychiatrist, the resident realized that this patient had reactivated feelings originally evoked by her mother, who had been intensely critical of her and guilt-provoking. As this young physician grew to maturity, the constant message from her mother was that her success in life was only possible because of the mother's self-sacrifice and that she had never done enough in return. The resident was experiencing this elderly patient as the mother she loved ambivalently and for whom she could never do enough. This countertransference response was the major reason for the physician's need to insure the best care in the ICU and the angry attack on the ICU staff when they refused her request.

Physicians' unconscious needs may thus produce patterns of behavior which ultimately are counterproductive.[12] Here are some examples: (1) The physician who must play the role of the omnipotent healer, who can "do no wrong." This is an attitude sure to ultimately bring the physician and/or the patients to grief. (2) The physician who must overly gratify his patients' every need, because he cannot tolerate their disliking him. As a consequence, he may try to anticipate what he thinks they will want to hear or have done, rather than what is truly in their best interest. (3) The chronically angry physician who may be reacting to an inability to gratify an unconscious need to be constantly in control of events or a feeling that he or she is not truly appreciated. (4) The anxious, perfectionistic physician who lives in fear of making a mistake, and burdens the patient with more tests and procedures than are really needed for fear he will miss something. He is unable to give them unqualified reassurance for fear that he could be wrong, and after all, how can you be absolutely certain about anything?

Dubovsky has summarized a variety of physician responses which usually suggest an unconscious conflict or countertransference reaction.[12] A modified version of his list follows.

Clues to the Presence of Countertransference

1. Experiencing any intense feeling greater than normal concern (especially anger, fear, guilt, disgust, sympathy, or sexual attraction)
2. Finding it difficult to pay attention to the patient; feeling preoccupied with other matters, drowsy or bored
3. Feeling unable to understand or empathize with the patient
4. Arguing with the patient
5. Feeling vulnerable to the patient's criticisms and becoming defensivc
6. Dreading the patient's visits
7. Feeling the patient doesn't really appreciate all you have done for him or her
8. Attempting to impress the patient with one's knowledge and prowess

9. Becoming excessively preoccupied with the patient as indicated by:
    a. repeatedly discussing the patient with others
    b. eager or unpleasant anticipation of the patient's next visit
10. Lack of concern about the patient
11. Departing from the usual routine with similar patients; for example, by consistently:
    a. talking more or less than usual
    b. seeing the patient earlier or later than the usual time
    c. cutting the patient's visit short or prolonging it
    d. failing to charge the patient

Whenever physicians experience such emotional responses or behavior, Dubovsky suggests that they ask themselves the following questions:

1. Are the doctor's feelings in direct proportion to the patient's behavior, or do they stem from the physicians's own personality conflicts?
2. Does an apparent lack of reaction, where one should occur, hide strong feelings?
3. Are there factors in the doctor's life, unrelated to the patient, that predispose the doctor towards such a strong reaction?
4. Does the patient remind the doctor of anyone in his or her life?
5. Are the physician's feelings characteristic of the way in which he or she responds to certain types of patients?
6. What does the doctor's reaction reveal about the patient?
7. Is the physician in danger of acting on his or her feelings?
8. Would consultation with a colleague help to clarify the physician's response and point out how to proceed?

Guidelines for Developing the Alliance

Sullivan provides a set of helpful guidelines in developing and maintaining a therapeutic alliance:[13] (1) Physicians need to understand the meaning of illness to their patients. (2) Doctors must understand what is going on between themselves and their patients. This requires an appreciation of the patient's perception of the physician and an understanding of their own responses to the patient. (3) Physicians need to recognize and accommodate to the patient's psychological needs and limitations and to accept them as they are. The following is a clinical example that illustrates several of these principles:

> An anxious 56-year-old male was admitted to the hospital for anemia and leukocytosis. The workup revealed chronic lympathic leukemia, an illness that may go on for years without producing much disability. The physician told the patient his diagnosis, explained its clinical course, and then explained that the patient's illness was mild and that he could expect at least ten good years before much difficulty. To his surprise the patient became suspicious, angry, and depressed. The physician felt unappreciated and upset.

On further exploration, the physician learned that to this patient, "mild" suggested that the physician was probably covering up bad news. Leukemia meant a certain and horrible death similar to that which he had seen his first wife endure. The ten-year prognosis meant death at a time when his son would be reaching mid-adolescence, when this lively and enthusiastic patient had hoped to enjoy the renaissance of his life.

The physician had not appreciated this patient's capacity to distrust physicians nor the effects of his wife's illness on his own perceptions of the illness. In addition, sixty-six did not mean constriction of activity or a reasonable life span to this man, whereas to the physician it did. The doctor and his patient obviously had quite different perceptions and expectations which the physician did not appreciate in developing his approach to this patient.

Nothing is ever static between people, particularly in the medical setting. The needs of patients will vary over time and with changes in the situation. The physician must be aware of the changing nature of the relationship. As anxiety and fear diminish, the patient may become more psychologically integrated and transference reactions may disappear or change. The physician needs to adjust the bedside or office approach accordingly. An authoritative stand may be useful for an acutely ill patient on the day of admission but may be inappropriate two days later or at a follow-up visit in the physician's office.

As we will examine in Chapter 2, some patients can regress under the stress of illness to demanding anger, clinging dependency, or self-destructive noncompliance. Although physicians can generally maintain clinical objectivity towards patients who are seriously psychologically disabled, such as the psychotic patient, they may have difficulty accepting these other types of behavior as forms of clinical disability.

Such patients can be a great burden to physicians. We are asked to relinquish the expectation of being appreciated and to accept such uncooperative, and at times, hostile behavior with equanimity. We may be asked to accept limitations on the quality of our medical care. All of this is not easy. The need to do a good job and be appreciated is strong, and we are all vulnerable to assaults on our self-esteem. Where there is a need to conquer illness, maintain illusions of power, or deny anxieties about death, the physician's own needs, conflicts, and countertransference responses will play a significant role in determining his or her reactions to patients. Our responsibility is to try and be aware of what is going on in ourselves so that we can identify such processes before they interfere with patient care.[14-17]

REFERENCES

1. Engel GL, Morgan WL Jr. The Clinical Approach to the Patient. Philadelphia, WB Saunders Company
2. Lewis JM, Usdin, G: Disease, illness and the interview, in Usdin O, Lewis J (eds): Psychiatry in General Medical Practice. New York, McGraw Hill, Inc. 1979, pp 3–22

3. Strain J: Psychiatric assessment in the medical setting, in Strain J, Grossman S (eds): Psychological Care of the Medically Ill: A Primer in Liaison Psychiatry. New York, Appleton, Century, Crofts, 1975, pp 11–23
4. Lipowski ZJ: Physical illness: The individual and the coping process. Psychiatr Med 2:91–102, 1970
5. Schmale, AH: Giving up as a final common pathway to change in health. Adv Psychosom Med 8:20–40, 1972
6. Jacobs S, Ostfeld A: An epidemiological review of the mortality of bereavement. Psychsom Med 39:344–357, 1977
7. Stein M, Schiavi RC, Camerino M: Influence of brain and behavior on the immune system. Science 191: 435–440, February 1976
8. Engel GL, Morgan WL Jr: The Clinical Approach to the Patient. Philadelphia, WB Saunders Company
9. Stunkard AJ: Obesity, in Arieti S (ed): American Handbook of Psychiatry, vol 4, ed 2. New York, Basic Books, 1979, pp 767–787
10. Bruch H: Eating disorders, in Arieti S (ed): American Handbook of Psychiatry. New York, Basic Books, 1973, pp 109–194
11. Jacobs JW, Bernhard MR, Delgado A, et al: Screening for organic mental syndromes in the medically ill. Ann Intern Med 86:40, 1977
12. Dubovsky SL: Psychotherapeutics in Primary Care. New York, Grune & Stratton, 1981
13. Crowley RM: Cognitive elements in Sullivan's theory and practice. Acad Psychoanal 8: 117–125, January 1980
14. Schontz FC: The personal meaning of illness. Adv Psychosom Med 8:63–85, 1972
15. Cassell E: Reactions to physical illness and hospitalization, in Usden F, Lewis, J. (eds): Psychiatry in General Medical Practice. New York, McGraw-Hill, Inc. 1979
16. Fabrega HJ: Culture, language, and the shaping of illness: An illustration based on pain. J Psychosom Med 20:323–337, 1976
17. Strain J: Psychological reactions to medical illness and hospitalization, in Strain J, Grossman S (eds): Psychological Care of the Medically Ill: A Primer in Liaison Psychiatry. New York, Appleton, Century, Crofts, 1975

BIBLIOGRAPHY

Arieti S (ed): American Handbook of Psychiatry, vol 4, ed 2. New York, Basic Books, 1979

Bird B: Talking with Patients, (ed 2). Philadelphia, JB Lippincott, 1973

Cassell A: The Healers' Art. Philadelphia, JB Lippincott, 1976

Drassman D: The problem patient: Evaluation and care of medical patients with psychosocial disturbances. Ann Intern Med 88:366–372, 1978

Dubovsky SL: Psychotherapeutics in Primary Care. New York, Grune & Stratton, 1981, pp 48–82

Engel GL: The need for a new medical model: A challenge for biomedicine. *Science* 196:129–135, 1977

Hyman MD: Social psychological factors affecting disability among ambulatory patients. J Chronic Dis 28:199–216, 1975

Kiely WF: Coping with severe illness. Adv Psychosom Med 8:105–118, 1972

MacKinnon RA, Michels R: The Psychiatric Interview in Clinical Practice. Philadelphia, W.B. Saunders, 1971

Sullivan HS: The Psychiatric Interview. Perry, HS Gawel ML (eds). New York, WW Norton, 1954

Jerry B. Finkel, M.D
Elizabeth Hegeman, Ph.D.

2

Working with Patients Who Present Special Problems

This chapter will explore a variety of clinical problems that interfere with adequate medical care and will suggest methods for dealing with them. The reader will find references in the bibliography for further exploration of these issues. These disparate problems have in common the capacity to evoke strong emotional responses in the treating physician. Many provoke anger, anxiety and guilt, and may cause the physician to perceive a patient as an onerous burden rather than as a difficult, clinical puzzle.

THE "DIFFICULT" PATIENT

Jerry B. Finkel, M.D.

The behavior of the "difficult patient" is usually the manifestation of an underlying personality disorder. A *personality disorder* is characterized by a chronic, maladaptive, inflexible pattern of perception, cognition, and behavior and usually also by impaired social and occupational functioning.

Personality disorders exist on a continuum of psychological integration and maturity. Four types of patients in particular evoke angry, even hateful feelings in their physicians: the *dependent clinger,* the *entitled demander,* the *self-destructive denier* and the *antisocial patient*. We will discuss each of these as well as several other personality disorder types: the obsessional, suspicious (paranoid), isolated (schizoid), and overdramatic (histrionic) patient. Finally, we will consider two additional types of problem patient: the hypochondriacal patient and the non-complaint patient.

Personality Disorder Types

The Overly Dependent, Clinging Patient

These patients suffer from an insatiable need for care. They are quick to express their gratitude, so the physician is easily seduced into the supporting role. Initially, there is pleasure in the feelings of power and uniqueness that this kind of patient can produce. Eventually, however, the feelings begin to shift as the patient's demands for attention escalate. The physician begins to realize that no matter how much is given, it never seems to be enough, since these patients appear to think of their doctor as an inexhaustible supplier of their needs. Emotional exhaustion begins to set in, followed by a growing resentment. As a consequence of this anger, the patient may be avoided, rejected, or referred to a psychiatrist. The patient usually perceives referral as the equivalent of rejection. Such a referral is doomed to fail.

In order to avoid this unfortunate sequence of events, these patients must be identified early in the relationship, for example, beware of patients who are too effusive in their praise. The overly dependent patient must be told early on that you have some specific guidelines for your practice that have been established to preserve your own energy and capacity for understanding. For example, the patient may be told that phone calls outside of office hours are for emergencies only (establish your definition of "emergency"). The patient is then free to accept or reject your rules.

Most patients will accept your guidelines. They will most likely also push to test the limits. It will be a lot easier for you, if you need only remind the patient of your earlier understanding. In the long run such early firmness is in the patient's best interest. To do otherwise is to set up the unfortunate series of events described earlier.

The Angry, Demanding Patient

These patients resemble the dependent clingers in their needs but differ in the methods they use to extract your support. Instead of flattery they use intimidation and guilt. They are never satisfied, withhold payment, and threaten law suits. Such patients are usually struggling with a conflict regarding their dependency on their physician, and the rage is a surface manifestation of this conflict. The angry outbursts usually cover their underlying fear that they will be abandoned. Their anger at being ill is directed at their physicians.

Patients in this category generally are diagnosed as having a borderline personality disorder; that is, they are unstable and immature, with a psychological organization somewhere between psychosis and a more integrated state.[2] Borderline patients are characterized by an impulsivity that is usually self-destructive in nature; intense, inappropriate hostility; marked mood shifts; feelings of emptiness; self-centeredness; suspiciousness; demandingness; and feelings of entitlement. They suffer from identity and gender disturbances and show patterns of intense, unstable, polarized, exploitative relationships. Physicians, nurses, family, and others are regularly idealized or denigrated by these patients, who have a tendency to experience significant others and themselves as if they were either all good or all evil. They have the bewildering capacity to then make rapid shifts in these evaluations. The capacity to see certain people as all good or all bad is a primitive psychological mechanism called *splitting*. These patients cannot see themselves or others in a coherent way. People are misperceived, and these perceptions are ever changing so that stable, meaningful relationships are impossible. Borderline patients also have almost no capacity to appreciate what is done for them and they denigrate much of the effort of their physicians, often with great hostility. It is no wonder that physicians often respond with increasing frustration, helplessness, dislike, and hatred.

Borderline behavior represents an angry demand for care and a return to a pain-free, anxiety-free state provided by a powerful and supportive authority, in this case, the doctor. Without these defenses, the patient runs the risk of overwhelming anxiety. Stress of any kind exaggerates these qualities in the patient.

How should one deal with this clincial problem, which elicits such strong emotional reactions? First, it is important for the treating physicians to know that their angry feelings are understandable. It is a great relief to a physician to know that he is not alone in responding so strongly. These patients make us feel helpless and unappreciated and often will not allow us to deliver adequate care. The result is anger and guilt. The difficulty is acknowledging the presence of these feelings and then dealing with them without acting them out, either overtly or covertly. It is possible to be angry, and through understanding, still carry out proper medical care.

To begin with, it is necessary to keep in mind that these patients are psychologically disabled and have limited control over their actions. Their provocative behavior must, therefore, be treated as a symptom. This can be accomplished without compromising personal integrity or principles of good medical care.

There are several things that can be done to reduce the patient's anxiety and promote better medical care. Groves has suggested the following treatment protocol for the hospitalized borderline patient.[3]

1. One physician should clearly be responsible for the patient's care. An ongoing relationship with the same staff member is essential.
2. The physician should maintain a professional, sympathetic approach. Too much closeness or distance frightens these patients. One should see them frequently, but visits need not be prolonged.
3. Nursing staff changes should be kept to a minimum.
4. Sympathetic limit setting on inappropriate behavior should be maintained. Behavior that is dangerous to the patient or others must be interpreted and firmly limited. Do it without anger and with an understanding of what is going on with the patient.
5. These patients need to feel entitled to the best of care. They fear unconsciously that you do not agree. When patients express their doubts regarding the quality of care they are receiving, avoid confrontations. Try responding that you agree that they are entitled to the best of care and that you will do all in your power to arrange that. You must try to help the patient understand that "the best of care" does not mean perfect care, which does not exist. You must acknowledge that the minor inefficiencies and inconveniences on which the patient focuses do exist, but then point out that they are not really going to affect the outcome of his or her illness. In this way, you avoid getting into an argument in which you need to defend your hospital or office staff.
6. When indicated, point out to patients that they are understandably angry at being ill, but that they are misdirecting their rage at those who are caring for him.
7. The patient must always be kept informed of his medical situation and of any changes in his diagnostic or treatment program.
8. Frequent staff meetings are necessary to discuss the effects of these patients' behavior. Borderline patients have the capacity to induce a wide range of reactions in the people who must work with them. If the patient's physician understands the behavior and can explain the patient's unconscious needs to the staff, the behavior will be more manageable. As you might expect, such patients will do badly in a situation where staff problems already exist.

Here is an example of a entitled demander:

> Mr. B, a 40-year-old married man, had been followed by his physician for six years for a duodenal ulcer. When under stress, he often discontinued his medical treatment and raged against his wife and children. He would

complain that he was not getting enough from life and express resentment that he was unappreciated at work and at home.

Impulsive and easily angered, Mr. B would denigrate most of his associates and speak of his wife as ungiving and uncaring. These attacks would evoke a great deal of guilt in her. The physician handled most of these crises calmly and supportively, never confronting the patient's feelings of entitlement. The rage usually subsided and the patient returned to his diet and medication.

On one occasion, a particularly violent argument occurred between the patient and his wife, and she threatened to leave home. He became enraged, began to drink and stopped his medical regimen. His ulcer symptoms flared up and he was hospitalized. His first words to his physician were "Your medicine has failed again. Isn't there anything else you can do for me?"

The physician was surprised by this attack and felt a wave of anger at the patient's apparent attempt to belittle him. When the patient persisted in attacking him, the physician had all he could to contain his resentment. He tried responding calmly, telling the patient that he was getting the appropriate treatment but that he had to follow medical instructions. His response, expressed in quiet tones, was, nonetheless, a muted, defensive confrontation. He was counterattacking to shore up his self-esteem. The physician would have done better by ignoring the patient's attack and sympathizing with his distress.

The patient heard the physician's response as a rejection. This confirmed for him that his physician cared little about him. He, therefore, stepped up his attack, comparing the doctor unfavorably to others in the hospital. The physician felt increasingly belittled and began to get tough, insisting that the problem was the patient's failure to follow instructions. The doctor gradually withdrew, spending less time at the bedside yet feeling guilty and anxious because he was not treating the patient well.

Since the patient showed different sides of his personality to different members of the staff, it was not long before the staff began to argue among themselves about his management. Some perceived him as a poor victim. Others saw him as a hateful complainer.

One day, in response to more complaining, the physician lost his temper. He told the patient that if he was that unhappy with his care, he didn't have to stay. The patient promptly signed out of the hospital.

The foregoing case demonstrates how difficult the borderline patient can be and how lost physicians and nurses can get in their own emotional responses. Had the physician not taken the patient's initial attack personally, he could have provided the emotional support the patient required, and the subsequent chain of events could have been avoided.

In the outpatient setting, these patients present special difficulties. There, the physician is often isolated and thus more vulnerable to the abuse of such patients. Always keep in mind that the patient's views, whether idealized or denigrating, do not represent reality. Reviewing such cases with colleagues can correct these distortions. Informal psychiatric consultations can also be useful. Therefore, if a patient is angry, demanding, and attacking and you are responding in kind, call someone and talk it over.

Deniers

Denial is a powerful tool that patients use to deal with overwhelming psychological stress. The degree of denial varies. For example, some patients may acknowledge the presence of their illness but apparently fail to appreciate the seriousness of the situation. Psychiatrists label this form of denial, *isolation of affect*. This behavior may not always interfere with medical management. Other patients may actually deny the existence of illness and thus seriously compromise their treatment. Denial is particularly frustrating in those patients who exhibit masochistic traits, the self-destructive deniers. These are the patients who appear to be suicidal in their persistent drinking, smoking, and other harmful behaviors. Actually many of these patients are using pain and self-destructive behavior to satisfy dependent needs, psychological mechanisms that are very different from the denial used to handle overwhelming anxiety. The physician needs to distinguish between these two.

Denial as a defense against overwhelming anxiety. Denial and isolation of affect are often appropriate defense mechanisms that allow patients to tolerate catastrophic illness. As long as denial does not produce self-destructive behavior, the physician does well to leave it alone. However, when denial interferes with medical management, it requires intervention.

Tactics need to be developed to help patients who use this defense to accept appropriate medical care. Direct confrontation, with a lecture regarding the seriousness of the patient's problem, usually increases anxiety, strengthens denial, and may rupture the therapeutic relationship. What is needed are techniques that reduce anxiety and mistrust while they raise self-esteem and hope for the future. In the author's view, it is not possible to diminish denial without simultaneously supporting the patient's self-esteem, since denial is often, in part, the result of a patient's real or imagined sense of humiliation and defectiveness brought on by his or her illness and hospitalization. A clinical example will be useful:

> A 60-year-old woman with a mass in her breast refused biopsy. She was in great pain. She denied the possibility of cancer and became suspicious and withdrawn. A review of her life situation revealed that she had lost all of her family and was in the process of being evicted from her apartment. She considered herself an independent and capable person, hav-

ing worked all her life, and she experienced her illness and hospitalization as humiliating and unacceptable. She denied that the mass could be malignant. She rationalized the fact that she was unable to leave her bed by explaining that the pain was caused by severe muscle aches. Despite two weeks of attempts on the part of staff to have her agree to the biopsy, she continued to strongly deny her illness.

The patient's physician became more and more anxious about her physical condition and pressed her, increasingly more bluntly, for permission to continue the workup and treatment. His frustration and annoyance were beginning to show. She continued to deny her illness. A physician from another hospital, whom she had seen for some years and whom she had trusted, was invited to speak to her. Soon thereafter the patient agreed to the biopsy.

What caused this woman to change her mind? In reviewing the interactions between physicians and patient, it became clear that it was probably due to a number of factors. First, the presence of the trusted physician reduced her panic. Second, she interpreted her doctor's calling in the other physician as a sign of respect and as a result, her self-esteem was raised; Third, her hopes were raised by the assurance from the trusted physician that if a breast malignancy were found, treatment would be available.

The two weeks of intensive concern and attention of the staff were probably also secretly enjoyed by the patient. This attention undoubtedly increased her sense of worth and made her feel more of an equal in relation to the medical staff. Parenthetically, the patient later confided to staff members that she had been frightened by her awareness that she was being given only palliative treatment. Thus it was becoming increasingly difficult for her to sustain her denial. In addition, the visiting physician, unlike the patient's physician, did not have to suffer helplessly while his patient's medical condition worsened. As a result, he was less anxious and could maintain a more empathic relationship. Too often in such situations patients are given an ultimatum by an angry, frustrated staff. This invariably increases anxiety and may force the patient to leave a physician's care.

Here is a second vignette:

A 40-year-old man presented in a general hospital emergency room with an acute surgical abdomen. The surgeon examined the patient and told him that the situation was critical. "We need to get you to the operating room immediately. You are in danger of dying." The patient, frightened and unsure of himself, told the surgeon that he did not want an operation because nothing was seriously wrong with him. The surgeon repeated his statement. "You must have this operation. Without it, you could die." The patient became enraged, denied any serious illness, but accepted admission to the hospital.

A psychiatrist was called and found that the patient was in a panic. The problem was compounded by the patient's long wait in the emergency room, the aloof manner of the clerk, and the fact that a total of four physicians examined him before anyone explained what was going on. He felt humiliated and belittled by this experience.

The psychiatrist sat by the bedside, addressed the patient by his proper name, and apologized for the administrative delays in the emergency-room. He tried to discuss the patient's medical illness but the patient insisted that his family and clergymen be present. The psychiatrist then mobilized family and clergy for an early morning visit. These maneuvers supported the patient, made him feel less frightened, and raised his self-esteem. Shortly thereafter the surgeon returned, sat next to the patient and quietly spoke to him again. "Mr. F, I appreciate your concerns about this procedure. I am very happy that you were able to discuss the situation with your family, and I am sorry about the way you were treated during the admission procedure. I hope that you will reconsider and allow me to try and correct your medical problem." The patient suddenly turned away, began crying, and agreed to the procedure.

Remember, do not allow your frustration to force you into issuing an ultimatum to patients like Mr. F. In most cases they will sign out against advice. We will discuss this problem at greater length later.

Self-Destructive Deniers. Self-destructive, noncompliant behavior can also be a patient's way of eliciting love and attention from others.[4] The behavior appears to follow a pain-dependent pattern. That is, self-destructive acts coerce significant caretakers into expressing their concern by responding angrily to the patient's behavior. Such responses may be poor substitutes for love and attention, but they satisfy the needs of persons who have been conditioned since infancy to expect attention only after they have suffered or engaged in destructive behavior. An enormous amount of attention can be obtained by suffering. Unfortunately, when masochistic behavior occurs in conjunction with serious illness, time sooner or later runs out.

When masochistic character traits are found in borderline patients, as they often are, they produce a formidable clinical problem. The physician, clinic, and hospital represent significant sources of caring to these patients. It is as if the clinic was personified in the unconscious and experienced as a parent. Self-destructive behavior may be rewarded by multiple admissions, consultants, special nurses, and the like. Such activities reduce anxiety by providing the illusion of security. However, this pattern leads to chronic noncompliance, which maintains both the illness and a difficult dependent relationship with physician and hospital.

It is interesting that some of these patients often anticipate staff anger and openly blame themselves for being so weak and self-destructive. They may alternate between claiming "victim" status in a difficult world and blaming and denigrating themselves. Both modes of behavior seek attention through suffering. Physicians respond initially with sympathy, but eventually they feel an increasing sense of helplessness as they experience the coercive control and rage of the patient. Sooner or later physicians are likely to respond with resentment and anger. There are also some fragile patients whose self-destructive behavior paradoxically reduces tension and leads to a feeling of well-being and integration.

How can the physician help these patients? Persistent self-destructive behavior is an indication for psychiatric consultation and treatment. This is easier when the patient sees the problem as the result of his or her own inadequacies. Patients who consider themselves "victims" may be convinced to see psychiatrists if the latter are presented as professionals with whom they can discuss specific problem-solving techniques for dealing with the patients' very difficult life situations. Physicians themselves should follow a protocol that limits self-destructive behavior. This includes setting specific limits and providing for continuity of staff and frequent visits. Treatment should be highly structured. Verbal and written instructions are important, as they help increase compliance. The physician should maintain a positive working alliance and try not to get into power struggles or feel personally rejected by the patient's destructive behavior.

In the case described next, self-destructive, denying behavior was gradually altered.

A 55-year-old man with chronic liver disease was readmitted to the hospital with acute hepatic decompensation brought on by a sudden increase in alcohol consumption. The patient had been an alcohol abuser for some years, but he at no time acknowledged his addiction. He claimed that he drank moderately because his job called for him to entertain clients. After a bleeding episode from esophageal varices, he agreed to stop drinking but started again six months later, again denying any serious alcohol problem. The patient's physician attempted to confront him but was rebuffed with angry denial. Accepting the fact that he was an alcohol abuser was too threatening to the patient, and further confrontation would have led to his resisting any further treatment. The staff decided instead to find out what stressors led to his binge drinking and attempt to work with him in these areas.

Review of the patient's history revealed considerable difficulty in his relationship with his wife. Additionally, he was in danger of losing his job because he was so argumentative and resentful. Crisis intervention and supportive therapy was begun and his wife was brought into the treatment. (These types of therapy are discussed in Chapter 3.) She agreed to reduce some of her demands during this period and accepted the idea of beginning couples' therapy when her husband was in better health.

Several months later, after the patient was discharged, he and his wife began seeing a psychiatrist in couples' therapy. Over the next year the patient's drinking decreased as the relationship improved, although he continued to drink whenever stresses increased. It became clear that his drinking was also used unconsciously as a weapon against his wife, upsetting her and demanding attention from her. Her anger was interpreted by the patient as evidence of her concern for him.

A review of this patient's childhood confirmed that he had obtained attention and care from his parents when he was sick, in pain or in trouble. At other times, he was essentially ignored. The patient had therefore been well conditioned to gratify his dependency needs through illness, pain and self-destructive behavior, even though his caretakers might be angry or critical of him.

Despite our best efforts, long-term compliance in self-destructive patients is poor. The physician's best tool is the maintenance of a positive working alliance in which the patient can be truthful in response to questions regarding compliance.[5] Remember, the patient is severely limited psychologically and is probably doing the best he can. The physician needs to understand that he can deliver only the medical care that the patient will accept.

Psychological change in these patients is very difficult to effect and requires long-term psychotherapy. Change occurs only in the context of a positive working alliance in which a corrective emotional experience takes place. In this milieu, patients can sometimes face their own hostility and dependency and give up the pattern of seeking security and acceptance through suffering.

The Antisocial Patient

Antisocial patients[6] have a history of chronic aggressiveness and rebellious behavior that often may be traced to childhood and adolescence. They are characterized by their inability to maintain a relationship or to perform adequately at work for a sustained period. There is a distinct lack of responsibility in their relationships as well as a failure to live always within the law. Desertion and promiscuity are common. These patients are often irritable, aggressive, assaultive, and impulsive, and they lack fixed short-term or long-term goals. Such patients may lie, cheat, and deceive those about them.

These patients evoke very negative feelings from most staff, and understandably so. The biggest problem, aside from noncompliance, is the possibility that real medical needs may be dismissed as another episode of deception. For example, a patient with sickle cell disease who had an antisocial personality was refused pain medication by staff because they felt, rather angrily, that he was feeding his drug habit. It is better to err on the side of allowing oneself to be exploited, that is, to assume that the claim is real. However, limits must be set in any medical situation, and antisocial behavior that is disruptive or dangerous requires intervention or transfer to an appropriate facility.

The Obsessional, Controlling Patient

Obsessional and controlling patients[7,8,9] are characterized by traits of orderliness, cleanliness, frugality, and intellectualization. They have restricted ability to express warm, tender emotions. They may insist that others follow their ways and remain unaware of the effect of their stubborn behavior on those about them. They are often indecisive and fearful of making mistakes. These patients ruminate and procrastinate, and are excessively devoted to work, often excluding pleasure at the expense of relationships. They strive for an anxiety-free state and attempt to reduce their anxiety by maintaining strict control of themselves and their lives. They can express stubborn oppositional behavior quite subtly. This can be understood as a repetition of early childhood oppositional behavior.

Illness threatens the obsessional patient's need for control. Under this stress such patients will seek as much knowledge as possible regarding their situation since this is their usual technique for dealing with anxiety. This search can lead to increasing pressure on their physicians to provide more and more information regarding diagnosis and treatment, as patients struggle to control their anxiety by convincing themselves that they and their physicians have all the facts needed to bring the illness under control. Unfortunately, the more these patients are told, the more they have to know. As this process unfolds the physician must deal with indecisive, hesitant patients who appear to be in constant doubt regarding every detail of medical management. The physician must learn to provide enough information to reduce anxiety without introducing extraneous detail that will serve only to make the patient more anxious.

Some obsessional patients are made anxious by the fact that they have now been forced to place control of their lives in the hands of another person. They will, therefore, seem to set up roadblocks to the full implementation of their physician's treatment plan.

Here is an example of the interaction between such a patient and his physician:

> The physician tells his patient that the diagnostic work-up revealed a duodenal ulcer and outlines the specific medication and diet required. The patient replies, "Thanks, Doctor, but are you absolutely sure I have an ulcer? Couldn't it be something else?"
>
> The physician, just a little perplexed, says, "Well, you know, we did all the usual blood and stool tests and x-rays, and the GI series definitely showed an ulcer.

The patient then says, "About that diet, is that really necessary? A friend of mine has an ulcer and his doctor doesn't have him on any special diet."

At this point, the physician is beginning to feel a vague sense of annoyance. He responds, "Well, it is true that there is a difference of opinion on the diet issue, but in my experience, the diet I described does help."

The patient then says, "Thank you, doctor, I am sure you are right. However, couldn't we postpone this treatment for the time being? I have some business trips scheduled and probably couldn't follow that diet."

The doctor is beginning to lose patience, does not quite understand what is going on between him and the patientn and responds, "Mr. Jones, you have a serious illness that needs to be treated, and I believe you need this medication and special diet now."

The patient responds, somewhat annoyed, "Thank you very much, doctor. I'll be in touch with you when I return from my trip." He leaves and is never seen again in the doctor's office.

This vignette demonstrates the patient's need to be sure he is getting just the right treatment, as well as his need for control. Although superfically quite respectful, the patient maintains a "Yes, but—" attitude. His apparent dismissal of the doctor's ideas leads to annoyance and anger on the part of the physician and an ultimatum that ruptures the therapeutic alliance.

Obsessional patients are unconsciously preoccupied with who has power over whom. Such patients seem incapable of a truly collaborative effort with others. The physician must act so as to give the patient a sense of retaining some control over his or her destiny. For example, if several courses of action are possible, these patients feel much better if they are allowed to decide which route they prefer to take. In the example above, a power struggle developed. It might have been avoided if the physician had been able to offer a choice between alternative diets or had more willingly agreed to a second opinion. Listen to your dialogs with patients. If you hear too many "yes, buts" from the patient, you probably have joined the power struggle.

Suspicious Paranoid Patients

Patients who exhibit signs of paranoid personality disorders are characterized by hypervigilance, secretiveness, and an unwarranted pervasive suspiciousness and mistrust with expectations of harm.[10] Such patients have a narrowly focused view of life and usually perceive most issues in polarized, black and white terms. They are often jealous and concerned with hidden meanings; they are hypersensitive, easily offended, and ready to counterattack. They appear cold and aloof.

Working with these patients can be difficult, because it takes very little to change what seems to be a positive alliance into a suspicious, guarded, hostile one. The physician must remain aware of this potential for sudden, apparently unprovoked changes in the relationship and must be prepared to deal with them. Such changes in the alliance can be interpreted directly and such an interpretation, if done in a properly supportive manner, can restore good reality testing. The primary rule in working with paranoid patients is to avoid power struggles. No matter how provocative the patient is, the physician must not be drawn into a verbal wrestling match.

Here is a clinical example:

> Mr. J had been followed by his physician for ten years for diabetes mellitus. He had always been a suspicious, distrustful man. His doctor learned to address him as Mr. J, maintained a respectful distance, and avoided confronting him regarding his recurring sense of outrage toward one person or another. The doctor listened sympathetically to his patient's distress and complaints. As Mr. J's diabetes worsened, his anxiety about his health increased.
>
> The physician communicated this state of affairs to the patient's wife when she called to inquire about how he was doing. When the patient discovered that his doctor had discussed his medical situation without his being present, he became enraged and agitated, accusing the doctor of colluding with his wife for reasons that the patient had not yet determined. Further evaluation of the marriage revealed it to be a highly ambivalent, difficult relationship. The stress of the patient's worsening health was increasing the intensity of his paranoid ideation. The unfortunate discussion with Mrs. J turned the working relationship with the patient into a nightmare.
>
> A psychiatric consultant advised the practitioner to reassure the patient directly regarding his illness and the physician's motives. The physician calmly and supportively said, "Mr. J, I can understand your distress. Your test reports now indicate that your diabetes is under control and you can go back to your usual work routine. I was in error in discussing your situation with your wife without your permission. I wanted to reassure her that you were doing well and to suggest some things that might be helpful to you."

The admission of an error in procedure reduced the patient's anxiety and, subsequently, his paranoid symptoms. His reality testing and the therapuetic alliance improved. Somewhat later, attempts were made to help the patient deal with his marital problems. Occasionally in such patients, however, reality testing will be distorted to the point of psychosis and appropriate antipsychotic medication may be indicated (see Chapter 7).

Isolated Schizoid Patients

The schizoid patient is characterized by the inability to form significant relationships and by an apparent emotional coldness.[11] Such persons appear to be indifferent to praise and criticism. They may appear somewhat odd, but their psychopathology is not severe enough to be called schizophrenic.

The physician should respect these patients' need for emotional distance and try to intrude as little as possible. Intimacy makes these patients very anxious. The physical closeness of diagnostic or hospital procedures can make for a very difficult situation. Such patients may leave medical care to restore distance between themselves and the health care providers. These patients require minimal contact and no unnecessary laying on of hands or conversation. They do require reassurance, and great care must be taken that nothing is said or done that will be perceived as rejection. This is difficult. A physician walks a narrow line between too much intimacy, which threatens the patient, and too much distancing, which may be interpreted as rejection. Remember, you are dealing with an anxiety-laden patient even though this may not be apparent from his demeanor.

Overdramatic Histrionic Patients

Histrionic[12] patients are overly dramatic and reactive, always needing to be center stage. Physicians experience these patients as shallow and superficially warm. They can be vain, demanding, self-centered, and manipulative. The female patient with a male physician can be overtly seductive or more subtly emphasize her helplessness and need for support. (The management of the sexually seductive female patient is discussed in detail in Chapter 4.) The male patient, especially when ill, may attempt to flaunt his "manliness" in the presence of female physicians or nursing staff. The physician must appreciate that hiding behind the superficial seductiveness is a very dependent, narcissistic, sometimes borderline patient.

Illness is perceived by histrionic patients as a defect which will make them appear unattractive or weak. As a result, they have an increased need to convince themselves and others that they are still attractive. Managing such patients should include a firm, supportive attitude with clearly established limits. These patients need to feel you like them. However, you must learn to enjoy their charm without becoming victimized by it. The difficult part for most physicians is to avoid getting swept up in the highly charged emotional atmosphere that these patients create. They usually respond well to a calm, supportive, reassuring manner, and they do not need the detailed medical review of their situation that the obsessional patient requires.

Other Problem Patients

In addition to the personality disorders, several other clinical problems give the physician great difficulty.

The Hypochondriacal Patient

Hypochondriasis is a psychiatric disorder characterized by a preoccupation with bodily malfunction and illness. DSM-III[13] lists the following diagnostic criteria:

1. The predominant disturbance is an unrealistic interpretation of physical signs or sensations as abnormal, leading to preoccupation with the fear of having, or the belief that one has, a serious disease.
2. Medical evaluation does not support the diagnosis of any physical disorder that can account either for the physical signs and sensations or for the individual's unrealistic interpretation of them.
3. The unrealistic fear or belief persists despite medical reassurance and causes an impairment in social or occupational functioning.
4. The disorder is not due to any mental disorder such as schizophrenia or affective disorder.

In most hypochondriacal patients, symptoms abate for periods of time, but the hypochondriacal pattern of reaction always reasserts itself whenever life stresses become overwhelming. Repeated medical workups are welcome, but reassurance alone provides at best only a temporary respite. These patients suffer a great deal. Their preoccupation with their physical state leave little room for much else in life. When hypochondriacal concerns are severe they may withdraw from relationships, becoming preoccupied with themselves and their physical complaints. Many see themselves as independent, well-functioning people victimized by bad luck in developing a physical illness that cannot be diagnosed and that renders them incapable of functioning normally. Others give up their independent, long-suffering facade and develop very passive, dependent, childlike behavior.

Hypochondriasis must be differentiated from depression and from schizophrenic states. The somatic concerns of the depressed patient are usually not a life-long pattern and have a discrete onset in association with a change in mood. The depressed patient will also manifest sadness, psychomotor retardation, lowered self-esteem, and sleep and appetite disturbances. These symptoms and the hypochondriacal preoccupation will disappear with adequate treatment of the depression (see Chapter 6). In contrast, hypochondriasis is characterized by a chronic remitting and exacerbating course that is unresponsive to the usual treatment of depression. Hypochondriacal concerns may also signal the onset of a schizophrenic reaction. Here the bodily preoccupations are usually more idiosyncratic and bizarre in nature and are accompanied by paranoid ideation.

The hypochondriacal patient uses illness as a defense against anxiety and unconscious dependency needs. The patient may be unconsciously demanding a dependent relationship without guilt. The illness leads to dependent gratification by the physician, since sick people are cared for and not much is expected of them. Such symptoms often camouflage a profound sense of inadequacy. Patients who cannot consciously accept their dependent needs can unconsciously use physical concerns and illness to solve this dilemma. They cannot give up their symptoms no matter how much coaxing and reassurance they get from physicians. Attempts to do so only increase their anxiety and strengthen their hypochondriacal defenses.

Hypochondriasis is a chronic illness in which the severity of the preoccupations is usually a barometer of the stress the patient is experiencing. Often such stress is a function of the degree to which the patient is required to act autonomously. For example, if the patient feels unloved, is separated from a spouse, or is asked to take on more responsibilities at work, his or her preoccupations may worsen, requiring more attention.

For the physician to respond with anger and/or a psychiatric referral is to miss the point of the illness. In most cases, such a referral will not be accepted by such patients, because they do not view their problems as psychological. The primary physician will remain the significant person in these patients' lives and must provide the needed psychological support. These patients will require frequent scheduled visits to the doctor in times of severe distress. Less frequent, but still scheduled, appointments are needed when the stresses are low.

Altman has stated that the goal of treatment should be to support the patient in a manner that minimizes suffering and requires minimal use of medical services.[14] After an initial careful medical evaluation, the physician should avoid being seduced into long and costly additional medical workups. Patients should be told that there is no evidence of a serious medical condition. Although they will not accept the notion that "There is nothing wrong," they will usually accept the statement that they do not have any life-threatening illness. To the hypochondriacal patient, there is a very big difference between "I've found nothing wrong with you" and 'I've found nothing that you need to worry about." Above all, patients must sense that you do not doubt the reality of their symptoms. They *are* real, even though the patient's concerns about them may be unrealistic.

As patients talk about their lives, support their attempts to tolerate pain and move toward independence. Try to open up a discussion of other areas in their experience by suggesting that life's problems can sometimes adversely affect the body. But do not persist in this approach if the patient is resistant to your suggestions.

Here is a clinical example:

A 47-year-old widowed mother of four had been followed for several years by her internist because of intermittent chest pain and preoccupation with her health. She was convinced she had serious heart disease, even though no data had ever been found to document this. During this period, she had been able to function reasonably well but lived with the fear that she would die soon. She consulted several other physicians, who also tried unsuccessfully to reassure her.

The patient had lost her husband ten years ago. Her chest pains began shortly thereafter. Prior to her husband's death, she and her husband had lived together in a stormy marriage for 15 years. During that period, the patient occasionally became preoccupied with a variety of somatic complaints but functioned reasonably well. Her husband was considerably older than she and had taken a dominant, authoritarian role in the family.

The patient had considered herself victimized by her husband's demands and felt ambivalent toward him throughout the marriage. When he died, she was forced to support herself and her children, which she did in spite of her fears. One year ago her pain had worsened, and now she was almost completely immobilized by her illness. This increase in her disability occurred at the time her son married and left home and her adolescent daughter became interested in boys. Because of the marked increase in her symptoms, the patient's son and daughter-in-law were considering moving back into the home to care for her. The patient had always tended to be angry and suspicious of others, and during the course of her illness she dropped the few friends she had. Her major activity became trips to her physician's office.

The physician initiated a series of conferences with the family. During these meetings, he tried to clarify for the patient's children what their mother's unconscious needs were and how they were played out through the physical symptoms. He was able to reassure them that she had no serious disease. Some way was needed to support the patient's need to be cared for and to reduce her fears of being alone. These goals had to be achieved without undermining the patient's own perception of herself as an independent woman victimized by illness and by life. The physician began by scheduling more frequent visits to his office and twice-weekly visits from the visiting nurse. Arrangements were made for the patient to live closer to her son and daughter-in-law, and a homemaker was assigned to visit her on a weekly basis. Another problem was her adolescent daughter, who was in conflict regarding her desire to go out with her friends and the obligation she felt to care for her mother. This resulted in rebellious behavior and failing grades at school. The daughter was referred to a psychiatrist for treatment.

In his later sessions with the patient, the physician gradually introduced the possibility that, although her pain was real, it was not cardiac disease and not likely to take her life. With the reduction in anxiety, the patient was able gradually to accept that her illness was not life-threatening. The ruminations over her health slowly decreased. She began to leave her apartment during symptom-free periods and developed some friends through church-related activities. Over the next year, there were occasional periods of exacerbation of her hypochondrial complaints when family stresses increased, but her overall level of functioning had improved.

The foregoing case history illustrates the use of physical complaints to obtain gratification for dependent needs. This patient's complaints were an expression of the anxiety raised by her children's increasing need for independence. The physician recognized the need to reduce her anxiety by becoming more of a "parent" through increased visits and reassurance. In addition he restructured her environment by moving her closer to her son and introducing a homemaker. This served to support her dependency needs as well. Finally, referring the patient's rebellious adolescent daughter for psychiatric consultation helped defuse a source of anxiety for the patient.

Noncompliant Behavior

Noncompliant behavior is the result of an exceedingly complex set of variables.[15] Patients come to physicians for advice. To refuse to take such advice, reflects the intense, usually unconscious emotional forces at work. Patients' intrapsychic conflicts, chronic personality difficulties, cultural issues, and the meaning of the illness all play a significant role. The physician's capacity to respond empathically without frustration is equally important. When patients fail to comply they are resolving some need or expressing some conflict through inaction. The physician needs to determine what such needs or conflicts are. For example, for some patients noncompliance is a way of getting the physician upset and angry, which reassures the patient that the doctor cares. The physician's basic tool is the capacity to understand what is going on in the patient's psychological world and to understand his or her response to it. Physicians who understand what is going on between them and their patients have room to maneuver and to deal with both their patients' and their own anxieties. The maintenance of a positive working alliance is the most important and central concern of the physician and the best way to insure compliant behavior. It is essential, as previously stated, that the patient be able to reply, "No," to the physician's question "Have you taken the medication?" At least one knows where one stands under these circumstances. The physician can then explore with the patient possible emotional sources of the behavior.

Some causes and remedies. Many noncompliant patients are self-destructive deniers or suffer from a borderline personality disorder (see previous sections in this chapter). For other patients, noncompliance may stem from resistance to the dependent role. For these people you must devise regimens that allow them to feel some sense of control. For example, a flexible diet is better than a rigid one to which the patient will not adhere. You may have to settle for a regimen that causes you some anxiety. This is preferable to one to which the patient cannot adhere at all or which causes the patient to further deny illness and perhaps even flee from all medical care. Remember, the relationship between physician and patient is the single most important factor in compliance to a medical regimen.

You can begin to explore the meaning of noncompliant behavior by suggesting that perhaps the idea of taking medicine is upsetting. Many identify such feelings if they are encouraged to do so in a nonpunitive manner. For example, they may tell you how frightened they are of having the same illness that killed one of their parents. This then provides you with the opportunity to allay the patient's anxiety with some realistic assurance regarding modern methods of treatment. Too often our tendency is to go in the opposite direction and try to motivate patients by reminding them how serious a problem is. Most noncompliant patients have been told the obvious medical facts. You must, therefore, learn to communicate the importance of following your regimen without producing panic.

Techniques for improving patient compliance, using educational and behavioral methods, have proved useful in some settings.[16] These include treatment contracts, mail reminders, graduated regimen implementation and the development of regimens based on each patient's personality characteristics. Reinforcement is used to change behavior in a gradual and systematic way. Unfortunately these techniques are of limited value where the psychological conflicts just described are present.

The threat to sign out against medical advice. In the hospital setting the threat to sign out against medical advice is a serious problem. A sick patient who threatens to leave the hospital against the advice of his physician is behaving irrationally. Only the strongest of emotions can produce this type of self-destructive behavior. The threat to sign out is the last desperate act of a patient who can find no other solution to deal with his or her intense emotional distress. Most patients prefer to resolve such crises, if given the opportunity.[17]

Patients who threaten to sign out are usually frightened, angry, or psychotic, and too often their physicians are unable or unwilling to acknowledge that they may have contributed to the problem. If the problem is to be resolved constructively, the physician must be able to ask dispassionately, "What is there in the hospital situation, including me, that has provoked the turmoil this patient is now experiencing?" Physicians must appreciate that it may not be what they have done but what the patient thinks they have done, since some of the patient's responses may stem from a transference reaction to the physician or the nursing staff. Obviously, the extreme dependent role of the hospitalized patient can evoke unconscious child–parent reactions. The physician can help the nursing staff to understand better what appear to be the excessive demands made by a frightened patient.

Such patients, dreading total dependency, may insist on having something done their way in order to reassure themselves that they still have some control over their lives. Unfortunately, it can become more important for the staff to establish who is boss than to understand the basis for a patient's stubbornness, thus leading to a confrontation. Such patients should be allowed to win the battle, for example, for a procedure change. Physicians may be concerned that patients will want to dictate their own treatment, but once patients are reassured that they are still in control of some aspects of their lives they are usually quite willing to allow physicians to retain the responsibility in really important matters.

A 34-year-old woman with an acute attack of Hodgkins disease was seen by the psychiatric consultant after she had dressed in street clothing and signed the Against Medical Advice form. She agreed to the consultation only to please her doctor.

The nursing notes described the patient's week in the hospital as punctuated by crying spells and requests for reassurance that she would not die. She also called her aged foster mother frequently on the telephone. The staff felt overwhelmed by this person's need for reassurance but found her likeable and made great efforts to comfort her. Her doctor, an intern, believed that her prognosis was very poor and had told the nursing staff that "she might not make it out of the hospital." He told the psychiatric consultant that he was afraid to give a young woman such a grave prognosis and had decided to avoid the issue until she asked.

The threat to leave the hospital occurred on the eighth hospital day. The ward staff had just dealt with a cardiac arrest when this patient asked for aid to get to the phone booth. An aide told her that she would have to wait. The patient began to cry and insisted on leaving the hospital at once.

The patient told the psychiatrist that she was terrified about the likelihood that she would die at any moment. She thought there could be no other explanation for the brief time her doctors spent with her. She became frightened of dying alone and decided to leave for home. She had been orphaned as a child and her foster mother was the only person she felt would see her through to the end. In addition, her foster mother's own well-being was a paramount concern of the patient's, for the mother was quite old. Being unable to telephone her mother provoked overwhelming anxiety in the patient.

The consultant suggested to the staff that they discuss her prognosis openly with her. This freed them from the burden of a "secret," which the patient had deduced from their unspoken behavior, and allowed the patient to seek and receive more emotional comfort from them. It was arranged that the intern would see her daily, even if only for a moment. The social service staff assisted the patient in planning for her mother's care. With the fear of abandonment and loneliness ameliorated and with planning for her mother under way, the patient had a calm course until her death in the hospital.

In situations where the patient is justifiably angry with the staff, a mere acknowledgement of the justness of the patient's complaint is usually enough to resolve the problem. It is when we are too "proud" or frightened to admit an obvious error that patients may feel that only a threat to leave the hospital or litigation will get them the attention or justice they believe they merit.

A 27-year-old woman with chronic sickle-cell disease and many previous uneventful hospitalizations suddenly threatened to leave against medical advice, to the surprise of her physician. He reasoned with her without success. Psychiatric consultation was then requested because the physician thought the patient had become "paranoid."

The psychiatrist first spoke to the nursing staff, who told him that the patient was a "crock" or a "junkie," who demanded more narcotics than she needed. The patient said that the nurses did not like her and that they deliberately made her wait for pain medication. She was furious with them and was going to leave for another hospital.

The medical student assigned to the patient felt that the nursing staff did give her less attention than the other patients. They were late with the analgesics because it seemed to them that the patient was asking for opiates when she appeared to be in no distress. The patient, in turn, had learned that she could not depend on getting medication when she really needed it and so asked for opiates when she felt only the beginning of pain. Patient and staff were increasingly distrustful and angry with each other. It was clear that the patient did not really want to leave but rather was communicating her frustration in the only way she believed was open to her.

In this case, the physician had failed to keep the nurses adequately informed about the patient's great need for analgesia. He, in turn, was not aware of the nurses' concern about what they believed was drug abuse and their consequent anger toward the patient. The psychiatrist suggested to the physician that he review the patient's medical situation in detail with the nurses and also point out to them that anxiety can actually add to the preception of pain. It was also suggested that the *prn* narcotic order be changed to a standing order, which the patient could refuse if free of pain.

With this increased understanding the hostility toward this patient cleared. Her total narcotic dose was one third less in the 24 hours following the consultation.

The threat to sign out can also be one manifestation of a psychotic decompensation. Effective management then requires an attempt to deal with the precipitating stress as well as the use of antipsychotic medication (see also Chapter 7).

A 39-year-old woman with severe cirrhosis and a history of an acute paranoid psychotic episode suddenly threatened to sign out because she

> believed the hospital food was poisoned. The staff promptly treated her with reassurance and phenothiazine medications, and she remained in the hospital. But she continued to eat only food brought in by her family and began to voice fears about God killing her for her sins.
>
> A psychiatric consultant was called, but he could not alleviate her fears. He suggested increasing her medication and feeding her by tube. When this was done the patient became actively suicidal, although she agreed to eat hospital food in preference to tube feedings.
>
> At a family meeting the doctor learned that the patient's kin had abandoned her because of her drinking. They had visited her in the hospital only at the request of her physician, to bring food when she was "crazy." Thus, when she could not eat hospital food, they visited daily, but when she was tube-fed they did not visit at all. This loss produced the despair and suicidal behavior. With this understanding, the patient's doctor was able to convince the family to visit her for medical reasons, even though they did not forgive her. Her delusions cleared rapidly and she did well after psychotropic drugs were withdrawn.

Patients with organic mental syndromes can become quite frightened by their inability to orient themselves to the new hospital environment. The hospital is usually a frightening place for the patient with an intact central nervous system. For the patient with an organic deficit, it can be truly terrifying. Our failure to recognize the deficit allows this anxiety to escalate, producing an "uncooperative" patient who may ultimately need to escape the strangeness of the hospital.

> A 49-year-old woman with a long history of alcoholism was admitted for evaluation of what her family thought was a partial loss of vision. Once in the hospital, the patient began to demand continuous attention and to refuse tests. She became quite angry about a proposed lumbar puncture and threatened to leave the hospital when pressed to have the test done.
>
> The psychiatric consultant found her to be disoriented to time and place and severely defective in recent memory. She was in a panic. The patient was told no further tests would be done for a while. Her bed was moved from a single room to the ward. A calendar, family pictures, and a radio were set up by the bed. Nighttime barbiturates were stopped. She responded to these changes with improved orientation and became quite cooperative. The lumbar puncture was then done without incident.

When all efforts have failed, and the patient is leaving against medical advice, the physician can remain an ally. The physician must resist the impulse to issue an ultimatum denying further care to the patient who leaves. It is young house officers who are most vulnerable to this impulse. They experience anxiety and guilt about their apparent failure to persuade the patient to stay. They become angry at the person who arouses these feelings and then resort to the threat to deny treatment. This is a punitive act that rarely dissuades the patient from leaving. But it can prevent the provision of adequate medical care in an outpatient setting, which may be all the patient can then tolerate.

PATIENTS FROM DIFFERENT CULTURAL BACKGROUNDS

Elizabeth Hegeman, Ph.D

Studies have found that physicians are often anxious, frustrated and uncomfortable when interviewing patients from religious or ethnic backgrounds that differ from their own.[18] There are good reasons for these feelings: the physician's job is much harder when it is not clear whether patient and physician have the same expectations about illness, treatment, and the nature of the physician–patient relationship.

Some physicians, and even some designers of training programs, fall into the trap of thinking that the physician should become thoroughly knowledgeable about the cultural patterns of all his or her patients. This unrealistic idea can burden health care workers unnecessarily. And it can lead to further misunderstanding if the physician acquires only stereotypical ideas and tries to apply them to individual patients. For example, a Puerto Rican patient with psychomotor seizures had to overcome the conviction of an emergency room physician, "knowledgeable" about Puerto Rican culture, that she was suffering from *ataque* before she could be successfully controlled on Dilantin. The physician was familiar with *ataque,* or the "Puerto Rican syndrome": an emotional disorder characterized by a sudden partial loss of consciousness that is accompanied by clonic or tonic seizures and at times by screaming or tearing of clothing. These acts are accepted by some Puerto Ricans as culturally appropriate on the occasion of grief or the sudden reception of bad news, or as a form of protest against maltreatment. Careful questioning about the onset of symptoms can help to distinguish *ataque* from a true seizure disorder.

It is much more useful for physicians to become aware of the *possibility* of patients' differing expectations and values, and to maintain a questioning, open stance in each situation. Spiegel has described how clashes of values can affect the treatment situation: if the physician holds the dominant American middle-class orientation toward future benefits and the patient comes from a culture in which present satisfactions are more important, they will disagree as to priorities in treatment.[19] The patient will be more interested in relief from pain, less interested in the possible side-effects of medication, and less likely to follow through in aftercare than the physician thinks he or she should be.

Not only does every culture have its own set of distinct values; every family constitutes a legitimate subculture. It would be ideal to have a "culture expert" on the staff of every health care facility, to sort out the cultural elements in patient–doctor misunderstandings, but this is usually not possible. Therefore, we must try to become more aware of the possible role of differing value systems. Here are some examples of important areas in which cultural factors can affect the treatment process.

The Meaning of Pain and Disease

Studies of ethnic groups show that they vary in their beliefs about the meaning of pain: some may feel that pain itself is the problem, to be eliminated by whatever means; some may feel that pain is unimportant except as a symptom of something that must be understood using all the tools of science; others may feel that pain is a trial to be endured so that the soul may be purified. These different attitudes can affect a patient's desire for medication and compliance with a regimen. Of course, within each such group there are individuals for whom the group norm does not apply.

Staff and patients may also differ as to whether suffering from pain should be openly expressed or dealt with stoically: particular patterns of behavior in response to pain are usually the product of early training. Patients brought up in households where it was important to control one's emotions will find it difficult to let us know how much pain they are experiencing. Problems begin when the expressive patient is viewed as a "cry baby" by a house officer brought up to suppress any signs of discomfort whereas the legitimate needs of the stoical patient are overlooked by the physician who expects someone in pain to let the world know about it.

Patients who feel in some way responsible for their own illnesses have an additional burden to face. Whether Christian Scientists who feel guilty for having allowed "mortal mind" to triumph, Ojibwa Indians who feel they have broken a supernatural rule, or smokers with lung cancer, such patients must now deal not only with the illness but with the guilt of "having brought it on themselves."

The stigma associated with certain diseases may interfere with a patient's motivation and follow-through in treatment. Many patients, for example, are unwilling to accept a diagnosis and referral for a mental problem, because, for them, intense shame is connected with a psychiatric diagnosis. However, many such patients *are* willing to accept psychiatric treatment by the primary care physician, provided a formal psychiatric diagnosis is not applied. Such patients may very well accept the notion that they are "nervous," "sensitive," or "upset" and may gladly accept help from their own doctors for this problem. Such an approach allows patients to be treated appropriately and avoids the need for them to seek treatment elsewhere, such as from neighborhood folk healers, who may diagnose spirit possession and administer herbs.[20]

What the Patient Expects of the Physician

As has been discussed elsewhere, all patients bring to their physician the conscious expectation that he or she will heal their illness, as well as various unconscious emotional reactions, reminiscent of their earliest child–parent relationships. Cultural factors also affect patients' expectations of their physicians. For example, patients whose families have lived in traditional rural communities for generations may have special needs for a more personal relationship than most physicians are prepared for. Such patients may seek a paternalistic connection with the physician as an honored authority who must be showered with gifts or invited to family occasions.

Patients raised in a setting in which the parental authority figures ruled by instilling fear in other family members are likely to be intimidated by their physician's comparable role. As a result, such patients are not likely to ask any questions regarding their physician's instructions. Thus they must be asked specifically if they have any questions about the treatment regimen. Since this may still not free them up to ask, they should be given a written outline of the recommendations. They should also be asked if the regimen will interfere in any significant way with their daily routine: for example, will it be possible for them to take pills four times a day?

Such patients also are not likely to call for assistance prn. Although they can be encouraged to make such calls, it is more realistic to spell out those circumstances in which they *must* call (only specific appointments will bring them back) for follow-up visits and regular checks-ups.

Decision-Making and Family Values

In many non-Western families, especially those from Mediterranean and Middle Eastern countries, one's identity as an individual and as a member of a family often merge. When a member of such an "embedded" family becomes ill, it may not be easy for the physician to know with whom he or she must deal. Patient and family may expect that everyone must be consulted before decisions are made. In such situations, it can be useful for the physician to appoint an appropriate person in the family to serve as liaison with the doctor, and to speak only with that person. If family members need to participate in the treatment, they can be given supportive assignments such as maintaining the patient's household and other daily tasks.

Sometimes a family's need for privacy will interfere with the taking of an adequate history. Illegitimate children, children from a previous marriage, and other so-called black sheep may be "forgotten" by family members when the physician inquires about familial illness. Thus it can be helpful to ask, "Does this man have other children?" and "Did your grandfather have other families?" The household may include members that the physician would never think of asking about: the unlikely diagnosis of cholera was facilitated in New York's Chinatown when a careful inquiry turned up the presence of two distant cousins who had recently arrived from Hong Kong. Physicians who make it clear by their directness and objectivity that they do not disapprove or look down on the family for such matters will make it easier for family members to provide a complete history.

In summary, the best way to improve rapport and to treat patients from different backgrounds effectively is not to endeavor to become an expert on the patient's culture but rather to feel comfortable in asking questions until one believes he or she understands what the patient and family expect of the physician. Of course, such an exploration mean additional time will be required. In the long run, such an investment of time should save time and improve the general level of care.

REFERENCES

1. Groves J: Taking care of hateful patients. N Engl J Med 298:883, 1978
2. Kernberg O: Object Relations Theory and Clinical Psychoanalysis. Jason Aronson, Inc. New York 1976
3. Groves J: Management of the borderline patient on a medical or surgical ward: The psychiatric consult's role. Int J Psychiatry Med 6:337–347, 1978
4. Thompson C: The interpersonal approach to the clinical problems of masochism, in Masserman J (ed): Science and Psychoanalysis: Vol 2, Individual and Family Dynamics. New York, Grune & Stratton, 1959, pp 31–38
5. Sackett DL: A Compliance Practicum for the Busy Practitioner, in Haynes B, Taylor D, Sackett DL (eds): Compliance and Health Care, Baltimore, Johns Hopkins University Press, 1979
6. APA Task Force on Nomenclature and Statistics: Diagnostic and Statistical Manual of Mental Disorders, (ed 3), Washington, D.C., American Psychiatric Association, 1980, pp. 317–321
7. Salzman L, Thaler FH: Obsessive compulsive disorders: A review of the literature. Am J Psychiatry 138:286–296, 1981
8. Schimel J: The power theme in the obsessional. Contemp Psychoanal 9:1–28, 1972–73

9. Kahana R, Bibring G: Personality types in medical management, in Zimberg, M. (ed): Psychiatry and Medical Practice in the General Hospital. New York, Int'l University Press, 1964
10. Diagnostic and Statistical Manual of Mental Disorders (ed 3), Washington, D.C., American Psychiatric Association, 1980, pp. 307–309
11. ibid, pp. 309–313
12. ibid, pp. 313–315
13. ibid, pp. 241–252
14. Altman N: Hypochondriasis, in Strain J, Grossman S (eds): Psychological Care of the Medically Ill: A Primer in Liaison Psychiatry. New York, Appleton, Century, Crofts, 1975
15. Sackett DL, Snow JC: The magnitude of compliance and non-compliance, in Haynes B, Taylor D, Sackett DL (eds): Compliance and Health Care. Baltimore, Johns Hopkins University Press, 1979
16. Dunbar JM, Marshall GD, Hovel MF: Behavioral Strategies for Improving Compliance, in Haynes B, Taylor D, Sackett DL (eds): Compliance and Health Care. Baltimore, Johns Hopkins University Press, 1979
17. Albert HD, Kornfeld DS: The threat to sign out against medical advice. Ann Intern Med 79: 888–891, 1973
18. Leifur D: Physicians' response to patients: A study of factors involved in the office interview. J of Fam Pract 6:1065–1073, 1978
19. Spiegel J: Some cultural aspects of transference and countertransference, in Masserman J (ed): Science and Psychoanalysis: Vol 2, Individual and Family Dynamics. New York, Grune & Stratton, 1959
20. Garrison V: Support systems of schizophrenics and non-schizophrenic Puerto Rican migrant women in New York City. Schizoph Bull 4:561–595, 1978

Jerry B. Finkel, M.D.

3

Psychotherapy in Medical Practice

Many people turn to their family physicians for help with emotional and family problems. Others present with medical symptoms in whose etiology and course psychological factors have played a significant role. Still others present with emotional disorders secondary to a medical illness. The physician's relationship with patients and families provides an ideal context for the diagnosis and treatment of these problems. All physicians practice the art of listening to and advising patients. Psychotherapy is essentially a refinement of this art, which every primary care physician practices daily but usually without conceptualizing his or her skills in these terms.

This chapter is an introduction to the kinds of psychotherapy physicians can use in everyday practice—skills that are necessary for good primary care. Expertise in psychotherapy requires an understanding of psychopathology, psychological development, and psychodynamics as well as supervision by an experienced psychotherapist. Medical practitioners who wish to pursue their interest in psychotherapy should seek and develop such a supervisory relationship.

The many forms of psychotherapy are based on a variety of theoretical hypotheses. The approach discussed in this chapter is based on the assumption of a psychodynamic developmental model in which children born with a genetically determined biology interact with family and others and pass through a variety of developmental stages, each with its own tasks and anxieties. Issues of trust, dependency, separation, competition, guilt, sexuality, and autonomy are dealt with by the developing person but may reemerge later in life if early development is disturbed by inadequate parenting and/or a variety of other stresses. Such a disturbance is usually associated with anxiety and misperceptions of self and others, so that relationships and a consistent positive sense of self are difficult. A second assumption of the approach discussed here is our ability to repress material so that it is out of awareness, in our unconscious; such repressed memories, desires, fears, and conflicts may still play a central role in shaping our lives even though we are unaware of them. Personality disorders are nothing more than chronic maladaptive ways of dealing with these misperceptions and unresolved conflicts. Similarly, the development of acute psychological reactions can be understood as a regression under stress around one or another of these same issues.

Psychotherapy is a talking treatment that differs from advice giving because it is based on the assumption that actions and feelings are not always logical but rather are derived from unconscious needs, fears, and conflicts and the defenses used to cope with them. Psychotherapy takes into account patients' misperceptions and the anxiety that even "good" advice may raise. The most ambitious category of treatment is psychoanalysis, in which an attempt is made to understand a patient's unconscious processes, heal old psychic wounds, and restructure personality in more adaptive ways. Analysis is a process of uncovering. Such work is difficult and time consuming. Some modified forms of psychoanalytic psychotherapy are more limited in their goals. Restructuring attempts are not a realistic goal for nonpsychiatric physicians and should be undertaken only by psychoanalytically trained psychotherapists.

Other forms of psychotherapy can be subdivided into crisis intervention, brief therapy, and long-term psychotherapy. These therapies are essentially supportive but are based on the psychodynamic assumptions we have outlined and can be skillfully practiced by physicians. This chapter will explore the principles of these supportive forms of psychotherapy.

THE ROLE OF TRANSFERENCE

At the heart of the psychotherapeutic process is the phenomenon known as *transference*. This term, as discussed in Chapter 1, refers to the patient's unconscious tendency to assign to others in the present environment feelings and attitudes that were originally linked with significant figures in the person's early life. For the psychoanalyst, transference provides an excellent opportunity to analyze the patient's earlier emotional responses in the context of his or her reaction to the analyst. For the primary care physician, however, the transference has a different use. Since the patient–physician relationship so closely parallels the early child–parent relationship, patients may react to physicians as they might have to their original parental figures. For most patients, this can be a powerful constructive force.

These early child–parent relationships can also produce negative transference responses, which can make for difficult patient–doctor relationships. A very positive transference also contains a potential for difficulty if unmodified by conscious reality factor; that is, if our patients expect us to behave like the ideal parent—to be omniscient, omnipotent, and to demand nothing in return. Unfortunately, we must fall far short of this idealized image. As previously discussed, most of our patients can deal with our human limitations, but some cannot.

The transference can thus be a powerful force for the relief of emotional pain in the patient's life. As a parent, you play this significant role with your own children. You lend a sympathetic ear, provide reassurance that you care about them, and somehow, almost magically, the distress is gone. You have the potential for similar cures in your relationship with many of your patients.

As noted earlier, physicians obviously are also susceptible to the transference phenomenon. When feelings related to early child–parent experiences are produced by patients in the physician they are called *countertransference* reactions. Physicians may find themselves becoming angry, authoritarian, detached, or overprotective with particular kinds of patients. The most difficult problem is recognizing that a countertransference problem exists (see Chapter 1).

Conducting psychotherapy requires being aware of the changing nature of the patient's transference reactions and the physician's responses to them.

THE PHYSICIAN AS PSYCHOTHERAPIST

Psychotherapy is usually perceived by physicians as requiring little if any significant action on their part. Since most physicians have difficulty accepting a relatively passive role in their professional lives, they tend to avoid engaging in such therapy. This fear of passivity is related to two factors: (1) our self-image as healers demands that we act; and (2) we believe that our patients expect action in return for the fee they have paid us. Once we grasp that listening can be an active form of therapeutic behavior, it can become a powerful tool in our armamentarium. Our listening time then becomes a commodity for which we can charge a reasonable fee.

The physician's role as psychotherapist may involve more than listening. For example, he or she may have to take the lead, encouraging a patient to discuss a particularly sensitive subject. The mere act of asking may often be enough. For other patients more active probing may be needed. Patients may need assurance that their angry feelings are justified or an indication that their guilty feelings are excessive. Patients made anxious by conflict may be able to think a problem through more easily by discussing it out loud in your office than by struggling with it alone and at home. You can ask questions that can help clarify the issues.

A good therapist tries to empathize with a patient; that is, the therapist develops the capacity to experience a problem from the patient's point of view. This ability to share the feelings of another person is used for the purpose of understanding. *Empathy* is not the same as *sympathy;* the latter is a less objective feeling of compassion for another's plight. A patronizing quality may accompany an excessive show of sympathy, and sympathy alone precludes any effort at greater understanding of all the factors that may have contributed to the patient's situation. It can thus prevent the patient from making any effort at self-change. Excessive sympathizing can also keep the patient from expressing any dissatisfaction with his doctor.

A medical practitioner should know how to deal with an acute crisis and how to provide effective support. The remainder of this chapter will describe some principles and techniques of crisis intervention, brief psychotherapy, and long-term supportive psychotherapy. At times pharmacologic intervention is required. The reader should consult Chapter 5 for further discussion of the use of drugs in anxiety states.

GOALS OF SUPPORTIVE PSYCHOTHERAPY

For well functioning patients presenting with regressive symptoms the goal is symptomatic relief with a return to a previous level of adequate function as quickly as possible. Severe regression requires crisis intervention techniques. In less severe adjustment disorders a brief period of psychotherapy designed to support, clarify, and facilitate adjustment to stressors is indicated.

For chronically symptomatic and disabled patients the goal is to maintain psychological integrity and the capacity for adequate functioning. Achieving this goal may be possible only with long-term supportive therapy, which at times can include crisis intervention and clarification of issues. Although not a direct goal, such supportive treatment can lead to maturational changes because of the nature of the therapeutic relationship and the material discussed and clarified.

PATIENTS IN CRISIS

Most people are able to deal with the stresses that life invariably produces. However, some patients under stress experience problems that are beyond their capacity to solve, and they become symptomatic and psychologically disabled. Anxiety, helplessness, shame, anger, and guilt may ensue. If the problem continues, the anxiety may reach the point where more serious psychiatric symptoms develop. How a patient reacts to stress depends on his personality integration and the circumstances of his life. The most common sources of crises are real or misperceived changes at work or in significant personal relationships that the patient feels helpless to reverse. Maturational points such as graduation, leaving home, taking a new job, marrying, and the like are a second major source of crises. Each of these events requires that the person advance to a higher level of functioning. A third source of crises are events that have symbolic meaning to the patient and that evoke severe anxiety. When in crisis, a patient can be viewed operationally as a child temporarily in need of a parent. The medical practitioner is uniquely equipped to play the parental role.

PRINCIPLES OF CRISIS INTERVENTION PSYCHOTHERAPY

The precipitating stress, the event or situation that has led to the patient's distress and disorganization, must first be identified. During the period of crisis the physician has great influence, as the patient is highly suggestible. The transference relationship is intense, develops rapidly, and gives the physician enormous emotional influence with the patient. Successful crisis intervention requires the development, maintenance, and exploitation of a strong, positive transference reaction. The physician becomes a parental figure and uses this to advise, motivate, and encourage the patient. This relationship may change rapidly as the crisis recedes, and the physician must be prepared to alter the nature of the therapeutic relationship as the patient's level of integration improves.

The physician must assess preexisting functioning and personality integration as well as the capacity of the family to support the patient during the period of crisis. Remember that patients continue to live in the same stressful environments that may have brought them to you in the first place. Often the presence of the physician and the promise of therapeutic intervention is enough to allow patients to maintain both their equilibrium and problem solving capacities, but keep in mind that some changes in the environment and social milieu may be necessary to prevent recurrence of the problem.

The goal of crisis intervention is the reduction of anxiety and the reestablishment of the previous level of functioning and equilibrium. This goal is accomplished by changing patients' perceptions of themselves, the crisis, and the events that led to it, and by offering solutions to their problems. During a period of acute crisis, the physician provides structure, gives advice, makes judgmental statements, provides alternative solutions, supports dependency needs, relieves guilt, manipulates the environment and support systems in useful ways, and does whatever is necessary to raise the patient's self-esteem. In this work physicians can be directive and can make statements that would be inappropriate in other forms of psychotherapy. For example, patients may be told that it is simply not true that they are incapable of resolving a situation or that they are absolutely right concerning some transaction with a spouse. Patients rely entirely on the therapist during this period and see the therapist as possessing the strength and wisdom to help them through the crisis.

Crisis intervention can be viewed in much the same manner as a medical emergency. The physician must be prepared to put aside other matters and to deal with the problem, which often takes considerable time to resolve. The physician will often need to work with family members and others. The patient's self-esteem is critical, and anything that is required to help maintain and improve it is helpful.

Although the techniques of crisis intervention can reduce the necessity for hospitalization, there are times when hospitalization is indicated, usually when there is no reliable family member to support and observe the patient. A psychiatrist should be called in consultation whenever there is evidence of psychosis or suicidal thinking.

Following the initial session, the patient may be seen as often as required. Try talking first whenever possible. Agitated or depressed patients may improve quickly after a short period of crisis psychotherapeutic intervention. Do not rush in with medications unless it is absolutely necessary, however, severely anxious, depressed, or disorganized patients must be provided with appropriate medication. Such patients require psychiatric consultation. The following is an example of effective crisis intervention:

> A 31-year-old man came to his physician's office feeling anxious and experiencing episodes of depersonalization. He felt depressed and complained that he could not concentrate at work and had become quite unsure of himself. These symptoms had been present for about a week. Two days before the onset, the patient and a friend were confronted in a park by a group of boys who suddenly attacked them. Frightened, the patient ran for help, returning with a policeman to find his friend bruised and beaten. The patient became preoccupied with the event, ruminating about his decision to leave his friend and go for help. He became increasingly withdrawn and depressed.
>
> The physician knew his patient as a successful young executive who had a history of good health and a high level of achievement. He formulated the problem as a guilt reaction to the patient's panic and abandonment of

his friend, with subsequent self-reproach, loss of self-esteem, and depressive symptoms.

The physician told the patient that the decision to find a policeman was an appropriate one. Staying would have meant that both he and his friend would have been hurt, and it was understandable that he would have decided in favor of seeking help. The physician reassured the patient that such feelings were a normal response and that the decision to seek help was the best one. Treatment was directed toward making the patient feel better about himself and reducing his anxiety and guilt. The doctor used his transference role as the wise parent to support the patient's rationalization to maintain his self-esteem. The patient felt considerably improved at the end of the interview. He was given an appointment for the next day. By that time, most of his symptoms had disappeared.

BRIEF PSYCHOTHERAPY

For less severe adjustment disorders in well integrated patients and for extended work beyond a crisis period, focused brief psychotherapy may be indicated to continue support, clarify issues, and facilitate adjustment. This sort of work is usually done on a once weekly basis of thirty minutes or more of uninterrupted time and may last up to six months. Therapy that extends beyond eight weeks should be discussed with a psychiatrist.

The role of exploration and clarification depends on the nature of the patient's psychopathology and the strength of the therapeutic relationship. A useful clarification is one that leads to better understanding with reduced anxiety and an increased sense of integration and well being. Clarifications that increase anxiety lead to defensive responses or further regression are not useful. Material that the patient is not able to accept or that reduces self-esteem raises anxiety and is not therapeutic.

This type of psychotherapy, therefore, requires empathy and listening with "the third ear." Patients often express thoughts and feelings in disguised ways; the empathic observer can identify them, but the patient does not. Patients may deceive themselves to avoid knowing. The task of the physician is to decide what material should be clarified for the patient, what should best be left alone, and when rationalizations and other defenses should be supported. This is quite difficult. The following example may help illustrate these points.

A 40-year-old woman presented with the complaint that she was having anxiety attacks and felt acutely depressed. These symptoms had been increasing for a month. The physician inquired as to what was going on in the patient's life at the time the symptoms began. Initially, the patient denied any significant events but a parallel history of the recent past re-

> vealed that her husband had begun a new business venture at that time, requiring him to leave town three days each week. The patient and physician agreed that her symptoms were related to her husband's new business venture and frequent absences. The physician considered what to say to her that would be useful. She was moderately depressed and not in crisis. He surmised that the patient felt threatened by her husband's new business and separation from her. She was no longer the center of his life and had become fearful and angry.

The physician considered several possible interventions—first, "Your symptoms hide your angry feelings toward your husband for leaving you so often."

Although accurate, this clarification was put aside because the physician felt the patient would not accept that she was so angry and demanding. She might respond to such an interpretation by denying it and by attacking the physician for his lack of understanding. Thus this intervention was discarded as an initial statement; it uncovered too much unconscious conflict and could raise the patient's anxiety and evoke defensive responses.

The physician considered a second alternative: "You need your husband a great deal. His separation from you is causing you anxiety and depression."

Again an accurate observation; the husband is experienced by this patient as a nurturing parent now rejecting and leaving her. This interpretation was rejected as nonsupportive because it prematurely exposed the patient's dependency needs and separation anxiety.

The physician searched for words that would not uncover these conflicts directly but would help the patient explain her symptoms in an acceptable way—that is, he sought an approach that would reduce her anxiety and strengthen her sense of self.

The physician commented, "It does appear that your symptoms are related to your husband's new business and frequent absences. You're a devoted wife who believes in a close marriage and you're apparently paying an emotional and physical price for that."

Notice that this interpretation supports the patient's self-perception that she is devoted and understanding, and that a good marriage is a close one without separation.

The immediate effect was relief and reduction of anxiety. The patient responded, "I love my husband dearly. I don't think he appreciates me and I'm getting sick over it."

The physician suggested they meet weekly to discuss the problem. During the next few weeks the patient gave more open expression to her anger at her husband for leaving home so often. During the next two months she acknowledged that his business ideas made sense and that she wanted him to be successful but that she couldn't tolerate the separations. The physician discussed the case with a psychiatrist who suggested he respond with an interpretation. "You care a great deal for him, but perhaps you are too possessive and this produces your conflict." This statement suggested problems of dependency and separation without using language that would belittle the patient. Telling a patient she is possessive is one thing; telling her she has excessive dependency needs is quite another. The patient agreed and accepted a referral to a psychiatrist for further exploration of these issues.

This case example demonstrates how empathy, timing, and language are the basic tools for good psychotherapy.

LONG-TERM SUPPORTIVE THERAPY

Some patients require a purely supportive form of psychotherapy, for example, patients with chronic pain or hypochondriasis. For this group the primary need is the gratification of dependency needs not adequately met in their personal lives. Physicians function as unconscious parental substitutes for these patients. In our society, the clergy sometimes share this role, but many of our patients find the doctor-patient relationship the more comfortable one from which to gain this support.

For example, hypochondriacal patients will use physical symptoms as the ticket of admission to the physician's office. This is not a conscious subterfuge. They truly experience the physical problem of which they complain. Many patients with chronic illness adjust to their discomfort or disability, however, for the patient with unmet dependency needs or a heightened sense of vulnerability, physical symptoms become socially acceptable reasons for calling upon the physician. The physician must do more than conduct a cursory exam, order another set of diagnostic tests, and reassure the patient, for the failure to identify the underlying emotional need and to act accordingly will produce a cycle of recurrent complaints, reassurance, and frustration for patient and physician alike.

Physicians usually have no difficulty identifying hypochondriacal patients when they think about this issue. The physician's problem is usually his unwillingness to accept the chronicity of the diagnosis or to acknowledge the effectiveness of just listening. As noted earlier, for many patients ventilation of their physical complaints plus an opportunity to share something of their personal lives with you is a truly therapeutic experience. To fail to acknowledge that is to deprive you and them of considerable gratification (see Chapter 2).

Principles of Long-Term, Supportive Psychotherapy

There are patients for whom a long-term relationship with a physician is essential for adequate functioning. Our knowledge of unconscious psychodynamics provides insight into the sources of a patient's chronic difficulty and may, for some patients, lead ultimately to a psychiatric referral. For most patients, however, the physician uses his knowledge of psychodynamics to devise a supportive strategy that consistently tries to reduce anxiety and raise self-esteem. This may require fostering rationalizations, reaction formations, and other defenses while gratifying needs. As noted earlier, the physician does not interpret the physical preoccupations of the hypochondriacal patient. To interpret them would lead to increased anxiety, denial, and a possible rupture in the therapeutic relationship. Instead, without mentioning dependency needs, the patient's need for parental support is gratified through office visits and supportive statements.

Long-term supportive psychotherapy requires support and intermittent crisis intervention therapy. These patients are vulnerable to regression under crisis. They cannot function autonomously and require a lifelong parental relationship. Each time the patient is seen, attempts are made to reduce anxiety and raise self-esteem. The primary care physician and the psychiatric consultant remain a team throughout the course of treatment.

Some patients demand dependent gratification through covert or overt hostility. They may subject the physician to negative, angry, denigrating statements. In spite of their seemingly low appraisals of the physician, such patients keep returning. Stay calm, assured, and helpful; these are people in need.

Listen empathically without rendering judgments, and help patients sort out and reevaluate realistically the alternatives to their life problems. Help them develop confidence in their own capacity to cope with life's stresses. Patients use psychotherapy as a sounding board to express thoughts and feelings that have frightened and confused them, shamed them, or made them feel guilty. They should be encouraged to talk about what is bothering them. This talking is a process of sharing problems and a mutual search for ways to resolve them. You do not have to have all the answers to the patient's life problems.

The frequency of visits can be determined only on an individual basis. Some anxious patients may require weekly visits; others may be seen biweekly, monthly, or even less often, depending on their needs. During periods of crisis, additional therapeutic sessions may have to be scheduled.

In general, psychotherapeutic sessions should run 20 to 30 minutes, but some patients may require more time. Try to listen for themes that emerge in the course of a patient's discussion, themes that he or she may be unaware of and need to communicate. The physician determines what needs to be clarified and what material requires a therapeutic strategy to reduce anxiety.

In the early stages of treatment the patient may feel guilty about discussing negative feelings about close family members. The physician must reassure the patient that this is a normal response and a part of psychotherapy. Remember to maintain the patient's privacy and privileged position. Do not communicate with family or friends about any material discussed without the patient's permission.

In the course of treatment, patients may change their conscious and unconscious response to the physician. At times such changes may be hidden behind a variety of symptoms, such as anxiety or acting out. *Acting out* may be defined as action that relates to a conflict between patient and physician. For example, a patient who misses an appointment because he or she "forgot" the date of the meeting may be expressing anger without being aware of it. Try to understand what is going on between the two of you, including your own emotional responses to the patient. The problem may be the patient's intense transference response to you or it may relate to nontherapeutic emotional responses on your part. The source of the anxiety must be identified and dealt with. Such feelings or behavior on the part of either patient or physician should be discussed with a psychiatric consultant.

Termination of Treatment

For many patients supportive psychotherapy will continue for life. Others may develop the capacity to function more effectively through their own personal growth, the healing effects of psychotherapy, and the therapeutic relationship with the physician. When you sense that the patient is less in need of psychotherapy, you can explore the possibility of decreasing the frequency of sessions. Always keep open the possibility of increasing the frequency of sessions or of restarting psychotherapy. The transference aspects of the relationship will continue even if a strictly psychotherapeutic relationship has ended.

The following case example illustrates many of the principles outlined above.

> A 35-year-old married woman with a 6-year-old daughter saw her physician in consultation because of a variety of complaints including headaches, muscle spasm, epigastric distress, and vague sensations in her chest. These symptoms frightened the patient, who felt she might have some serious, if not fatal, illness. The symptoms began when the patient's husband announced to her that he was unhappy and considering a separation. She became increasingly angered and demanded that he remain at home with her and their daughter, especially now that she was ill. The physician evaluated her medical status and could find nothing significant to explain her symptoms except her obvious anxiety. She appeared demoralized, though not depressed, and was quite concerned over her marriage. How-

ever, she was unaware of the effects of her demands and hypochondriacal concerns on her husband, who by this time was considering divorce.

The physician felt that the problem was clearly a reaction to the stress in the marriage and this patient's immature personality integration and approach to the marital relationship. The patient had idealized her husband as a powerful paternal figure who would care for her and love her in a rather static unchanging way. That, indeed, was how the courtship went. She began experiencing minor physical complaints a year after she was married.

When the husband was interviewed by the physician he expressed his concerns for his wife's health and his increasing feelings of inadequacy regarding his ability to give her what she needed emotionally. He was very involved in his business and was meeting men and women who were as excited as he by the prospects of success, mastery, and the enjoyment of life. His wife, on the other hand, preferred a cocoon-like existence.

The physician saw both wife and husband five times. These sessions were characterized by the wife's incessant complaints, and little progress was made. It seemed clear to the physician that there was little room to maneuver; the husband had clearly outdistanced the patient emotionally and was no longer happy in the marriage. Shortly thereafter the husband left and, although he maintained a cordial relationship with his wife and a close, involved relationship with his daughter, he never returned. Eventually, they divorced.

The physician had consulted a psychiatrist for advice on several occasions, and both felt that supportive psychotherapy was the appropriate treatment for this young woman. During the period immediately following the separation, the physician saw this patient several times weekly for 20 to 30 minutes and listened empathically to her grief and concerns about going it alone. He reassured her again and again that there were no serious medical problems when she became frightened by her physical symptoms. She was also unsure of her ability to handle her daily routine and the problems of bringing up her young daughter. In fact, she was doing quite well and needed to be reminded of that. She was angry at her husband and spent many sessions expressing her rage and resentment. The physician listened empathically and commented that he could understand how much pain she was in and how disappointed she was.

No attempts were made to analyze either her sense of entitlement or her dependency needs in the relationship and how these factors underlay her hypochondriacal concerns. Gradually the patient's mood lightened, and she continued her life without her husband. She found a part-time job and began seeing other men. At her suggestion, sessions were reduced to once weekly. Each session generally began with the patient anxiously discussing her physical symptoms. Then she would express her feelings of guilt and her conviction that she had been a terrible mother and an awful wife, and she would repeat her fears for the future. The physician would respond by reassuring her again about her health and by finding constructive things in her relations with her daughter and others and generally in her life. Thus he reassured the patient that she was handling herself and her daughter in a reasonable way, much to her relief. The physician's comments were communicated in a calm, supportive, and friendly way that supported her need for an all-knowing, wise, paternal figure. This work continued in pretty much the same way for a period of eighteen months. At six-month intervals, the physician consulted the psychiatrist for advice concerning his work with this patient.

At the end of the 18 month period the psychiatrist felt that the patient was integrated enough for the physician to begin to explore why she felt so frightened and anxious and was so self-denigrating. An exploration of her developmental years and early adult relationships ensued. Again, no attempt was made at interpretive work although the patient was able to make many constructive connections herself. The transference relationship with the physician was initially one of her idealized father but over the next year gradually changed as the patient felt increasingly disappointed that she was not getting enough care and love from the physician. She gradually recognized that this was a repetition of what she had felt with her husband. Now both physician and psychiatrist felt that she had reached the point where she could benefit from a more analytically oriented therapy. She had become increasingly curious about these emotional patterns and accepted a referral. The physician maintained his normal medical relationship with the patient thereafter.

This chapter has offered some introductory principles of psychotherapy in medical practice. Obviously, each individual requires an approach tailored to his or her needs and problems. This is especially true for patients in the pediatric, adolescent, and geriatric age groups and for patients who have family difficulties or sexual problems; later chapters deal with all of these issues. Readers who are interested in undertaking psychotherapy with patients should consider developing a supervisory relationship with a trained psychotherapist. The following bibliography will also prove useful. Those titles marked with an asterisk are recommended as initial reading.

BIBLIOGRAPHY

*Aldrich CK: Office psychotherapy for the primary care physician, in Friedman DX, Dyrud JE (eds): American Handbook of Psychiatry, Vol. V, 2nd Edition. New York, Basic Books, 1975

Balint M, Balint E: Psychotherapeutic Techniques in Medicine. London, Tavistock Publications

Bruch H: Learning Psychotherapy. Cambridge, Mass., Harvard University Press, 1974

*Dubovsky SL: Psychotherapeutics in Primary Care. New York, Grune & Stratton, 1981

*Enelow AJ: Elements of Psychotherapy. New York, Oxford University Press, 1977

Erikson EH: Identity and the Life Cycle. Psychological Issues, Vol. I, No. I. New York, International Universities Press, 1963

Fishman C, Nadelson T: Crisis Intervention in Psychosomatic Medicine
Fromm E: The Forgotten Language. New York, 1951
Havens LL: Approaches to the Mind. Boston, Little Brown, 1973
Kaliner R: Psychotherapy in psychosomatic disorders. Arch Gen Psychiatry 32:1021–1028, 1975
Karasu TB: Psychotherapy of the medically ill. Am J Psychiatry 136:1:1–11, 1979
*Kolb L: Psychotherapy in medical practice. Texas State Journal of Medicine 57:558–562, July 1961
Linn L: Basic principles of management in psychosomatic medicine, in Wittkower ED, Warnes H (eds): Medical Department. Hagerstown, Maryland, Harper and Row, 1977
MacKinnon RA, Michels R: The Psychiatric Interview in Clinical Practice. Philadelphia, W.B. Saunders, 1971
May R: The function of myth in sickness and health, in Witenberg E: Interpersonal Exploration in Psychoanalysis. New York, Basic Books, Inc., 1973
Mott J: Brief psychotherapy in medical practice, in Balis GU, Wurmser L, McDaniel E, Grenell RG (eds): The Psychiatric Foundations of Medicine, Vol. 5, Psychiatric Clinical Skills in Medical Practice. Boston, Butterworth Publishers, Inc., 1978
Penna M, McDaniel E, Gallahorn GE: Crisis intervention and supportive techniques in patient management, in Balis GU, Wurmser L, McDaniel E, et al. (eds): The Psychiatric Foundations of Medicine, Vol. 5, Psychiatric Clinical Skills in Medical Practice. Boston, Butterworth Publishers, Inc., 1978

Lila J. Kalinich, M.D.

4

The Management of the Female Patient

In an era in which women are questioning all institutions that influence cultural norms, medicine has not been spared. Organized women's groups have become increasingly critical of the medical establishment,[1] largely for its apparent failure to allow women to participate in a reasonable way in making decisions about their own health care.

Such criticism is especially severe when one medical approach or the other involves risk. For example, women are still angry about the demonstrated adverse effects of using diethyl stilbestrol (DES), the Dalkon shield, and oral contraceptives. One can argue that these effects were not predictable. However, women are tending to interpret revelations of this sort as signs of medicine's more general insensivity to the needs of women.

A growing literature[2] concerns itself with the female patient's need for a more effective voice in dealing with her physician. Much of this literature, in the spirit of patient advocacy, has been written expressly for women, providing them with much needed information. Rather little has been written for physicians who might be interested in enhancing their understanding of the uniquely feminine issues that shape the woman's experience of being a patient. The aim here is to do just that: to clarify why some women do not speak out, and why others who have still feel that they have not really been heard.

The author wishes to acknowlege the inspiration provided by Mildred L. Bowen, M.D. (Western Reserve Medical School, 1926)

THE DOCTOR–PATIENT RELATIONSHIP

More and more women are emphasizing the social and psychosexual aspects of their roles as patients, scrutinizing and challenging the assumptions that seem to underly the delivery of health care. Among U.S. physicians, 93 percent are men; but women, on the average, make 100 percent more patient visits than men (if visits of mothers to pediatricians are included).[1] As a result, women often view the doctor–patient relationship as a special case of the phenomenon of women dealing with men: a heterosexual relationship with all its attendant complexities, the implications of which vary depending on a woman's self-perception, aspirations, and reaction to the medical model.*

The physician, since Hippocrates, has had to bear both the burden and the reward of occupying a very special place in society. He has been privy to the magic of disease and cure. He has been expected to act as a kind of parent surrogate, to foster the belief that there remains someone to nurture and protect us even after the (psychological) death of our parents. That the doctor–patient relationship has tended to take on an authoritarian form is, therefore, no surprise. And this form worked relatively well in a culture where roles and role expectations were clearly defined. Today's blurring of those boundaries has introduced confusion for both the woman and her doctor, leaving each at a loss as to what the other wants and needs.

Recent articles have very pointedly addressed the issue of sexual prejudice in medical training, diagnosis, and patient management. Howell, for example, discusses the attitudes toward both female students and patients in medical teaching.[3] The bawdy, club house atmosphere has encouraged an occasional pin-up to find its way into the anatomy lecture, communicating the clear message that women are still to be disparaged. Women patients are often unfairly portrayed as hysterical, nagging, or trivial in their complaints. When diseases of psychogenic origin are discussed, the hypothetical patient is almost routinely referred to as female. Further Howell cites issues of even greater consequence, such as a high rate of hysterectomies performed without proper indication; the failure of most physicians to do routine breast exams despite the fact that breast carcinoma ranks second as a killer of middle-aged women; and the frequency with which the pelvic exam is omitted from the routine hospital admission physical.

---

*To underline this conception of the doctor–patient relationship, the male pronoun will be used in reference to the physician throughout most of this chapter.

It is true that the failure to perform these examinations may reflect the male physician's discomfort with sexually related procedures more than disparagement of women as such. Nevertheless, the consequences are the same, and women as patients are in a vital way medically short-changed.

In a similar vein, Lennane and Lennane question the emphasis on the role of psychogenic factors in female disorders.[4] In spite of empirical evidence that implicates organic causes in primary dysmenorrhea, nausea of pregnancy, and pain in labor, assumptions about the psychogenic origins of these difficulties have led to irrational approaches to management. According to these authors, this willingness to emphasize psychogenic factors in women reflects a moralistic infantilization of the female patient.

Physicians have often been inclined to assume psychogenic causes for other somatic disorders in females. A woman physician, in general practice for fifty years, told the author of several cases in which pulmonary and renal TB in women had initially been diagnosed as "hysterical." She doubted that this diagnosis would have been made in males. Without question, men have also been subject to misdiagnosis and bad medical practice. However, the abuse of the psychogenic explanation for physical symptoms does seem to be more likely to occur as part of the special experience of the female patient.

THE CONTEMPORARY WOMAN

The most common complaint of the contemporary woman is that her doctor does not take her seriously. Anecdotes reported by Luy illustrate the physician's tendency to infantilize and patronize his female patients.[5] For example, in response to a question such as "What's an erosion?" a doctor may reply, "Nothing serious—don't worry about it." When the author herself was a medical student, she visited a gynecologist who told her, "your little girl organs are okay." Kaiser and Kaiser, in their article, "The Challenge of the Woman's Movement to American Gynecology," remind their readers that women come to their practitioners in a state of vulnerability, often feeling low and willing to be dependent. It is often tempting to respond with the proverbial pat-on-the-head, "leave the worrying to me" attitude, thinking that this is what the woman wants. In the past such a response might have been sufficient. Women felt comforted by the implication that someone was really willing to take total responsibility for them and physicians were spared the time and effort required to communicate medical information adequately. Of course, some physicians treat all their patients this way, but it is probably true that physicians are more likely to relate to female patients in this manner. More women these days are infuriated by such an attitude. They are demanding that they be treated as partners in their own care.

In most cases, this unconscious concept of women revealed by this physicianly–fatherly attitude is more annoying than harmful, more benign than malignant. But some of its manifestations are more egregious than others. A woman recently described an interaction she had had with her mother-in-law's oncologist. In response to her questions about medications, the doctor replied, "When you have gone to medical school, studied biochemistry and pharmacology, and gotten your degree, I will spend my time trying to answer your questions. Until then I have more important things to do." The same physician answered these questions immediately when asked by the woman's husband, who was no better equipped to comprehend the answers than his wife, a Ph.D. The woman herself, dumbfounded, never said a word.

It is telling that such anecdotes have remained largely within the confines of oral history. Women have been unable to confront their physicians with their dissatisfaction face to face. They have stored their resentment, ventilated to friends, and in the extreme, gone elsewhere for care. The need for self-assertion in such a confrontation has been and remains a source of great conflict for women. With roots in both cultural stereotypes and individual psychologies, this conflict is sometimes more tumultuous in the woman striving for gratification in less traditionally feminine ways. The career woman, for instance, is especially sensitive to being seen as aggressive, pushy, unpleasant, or unfeminine, when feminine has often meant quiet, passive, compliant, and trusting. She fears that questioning her physician may cause him to have a negative opinion of her. It may also make her see herself in a less favorable light. Such a woman therefore refrains from calling her physician with questions or physical complaints. She fears that she will be "bothering" him and that he will become annoyed and retaliate by taking her less than seriously when she really needs him. A pediatrician recently commented that routinely, mothers who call him apologize for disturbing him, whereas fathers almost never make such apology.

The woman's reluctance to assert herself can become confused with conflicts over being dependent on her doctor. Greenberg and Fischer, investigating the issue of willingness to adopt a sick role, found that middle class women concerned with issues of autonomy and independence were more inclined to delay seeking medical attention than were their traditional sisters.[7] Although this was understood to be partly because these women had a greater sense of bodily integrity, their negative expectations of the doctor–patient relationship made their contribution as well. The perceived threat to independence weighed more heavily on their minds than the threat of physical disability.

The consequences of the neglect of patient participation in their own health care are potentially very serious. Such women may ignore simple preventive measures such as Pap smears and breast exams. They may fail to consult an obstetrician for prenatal care early in pregnancy. They may ignore follow-up visits after surgery or illness. Or, they may stop medication before completing a full therapeutic course. This behavior in the past was typical of the indigent female patient—especially in a clinic setting—or of male patients unable to accept the notion that they were ill and dependent. Now some middle class women seem to be responding in a similar way as a manifestation of their perception of the health care system.

More and more women are, therefore, turning to female physicians. To have had a menstrual cramp is to know one. These women expect that the issues so central to their lives will not be minimized by a woman doctor. However, the majority of women continue to see male physicians. It is, therefore, essential that such physicians become more aware of the concerns of female patients, and of how preconceived attitudes may unwittingly affect the behavior of both physician and patient.

Physicians must try to be tolerant of the contemporary woman's questions, even when they seem somewhat lengthy and tedious. Spending the extra time to make both the patient's disease and its treatment as comprehensible as possible will often spare both doctor and patient difficult times. Further, physicians must not unnecessarily conceal areas of ambiguity just to minimize the patient's anxiety. The contemporary woman will notice the physician's lack of clarity and misinterpret it. She can tolerate a frank discussion of the limitations of medical knowledge better than she can tolerate a feeling that she is being patronized. Finally, physicians must remember that the independent, noncomplaining, contempory woman merits some extra concern in that she is probably working overly hard to conceal the depth of her distress, pain, or fear. She is tending to wait too long to utilize her doctor's services. She, more than others, needs to be encouraged to seek help, to allow herself to be a bit more dependent. She needs to know that she will not be seen as a troublesome little girl or a nagging woman if she does.

THE TRADITIONAL WOMAN

One of the results of the traditional woman's willingness to assume an unquestioning and passive attitude toward her doctor is that she often acts like a child. Her vision of the physician as an omnipotent, omniscient figure who can care for her without requiring her collaboration, combines with the stress of illness to foster a psychological regression. Some of this is necessary for a healthy adaptation to illness and hospitalization. However, such a regression can go to an unhealthy extreme.

Infantile and demanding behaviors can emerge. The woman may unconsciously pressure her doctor to do more for her than he can. For instance, she may communicate her wish for a magical cure or make subtle demands for more attention. The physician is thus made to feel inadequate, guilty, and finally enraged. Some women may resort to seductiveness in an effort to make an impact on their physicians and retain some sense of control. Others, defending against sexual feelings, will, like their contemporary counterparts, fail to request what they need. One woman recently reported that she could not remind her physician to do a breast exam because it approximated a sexual fantasy.

The traditional woman may also become diffident and suspend the operation of those faculties necessary for self-observation and good judgment. It is not unusual for such a woman to leave her doctor's office wondering why she behaved like a child or why she failed to provide him with important information. For instance, an elderly woman seeing a consultant for her hiatus hernia listened to him, agreed compliantly with his treatment plan, and only later realized that the medications he suggested were the same as those she had been taking and from which she had gained no relief.

Overcompliance can complicate history taking significantly. Trying to please her doctor, a woman may be overly inclusive on the review of systems; or, conversely, she may neglect to report something vital for fear of being trivial. The point is that often, in an effort to be a "good patient," she fails to use her common sense. And the woman may be left with a profound sense of humiliation when she realizes that she has presented herself so foolishly.

In a certain sense it is evident that the physician should be most concerned for the traditional woman. She is less accustomed to observing her own reactions and formulating her own opinions. She is less likely to notice just where the doctor–patient relationship breaks down, less likely to be able to articulate her complaints or to seek alternative care.

While with the comtemporary woman the doctor must acknowledge and respect her expectation that she be treated as an equal, with the traditional woman he must work especially hard to encourage her to feel that she is entitled to think along with and question her physician. He must ask her, for instance, at the end of a visit, if she has understood her instructions. He should invite her to call should any questions occur to her at home, reassuring her that the stress of being in the office often makes it difficult for patients to think clearly.

THE SEDUCTIVE PATIENT

Occasionally a female patient will engage in overtly seductive behavior. Although, in some cases, women without adequate sexual satisfaction in their lives may find the intimacies of the physical exam erotically stimulating, the motivation for seductive behavior is rarely sexual. At times, the woman finds that the male doctor unconsciously fulfills a fantasy of an omnipotent male protector who can be won sexually. At others, she attempts to convert the anxiety-producing doctor–patient relationship into a more familiar and less threatening one by sexualizing it. Clearly, the patient is responding to the physician's role rather than to him personally.

In most situations, maintaining a professional distance in the relationship is sufficient to indicate to the patient that her advances are ill-directed. Any behavior on the doctor's part that is flirtatious, casual, or provocative will only aggravate the problem. Should it become necessary for the physician to be more direct, he should remind the patient that she has come to him for medical consultation because she is in need of care; that although for the moment she might feel otherwise, she needs a physician rather than a lover; and that her interest is related to his professional role rather than to him. The physician's willingness to gently and clearly outline the boundaries of the relationship will ultimately provide relief, despite the fact that some women will react with embarrassment or pique. If he is neither judgmental nor self-righteous, the patient will be able to remain in his care with no lasting loss of face.

WOMEN WHO CHOOSE WOMEN PHYSICIANS

There are two groups of women who often pose problems for the woman physician. One group selects a female doctor because she gains a sense of comfort from the false assumption that all women are alike. Their belief that the female doctor universally shares their attitudes leads them to expect an almost automatic compliance with their demands. When the physician does not comply, they may respond in a betrayed and angry way, sometimes becoming frankly manipulative. The other group perceive only men as having genuine authority and may seek the care of a woman in an unconscious attempt to avoid an authority figure. In this case a woman, *any* woman, will be perceived as a peer at best and therefore more subject to the patient's whim and will.

The woman physician must be tolerant of the presumptiousness and disdain for women that is implicitly communicated by the second type of patient. It is easy to become angry and insulted under these circumstances. But it is imperative that these mistaken notions be treated as carefully as the disease. With the first type of patient the woman doctor must not abandon her own sense of professional decorum because of the "at home" quality of the patient. The doctor herself will later become surprised and upset when she confronts the rage of this formerly friendly patient should she not yield to the patient's demands. With the second type of patient the woman physician may react with irritation precisely because she secretly shares the idea that women cannot wield true authority. She must remind herself that medical authority is determined by knowledge rather than gender.

THE UNIQUELY FEMININE ISSUES: DEVELOPMENTAL LANDMARKS IN HEALTH AND DISEASE

For both men and women, the experience of the body is a powerful organizer of the personality and the sense of self. A look at the dawning and development of the woman's sense of biological femaleness clarifies to some extent the origin of some of the traits described above.

Reactions to menarche are often of a traumatic nature. Blood is associated with injury and pain; the flow and its hygienic consequences are linked to dirt and messiness—in effect, they are anally tinged. The exploration of the genitals, unavailable for real looking, is often fraught with anxiety and confusion. Controversial Freudian theories aside, each child must attempt to assimilate and integrate some notion of its physical self. And for the girl child a picture of herself as damaged, dirty, and most of all, unable to control what comes out of her body, is often part of her self-concept. In the best circumstances, the reality testing provided by maturation in a supportive environment comes to temper this picture. Even so, the rudiments of it remain to influence the woman's subsequent reactions to somatic and psychological distress. Later, these reactions are compounded by heightened sexual feelings, themselves often experienced as a threat to the woman's sense of control.

Menstruation

It is easy to see that menstruation remains a potential monthly threat to the woman's sense of integrity. She often feels that her aggressive feelings, especially, are leaking out everywhere; and she and others in her world usually regard the expression of such feelings as unfeminine and unacceptable. Her premenstrual moodiness diminishes her self-esteem, which is often further lowered when those close to her regard her anger over realistic issues as unjustified simply because she happens to be menstruating.

The physical sensation of bloating heightens a woman's perception of her body as something out of control. Her image of her body changes from the beginning to the end of the menstrual cycle. The result is a certain instability in her mental representation of her physical self which only heightens a feeling of physical vulnerability.

For many women, menstruation is further complicated by the occurrence of dysmenorrhea and/or the premenstrual syndrome. Until recently, primary dysmenorrhea and the premenstrual syndrome were considered by most physicians to be an exaggerated response to normal physiological processes. Afflicted women were seen as rejecting of the "feminine role." Women with these complaints were often made to feel guilty or inadequate. Their requests for treatment were dismissed.

The discovery during the past decade of a physiological explanation and an effective treatment for dysmenorrhea has brought many sufferers of dysmenorrhea "out of the closet." Recent figures therefore reflect more accurately the high prevalence of this condition.[8] It is now even more important to ask routinely about both dysmenorrhea and the prementrual syndrome.

Primary dysmenorrhea is related to elevated levels of prostaglandins in the endometrium and menstrual fluid. This is thought to result in hyperactivity of the myometrium with associated uterine ischemia and painful cramping. The release of prostaglandins into the systemic circulation probably explains the symptoms that accompany dysmenorrhea: diarrhea, faintness, dizziness, and headaches. All of these are relieved in 60 to 100 percent of patients by a group of prostaglandin-synthetase inhibitor drugs which include mefenamic acid (Ponstel), naproxen sodium (Anaprox), and ibuprofen (Motrin). Table 4-1 provides dosage recommendations for these drugs.

The development of an effective treatment for dysmenorrhea and the acknowledgement that its orgins are somatic rather than psychogenic has focused attention on the premenstrual syndrome, for which an etiology and a consistently effective treatment have yet to be determined.

Table 4-1
Dosage Recommendations for Prostaglandin-synthetase Inhibitor Drugs

Drug	Initial Dose	Subsequent Dosage
Mefenamic acid (*Ponstel*)	500 mg	250 mg q. 6 hr prn
Naproxen (*Anaprox*)	600 mg	300 mg q. 6 hr prn
Ibuprofen (*Motrin*)	550 mg	275 mg q. 6 hr prn

The term premenstrual syndrome (PMS) encompasses a variety of physical, mood, and behavior changes that regularly occur in the late luteal phase of the menstrual cycle and are relieved by the onset of the menses. Most women experience some recurrent premenstrual physical or emotional changes. The spectrum of severity is very wide, with mild symptoms reported by the majority of women. However, in 20 to 30 percent of women symptoms are more severe and may even be incapacitating. Within this group there may be premenstrual deterioration of interpersonal relationships, marital discord, child abuse, work absenteeism or inefficiency, and an increase in accidents, psychiatric admissions, and suicide attempts.

The most common manifestations of PMS are breast swelling and tenderness, abdominal bloating and edema of the extremities, fatigue and depression or irritability and tension, appetite changes, cravings for sweets and salty foods, headaches, bowel changes, and acne.

The following have been suggested to explain the pathogenesis of PMS: a high estrogen-progesterone ratio, estrogen excess, progesterone deficiency, vitamin B6 deficiency, hypoglycemia, fluid retention, increases in prolactin, aldosterone, vasopressin, or angiotensin, increased monoamine oxidase activity, serotonin deficiency, and prostaglandins. Recent theories suggest that withdrawal from the central effects of the neuro-peptides β-endorphin and α-melancocyte-stimulating hormone produce a variety of neuroendocrine changes within the brain-hypothalamus-pituitary axis. Mood and behavior changes may result from the effect of these peptides on neurotransmitter function. Treatment studies based on these theories have yielded inconclusive results.[9]

In the absence of a better understanding of pathogenesis and the development of specific treatments for PMS, treatment must be supportive and symptom oriented. Physicians can be therapeutic by recognizing and acknowledging the validity of the complaints. The following are suggestions for the management of patients with PMS.

Education. Patients will feel more in control and therefore better able to tolerate the sudden cyclical changes they experience if they are prepared for them and are taught how to reschedule their daily activities accordingly. They should be advised to keep a monthly calendar so that they will anticipate difficult days. Some patients may need "permission" to take it a bit easy during the premenstrual period. They should be encouraged, for example, to take time for a nap, arrange for a baby-sitter, etc. They should not schedule a large dinner party or an important business meeting. They should understand that it may be particularly difficult to diet at that time. Pointing out the organic etiology of the syndrome will help minimize whatever sense of inadequacy they might feel regarding these transient changes in functioning.

Diet. Reduction or omission of caffeine-containing beverages and chocolate may be helpful in minimizing two of the most common premenstrual symptoms, breast tenderness and irritability. A low sodium, low carbohydrate diet, and reduction of alchohol intake may also alleviate some PMS symptoms.

Diuretics. Mild diuretics premenstrually may make women who complain of severe bloating and edema more comfortable.

Vitamin B_6. A trial of supplemental Vitamin B_6 in daily doses of 100 mg has been reported to be helpful in some cases. The rationale for this treatment is based on the role of Vitamin B_6 as a co-enzyme of the metabolism of the neurotransmitters dopamine and serotonin.[10]

When symptoms remain severe or incapacitating after supportive measures have been suggested, one or more of the following treatments should be given a therapeutic trial.

Benzodiazepines given premenstrually may be helpful for the anxious, irritable patient. They will not help the depressed patient. The most common type of premenstrual depression is an atypical form with lethargy, hypersomnia, and hyperphagia. Small doses of amphetamine (5–10 mg/day) may alleviate these symptoms if given during the premenstrual period. Benzodiazepines and amphetamines should *not* be given to patients prone to substance abuse.

Some studies have reported that women with affective illness have a higher incidence of PMS, and their depressive symptoms may be exacerbated premenstrually.[11] In such situations, treatment of the depression with antidepressant medication will be helpful in reducing the severity of the PMS.

It is important to consider that exacerbations of migraine, epilepsy, asthma, depression, and psychosis may occur premenstrually and cyclical variations in dosage of medications used to treat these patients may be necessary. Some women who are being treated with drugs such as phenothiazines, methyldopa, or reserpine may have worsened PMS symptoms because these drugs stimulate prolactin secretion.

It is critical to recall, when all is said and done, that women do have a psychology that reacts to their biology. Sometimes those old interpretations regarding oedipal conflicts and feminine role rejection have their place. Women with profound PMS and/or dysmenorrhea have been significantly helped through pschotherapy or psychoanalysis. The physician should therefore explore the possibility that marital and other conflicts may be present, and refer such patients for psychiatric consultation.

The First Pelvic Exam

The introduction of the adolescent female to the pelvic exam is often a critically sensitive event. The young woman is routinely frightened of her first vaginal penetration, even if by a speculum. Clearly the pelvic exam was and still is linked to the induction of adult genital sexuality. It is very important that the examining physician treat this event with the care and respect that it merits. The presence of a female nurse or aide often provides a measure of comfort for the patient and protection for the physician. Even this arrangement, however, does not entirely eliminate the potential for emotional trauma, and the physician must not be fooled by the modern adolescent's show of nonchalance. Despite the current social pressure to act as though it were otherwise, sexuality is today as conflict-laden and frightening for the adolescent as it ever was.

If, on the other hand, the adolescent girl reacts with extreme sensitivity to the examination of either the genitalia or the breasts, the physician should be alert to the possibility that this youngster may require special assistance with the stresses of puberty. In some cases a referral to a female physician may suffice. In all cases an effort should be made to assess the adolescent's overall social, family, and sexual adjustment. This information will help determine whether a patient requires psychiatric referral (see also Chapter 11).

Disease of the Reproductive Organs

Disease of the reproductive organs can generate a host of complex responses, which are often contingent on the degree to which a woman is at peace with her sense of her feminity, sexuality, and life role. Disease can reawaken the unconscious sense of being intrinsically damaged. A woman may find herself struggling with the notion that reproductive tract disease is a punishment, either for sexual activity, or her daring to be different from the kind of woman that the culture encourages.

Hysterectomy

As a surgical procedure, the hysterectomy ranks second only to the tonsillectomy in frequency of performance.[2] Reactions to a hysterectomy can be especially complex. The uterus often serves as a kind of focus for the formation of feminine identity. Although the loss of a body part is always emotionally shaking, no other internal organ is assigned this kind of significance. Hysterectomy can result in clinical depression. Women express a feeling of being empty inside, having a space that cannot be filled up. Sometimes sensations similar to the "phantom limb" are described. In many cases a time of grieving is required to cope with the loss of whatever part of womanhood the uterus represented. Fears that hysterectomy will diminish sexual responsiveness are common, especially among the lower class or the poorly educated. It is not unusual for women in these groups to be viewed as no longer sexually adequate and to be rejected by their husbands. In general, the more passive and dependent the woman, and the more stereotyped her sex role behavior, the more prone she is to a morbid reaction to hysterectomy. Kaltreider and Horowitz documented that the persistence of a wish for future children correlated with a poor clinical outcome.[12]

Even a woman who seems to adjust well initially to a hysterectomy may later show evidence of distress. Although not necessarily clinically depressed, she may describe intrusive thoughts and memories about the procedure that she finds highly unwelcome. These thoughts shake a part of her that would prefer to deny the significance of the surgery.

The physician can sometimes predict a problematic response to hysterectomy during a preoperative interview with the patient. He should explore disappointed hopes, fears, and fast-held myths about the surgery and its effects. A similar interview with the husband should be part of the routine management of a hysterectomy. Simple clarification can often allay significant anxiety. However, unconscious ideas and conflicts about the uterus can continue to distort a couple's understanding. If information does not seem to make a difference in at least tempering the fear, it is wise to be on the alert for a postoperative pathological response. Allow for a period of grieving postoperatively, considering the possibility that the patient may have a delayed reaction. Encourage her to verbalize feelings and thoughts about how she has changed. Monitor her functioning both in her ordinary routines and in her relationship with her spouse. Watch for signs of depression with marked fatigability, anorexia, and sleep problems. If despite your efforts, the patient continues to be troubled at the time of her followup visit at three months, refer her to a psychiatrist.

Pelvic Pain

The evaluation and treatment of pelvic pain remains a somewhat controversial and clouded area. Even the recent literature implies that psychogenic contributions have not been given sufficient credibility. This is remarkable, given the tendency, described earlier, to emphasize psychogenic factors in women patients with genuine organic illness. A study by Beard et al., in 1977, concluded that "psychosomatic disturbance must be recognized as a bona fide cause of pelvic pain,'' and it expressed the hope that unnecessary surgery might be avoided.[13] Beard et al. found that the group of women with pain and a negative laparascopy were significantly more denigrating toward themselves and their partners, and less orgasmic. These findings are in essential agreement with the findings of a study conducted in 1960.[14] But these earlier authors went on to state that ''patients with pelvic pain were unable to establish and preserve that (unconscious) sense of feminine identity which permits the unhampered execution of feminine functions (homemaking, relating affectionately to a husband, performing sexually, menstrually and gestationally).'' Note that this description of feminine function contains no reference to genuine personal pleasure or growth.

Friederich, in an illuminating paper, describes the typical history of a woman inclined to express the pain of her life experience through pelvic pain.[15] Such women tend to have disturbed childhoods, frequently with a history of violence and physical abuse. From an early age, pain has been no stranger to them. One parent was often neglectful, alcoholic, or promiscuous. Frequently, the woman marries early to get away from home, only to recreate, with her spouse, aspects of her life with her parents. With her husband, as with her parents, she inhibits the expression of her rather enormous rage in order to avoid even greater abuse or rejection. When angry feelings are evoked, she may develop pain instead.

Taking a careful history may provide data that can help the physician to distinguish the woman likely to have psychogenic pain from the woman with organic illness. In addition to the factors described above, it is not uncommon to find that complaints referrable to the pelvic area were present from childhood. Thus a careful chart review alone may avert unnecessary surgery. Further, the physician may discover that the woman is sufficiently gratified and supported by his willingness to listen to her so that the pain recedes in significance. Though it may not disappear, its presence may not concern her as much.

Some feel that psychotherapy is not likely to help this group of patients, that their conflicts are too overwhelming for direct exploration. Although some patients may be resistant, psychiatric evaluation and treatment should nonetheless be considered. The outcome of therapy depends as much on concurrent areas of strength, such as motivation and capacity for flexibility and change, as it does on the nature of the psychopathology alone. In a word, it seldom hurts to try. The referral to the psychiatrist must, as always, be made with tact. It is not necessary to emphasize the psychological basis of the symptom. One can simply point out to the woman that living with chronic pain is enough to send anyone to a psychiatrist; that she might benefit from talking to someone about it (see also Chapter 19).

Sexual Problems

Scully and Bart, in an illuminating review of 27 gynecology textbooks written since 1943, have demonstrated the failure of the authors and their publishers to integrate the work of Kinsey and of Masters and Johnson into their understanding of female sexuality.[16] Even some of the most recent books suggest that women be instructed to organize their sexual needs around their husbands and to deceive the latter when sexually unsatisfied. Certainly a notion that women themselves have sexual appetites that deserve satisfaction seemed lacking. Such attitudes, even when only implicit in a physician's training, must influence his perception of his female patients' sexual lives and will negatively affect his ability to counsel a woman who comes to him with sexual problems and questions.

Some women have comprehended all of this, at least unconsciously. As a result, sexually active women have often avoided their physicians. Young, unmarried women have risked pregnancy to avoid the embarrassment of asking for birth control advice and the humiliation of being seen as indecent. On the other hand, some women keep silent about their failure to achieve orgasm because of their fear of the denigration of being labeled "frigid."

Patients' perceptions of their physicians' attitudes clearly can greatly influence the patterns of treatment of venereal disease, considered epidemic today. If a woman feels shamed for sexual activity, she will certainly feel ashamed for having contracted VD. If she is unable to discuss her sexuality openly she may be inclined to avoid treatment for venereal disease until serious damage has been done. Encouraging the female patient to have a healthy attitude toward her sexuality will help prevent this kind of neglect. Such encouragement can be offered during routine visits simply by remembering to include sexuality in a review of systems. Providing the opportunity to talk about sex in a relatively neutral way sanctions its discussion should a problem arise.

Many physicians have received inadequate training in all aspects of human sexuality. There have been recent efforts to correct the deficiency. Chapter 9 deals with these issues in both male and female patients.

Pregnancy

Pregnancy and childbearing are issues at the core of every woman's life. Many decisions that she makes turn, in some small way, on the question of whether or not she will conceive. Can she? Will she? When will she? With whom? Even career decisions are often made in opposition to the press of pregnancy. The consideration may have a positive or negative valence, but it is almost never without charge. And this too clearly reawakens the concern about what comes out of her body. The girl child has to cope not only with the question of where babies come from, but with the mystery of how they get out of her as well. What hole in her body is large enough to accommodate this wondrous transit? This question often persists as a vague and awesome fear in the adult nulliparous woman, despite factual knowledge of anatomy.

The physical changes of pregnancy frequently portend a threat to the woman's sense of self and bodily integrity. The changes in the body often stress an already precarious body image. The stronger the woman's defensive need for control, the more threatening the changes. One woman, nearing her fifth month of pregnancy, became acutely depressed when she "popped." She had carefully guarded her weight and had continued all her vigorous athletic activities. Retrospectively she said she realized she had carried the fantasy that she would "beat this thing," that, through the exercise of her will, she could magically escape the transformations that other women experience. Others simply submit to the pregnancy and let it take over, feeling the helpless victims of their own bodies. Such an attitude may be manifest in undisciplined eating and salt ingestion, excessive weight gain, failure to exercise, and an unwillingness to participate actively in labor and delivery. Pregnancy seems to be only a more dramatic repetition of the dyscontrol of earlier biological events.

Pregnancy has the capacity to stimulate and bring to consciousness a woman's most primitive and animistic thoughts. Every superstition and old wives' tale presents itself with new life. Bibring, beginning in 1959 what was to be a long-term study of psychological processes in pregnancy, noted that diagnostic interviews conducted with women in a prenatal clinic showed that a great number of expectant mothers appeared as though they were either borderline or arrested psychotics.[17] They demonstrated magical thinking, premonitions, depressive reactions, primitive anxieties, and paranoid mechanisms, often associated with responses to their own mothers. On the basis of these data, Bibring came to understand pregnancy as a developmental crisis with a psychic disequilibrium common to all women, a formulation substantiated by her later work.[18] Bibring also found that in pregnancy, dependent and hysterical women were more inclined toward regressive tendencies; obsessional women became even more controlling.

In general, a woman's adaptation to her pregnancy will be more favorable, regardless of the particular nature of her conflicts, if she can feel the master of the experience rather than its victim. Information and education will help her to predict some of the transformations she will undergo, enhancing her sense of being in control. Answer her questions and encourage her to read. Use prenatal visits to discuss forthcoming stages of pregnancy and the delivery. Lamaze and other natural childbirth training classes are very useful in that they communicate the notion that the mother's participation in labor and delivery is crucial. This is often far less frightening than the thought that her role will be only a passive one. Keep in mind, however, that some women will use their ability to deliver without the help of anesthesia as a test of strength, or as a measure of their willingness to make the sacrifices necessary to be a good mother. These women will tend to feel disappointed, defeated, and depressed if they require any form of medication, anesthesia, or a Caesarean-section. Use prenatal visits to help the expectant mother to be prepared for the contingincies of labor and delivery, emphasizing that natural childbirth methods are to be used to assist her rather than to evaluate her capacities as a woman.

Fathers who plan to participate are often as anxious about labor and delivery as the expectant mothers. The anticipated event arouses fears and primitive sexual theories in them as well. They worry about the health of mother and baby. They worry about how distressed they will be by the rawness of the birth process, the pain, the blood, the procedures. They feel pressured to play the role of the strong male at the very time they are feeling stressed themselves. Acknowledging and exploring the husband's anxiety about helping his wife through labor will help him to be a more effective, less frightened labor coach.

Some men, despite information and support, fear that they will be overwhelmed by observing and participating in the birth process, and a few of them, in fact, will. In those cases, help the husband to graciously decline or withdraw to the waiting room. Help him to see his reluctance or inability to participate as something other than a masculine failure, and help his wife to overcome such a perception as well.

Motherhood

Women are beginning to learn that modern medicine may have inadvertently interfered with the establishment of crucial aspects of the mother–child relationship. Until recently, breast feeding was largely discouraged. Hospital practices designed to minimize perinatal morbidity and mortality may have served to obstruct critically timed events in the bonding process. Routine use of general anesthesia and rigid nursery rules and feeding schedules have all served to separate mother and newborn in the first few hours and days of life. Recent studies have shown that these separations may well have adversely affected maternal attachment and performance. Klaus et al. found that if a mother had merely 16 additional hours of contact with her baby in the first three days of life, she showed more evidence of spontaneous touching and more reluctance to leave the child.[19] These authors concluded that those first days encompassed a "maternal sensitive period." Others believe that the sensitive period in fact is contained in the first twenty minutes.[20]

Now through the willingness of women and their obstetricians to use the Lamaze and other methods of natural childbirth as well as partial or extended rooming-in, mothers are rediscovering the intensity of that early bond. As it is, motherhood has a way of facilitating and freeing a woman's assertiveness from conflict. A woman often discovers a new capacity for militance in the service and protection of her child. The mother who has held her infant in her arms for the first twenty minutes of life and who breast feeds has had more exposure to her baby during the hospital stay than in the recent past. This mother may discover that she has considerable difficulty following advice in certain areas. She may find that she is unable to let her child cry so readily as is considered prudent by some. For a good portion of the first two to three years of her child's life she may experience significant anxiety about leaving him or her with a sitter. Often this kind of mother is viewed as neurotic, overly anxious, and overly attached, and as somehow satisfying her own dependent needs. The reality may be the opposite. She may in fact be responding to a precise imprinting. The more detached, cavalier mother is perhaps a medical–cultural aberration. The most recent attachment literature is beginning to note that fathers are also deeply affected by early exposure to their infants.[21]

This is not to say that some mothers are not neurotic, overly anxious, and overly attached. But even these women are responding to a kind of internal programming that is not so easily overcome. Parenting an infant taps the most primitive and least well controlled emotional responses. It requires a patient ear and a very methodical approach to the allaying of anxiety. Women need to be able to ask a multitude of questions. They require prenatal counseling. They need to be forewarned that the early weeks will be emotionally exhausting and hardly blissful. And they often need, in the absence of the extended family, basic instruction in mothering. Fathers too must be counseled about their reactions to the newborn. It is not uncommon for them to react with jealousy and resentment, as though the infant were a sibling competing for the attention and affection of their wives. Such a reaction can create personal agonies and extreme marital tensions that can sometimes be abated by a few sensitive words of warning during a prenatal talk.

MISCARRIAGE AND STILLBIRTH

It is understandable that our first reaction when faced with a patient and her family who have experienced this tragedy is to try to offer words of reassurance and encouragement. They are quickly told how common miscarriage is, and reassured, if possible, regarding the likelihood of future successful pregnancies. This information is useful and should be provided. However, the patient's need to grieve is often overlooked.

Patients who have experienced this loss complain that they were not offered the opportunity to ventilate their feelings. As a reaction to the discomfort they feel, friends, family, and medical staff tell them overtly or covertly that they expect them to "get over it." They can be made to feel inadequate if they grieve "too long." Husbands are encouraged "to be strong and supportive," which can be translated into a need to conceal their own feelings of grief. They must be helped to weep with their wives, so that these women understand that their husbands, too, experienced the tragedy of this loss. The husbands must be reassured that weeping is not a sign of weakness.

The birth of a stillborn child poses special problems. The mother is usually on an OB floor. A busy staff may overlook the fact that this patient has lost a baby. A sticker on the chart to that effect can serve as a reminder and prevent someone from making a remark which can be experienced as unfeeling. The parents of a stillborn child may wish to see and hold the baby, and they should be given that opportunity. Some women even express a wish for a photograph of the dead baby. It seems to be very important they have something concrete to verify the existence of the being they knew so intimately in utero. The funeral service issue should be discussed openly with both parents and, if the mother requests, the funeral should be delayed until she is able to attend.

The loss of the child will be felt by the couple for some time. It is thus important to schedule a follow-up visit with them about two weeks after the neonatal death. Initially, they will experience the grief. Just listening is all that is required here. Doctors tend to be uncomfortable with what they feel is a totally passive role. Actually, a good listener is engaged in an active process. Doctors also tend to become uncomfortable in the presence of a weeping adult. A common reaction is to get the patient to stop as quickly as possible. Try to avoid that. It only makes the patient feel guilty or inadequate "for having broken down." As an unconscious parental substitute, the physician's quiet acceptance of the tears can be very therapeutic.

Sometime in the near future, the patient and her husband will have to decide about future pregnancies. Here your best medical judgement regarding the risks will be needed. You will be more effective in this role if the couple feels that your earlier reactions demonstrated a true understanding of what they have been through. A movement to start self-help groups for such couples has begun. It is worth exploring the feasibility of such a program at your hospital. *

THE UNWANTED PREGNANCY—VOLUNTARY ABORTION

The unwanted pregnancy always raises the question of how and why the woman conceived. There are very few truly accidental conceptions: more often than not an unconscious wish to become pregnant colludes with circumstance to allow impregnation. For instance, a woman may want to have a child while her husband does not. She may simultaneously comply with her husband's wishes and her own by using a diaphragm with an insufficient amount of spermicidal jelly. No doubt such behavior accounts for a good number of the "diaphragm babies" that are born to this world.

The above example is a relatively simple one. Often the motivations are more complex. They can range from a need to prove that one cannot become pregnant to a need to prove that one can. Keep in mind that psychologically, becoming pregnant may have a vastly different meaning than carrying and/or delivering a child. And the need for the former does not necessarily imply a need or a wish for the latter.

Exploring the motivation for pregnancy becomes especially important in the woman who has repeated voluntary abortions. One 18-year-old unmarried woman hospitalized for her fifth voluntary termination of pregnancy revealed just how complicated the psychological influences can be. Although she consistently told the obstetrical house staff that these conceptions were all "mistakes" she tearfully acknowledged to the psychiatrist that each time she became pregnant she had secretly hoped for it but later realized she could not tolerate actually having the baby. She believed a baby would help her with her feelings of loneliness. She herself was the oldest of five children. Her mother was chronically psychotic and delegated much of the responsibility for the care of the younger children to the patient. The patient recalled one occasion when the mother set fire to their apartment in an intentional effort to kill all of her children. The patient believed that through abortion she herself had killed

---

* One such program is the *Hoping Program*, at Edward W. Sparrow Hospital, Lansing, Michigan, 48912.

five children. Through the psychiatric interview it became clear that the patient's behavior was very much linked to her effort to cope with her mother's homicidal wishes toward her children. The patient, however, was unaware of the ideational connection. She only knew that she felt like a "murderer," suffered from terrible guilt, and was convinced that God would punish her. In this particular case, as one obstetrical resident nicely put it, "Psychotherapy was the birth control of choice."

Although it is in vogue these days to minimize the feelings of anxiety, guilt, and depression that accompany the voluntary abortion, many women are very much at risk for a painful if not morbid reaction. This is especially true of the teenager who has not yet integrated her adult sexual functioning. She may still feel more like a child than a woman and often, therefore, identifies with the aborted fetus. Such an identification will intensify her negative and self-punitive feelings. Assume in all cases that abortion is a conflict-laden procedure, one which can be experienced as frightening and intrusive. Sensitive support is required. The physician should be available for emotional support subsequent to the abortion as well. If, despite your help, there is no significant improvement in the patient's anxiety or depression, refer her for psychiatric consultation.

At times the doctor will see a truly naive or ill-informed woman. In these instances he must provide the necessary contraceptive information.

Menopause

It is commonly known that menopause can be a time of crisis for the middle-aged woman. It is a time of physiological, psychological, and often social change. Hormones are in flux, menses stop, and some women complain of dizziness, palpitations, and depression. Here again the women who appear most vulnerable to menopausal distress are those who have defined their lives and sex roles traditionally and have been, perhaps, overly involved in their children. The departure of their children often coincides with the involution of their child-bearing function. Kraines systematically investigated menopause and found that most women do not experience menopause as a time of stress.[22] She went on to suggest that women who seek medical help for menopause are in fact a different group, varying from the majority of middle-aged women in their physical and emotional reactions to stress.

The women who do require help will seldom be able to articulate just what they need. They may focus on physical symptoms such as hot flashes simply to justify an appointment to see the doctor. This may be more an expression of a wish to be cared for than a request for medical attention and medication as such. Often an examination and the reassurance that menopause is time-limited and is "going fine" is all that is needed. The physician should offer the patient the opportunity to discuss her mood and to complain if she wishes.

He should watch for signs of a serious depression such as weight loss, sleep disturbance, and delusions of guilt and/or persecution. The latter group of symptoms should be treated as outlined in Chapter 6, on depression. Replacement therapy with hormones will not help the depression.

Rape

Rape is a very special potential problem of the female patient. The victim remains vulnerable to pregnancy, venereal disease, and acute and chronic psychological consequences. Until very recently, systematic and informed help has been unavailable to the rape victim.[23] The mythology of rape has proclaimed that the seductive woman has invited her assault. Because of this, women have often avoided seeking medical and psychological attention. If their own sexual lives have included fantasies of submitting to an overpowering sexual partner, they may feel inclined to believe they really were "asking for it." In this case, their sense of guilt (conscious or unconscious) will make them shy away from badly needed care. In that such submissive fantasies are extremely common in adult female sexual life, the physician must be keenly aware of how they can influence the woman's response to rape. He must remember that rape is an act of violence, not an act of sex; that a fantasy of submitting by consent is vastly different from being forcibly entered.

The physician must acquaint himself with the procedures necessary to evaluate the rape victim accurately. "Rape Kits" are now marketed by pharmaceutical houses to aid in the systematic examination of the genitals and vaginal vault, necessary for both medical and legal reasons. Further, the physician, rather than being judgmental, must be available for sensitive support. This is especially important in view of some of the long-term sequelae of rape, which include depression, phobias, paranoia, sexual difficulties, and diminished functioning in ordinary life activities. He must take the woman's claim seriously, saving his suspicions for later. Believing the woman can never cause her psychological harm; not believing her can. Remember that if a woman is so disturbed that she needs to feign rape, having trusted her will in no way significantly contribute to her disturbance. However, challenging the claim of a woman who has been raped can and will enhance the trauma. Look for signs of guilt in the woman, even if the rape has been documented, and encourage her to verbalize this feeling. Airing it will help the woman comprehend its irrational nature. Schedule follow-up visits to measure how the woman is coping. Do not hesitate to refer her for psychiatric care if she remains overwhelmed by the event.

In recognition of the complexities involved in managing the rape victim, hospitals are now developing rape teams, comprised of gynecologists, psychiatrists, legal advocates, social workers, and nurses. It is clear that the woman who is raped requires multifaceted and experienced care.

CONCLUSION

The physician treating the female patient must remember that each woman is finally a unique individual. However, if the physician keeps the following points uppermost in mind, he will increase his sensitivity and will be more likely to make the correct personal diagnosis.

1. Women, even aggressive women, are somewhere conflicted over asserting themselves. If a woman is overly demanding, consider first her fear that she will not be taken seriously or even heard.
2. The rational, independent, trouble-free female patient may call for some extra concern and attention. She is probably using your services too little, reluctant to be a bother, afraid that her dependency on you may make her think less of herself.
3. The traditional woman can create problems for her physician by being too willing to be dependent. She may fail to articulate sufficiently her symptoms and/or needs. She may sexualize the relationship or come to make excessive demands. A more active and responsible alliance with her doctor should be encouraged.
4. A woman often feels that her body is not entirely her own. It is often uncontrollable and may betray her. She can, as a result, become excessively controlling or excessively passive and helpless in her presentation. Remind yourself of this as you encounter, for example, the depression of a woman with vaginal bleeding, even when the cause is not serious. Consider it even as you approach the obese woman who is so hopeless about the prospect of controlling her weight.
5. The first pelvic exam is always a monumental and frightening event for the adolescent. Do not be fooled by a sophisticated facade. Sexuality always will be a source of enormous anxiety.
6. Pregnancy and the adjustment to the arrival of children are normative crises in a woman's life. Do not prematurely diagnose a woman as

disturbed simply because of the presence of travail in her life as she faces these events. Wait to see the final product of her psychological negotiations and support her and her mate during the time of crisis itself. Listen more carefully to the instincts generated by healthy maternal attachment. Be more patient—even with the neurotic behavior of the new mother.

7. The more rigidly stereotyped the woman's sex roles, the more potential there is for psychological hazard at each developmental step. This is especially true at the time of menopause, when the woman must begin to confront the prospect of old age and death and evaluate the substance of her life as she has lived it. For many women menopause is experienced as a liberation.
8. Rape is always a violent assault, a source of humiliation and trauma, and it is never invited. Expert help is required.
9. Whenever possible, include the patient's sexual partner or mate in counseling. Do not underestimate the role of the primary physician as educator.

References

1. The Boston Women's Health Book Collective: Our Bodies Our Selves. New York, Simon and Schuster, 1976
2. Notman M Nadelson C: The Woman Patient, New York, Plenum Press, 1978
3. Howell MC: What medical schools teach about women. N Engl J Med 290:304–307, 1974
4. Lenanne KJ, Lenanne RJ: Alleged psychogenic disorders in women—A possible manifestation of sexual prejudice. N Engl J Med 200:288–292, 1973
5. Luy ML: What's behind women's wrath toward gynecologists. Modern Medicine, 42:17, October 14, 1974
6. Kaiser BL, Kaiser H: The challenge of the women's movement to American gynecology. Am J Obstet Gynecol 120:652–665, 1974
7. Greenberg RP, Fischer S: The relationship between willingness to adopt the sick role and attitudes toward women. J Chronic Dis 30:29–37, January 1977
8. Svanberg L Ulmsten U: The incidence of primary dysmenorrhea in teenagers. Arch Gynecol 230:173–177, 1981
9. Reid RL, Yen S: Premenstrual syndrome. Am J Obstet Gynecol 139:85–104, 1981
10. Adams PW, Rose DP, Folkard J, et al: Effect of pyridoxine hydrochloride (vitamin B_6) upon depression associated with oral contraception. Lancet 1:897, 1973
11. Wetzel JN, Reich T, McClure JM, et al: Premenstrual affective syndrome and affective disorder. Brit J Psychiat 127:219–221, 1975
12. Kaltreider N, Wallace A, Horowitz M: A field study of the stress response syndrome. Young women after hysterectomy. JAMA 242:1499, 1979
13. Beard RW, Belsay CM, Lieberman BS, et al: Pelvic pain in women. Am J Obstet Gynecol 128:569–570, July, 1977

14. Gidro-Frank L, Gordon T, Taylor HD: Pelvic pain and female identity: A survey of emotional factors in 40 patients. Am J Obstet Gynecol 79:1184, 1960
15. Friederich MA: Psychological aspects of chronic pelvic pain. Clin Obstet Gynecol 19:300–406, June, 1976
16. Scully D, Bart P: A funny thing happened on the way to the orifice: Women in gynecology textbooks. J 78:1045–1050, 1973
17. Bibring G: Some considerations in the psychological processes in pregnancy. Psychoanal Study Child 14:9–44, 1959
18. Bibring G, Dwyer T, Huntington D: A study of the earliest mother–child relationship. Psychoanal Study Child 16:113–121, 1961
19. Klaus MH, Jerauld L, Krezer N, et al: Maternal attachment: Importance of the first post-partum days. N Engl J Med 286:460–463, 1961
20. Lozoff B, Brittenham G, Trause MA, et al: The mother–newborn relationship: Limits of adaptability. J Pediatr 01:1–2, July, 1977
21. Sosa: Maternal–infant interaction during the immediate post-partum period. Adv Pediatr 25:451–461, 1978
22. Kraines RJ, cited in Bart P, Grossman M: Menopause, in Nadelson C, Notman M, (eds): The Women Patient. New York, Plenum Press, 1978
23. Schuker E: A treatment program for rape victims. Alaska Med 20:48–55, 1978

Philip R. Muskin, M.D.
Donald S. Kornfeld, M.D.

5

The Management of Anxiety

Fear and anxiety bring most patients to your office. They come because they are concerned that a symptom may have serious consequences: they want reassurance that the headache is not a brain tumor, the chest pain is not a heart attack. Fear and anxiety motivate the patient to come for his annual physical. Fear and anxiety are the common denominators in all our clinical work. It is essential, therefore, for us to understand the varied forms they can take and how best to treat them.

For example, it can be important to understand the role anxiety and fear play in determining when our patients come for help. Often enough the decision to call for an appointment is influenced by nonmedical factors. Serious illness in a friend, a death in the family, problems on the job, can all consciously or unconsciously contribute to the symptom itself or the decision to call for help. Understanding the role anxiety plays in our patients' complaints will influence our management of their care. The parallel history taking technique described in Chapter 1 will be helpful in detecting the sources of anxiety in patients who are themselves unable to make these connections.

Conversely, anxiety regarding serious illness can cause a patient to deny the presence of a symptom and thus delay an office visit. An awareness of the delay and an understanding of its basis should help in management. This type of patient will need lots of reassurance to keep the anxiety at a tolerable level and prevent flight from treatment. The management of denial is dealt with in greater detail in Chapter 15, on the surgical patient, and Chapter 2, on the difficult patient.

A certain amount of anxiety is a necessary concomitant of life. The "nervousness" that students feel before an exam or that patients experience in your waiting room is "normal" and requires no treatment. In fact, a certain amount of anxiety has been shown to improve performance in a variety of tasks. We must help our patients to understand this so that tranquilizers are not abused. However, tranquilizers and a variety of psychotherapeutic techniques can be used judiciously to reduce excessive anxiety. The strategy best suited to specific situations will be discussed.

SITUATION-DEPENDENT ANXIETY AND FEAR

Fear and *anxiety* are often used interchangeably in everyday speech. However, psychiatrists make a helpful distinction. *Fear* is defined as a reaction to an actual, current, external danger; *anxiety* describes a reaction to an unconscious stimulus. In many situations the "nervousness" (a term patients are even more likely to use) that the patient feels represents a response that combines both conscious and unconscious reactions, that is both fear and anxiety. The patient is usually unaware that some previous experience or perception is contributing to the way he feels.

> A 36-year-old woman came to her physician complaining of insomnia and anorexia. She quickly became tearful and told him that after 15 years of marriage her husband had recently left her for another woman. She felt unable to cope with her household responsibilities and her two children. She was living in an almost constant state of anxiety. She could not imagine how she could survive on her own.
>
> The physician was initially shocked to find this patient, whom he had always thought to be quite an effective person, presenting herself as so completely helpless. He shared this observation with her, and this led to a discussion of her distorted perception of her self-worth. Apparently she had unconsciously perceived her spouse as a parent substitute and now without him felt as panicked as a child suddenly without parents. The physician's comments regarding his perception of her and her newfound awareness of her distortion of reality did provide some relief of her symptoms. However, they agreed that further psychotherapy would help her to understand this distorted self-image better and to modify it.
>
> Of course, the dissolution of a marriage is a frightening situation, but for this patient the emotional response carried a mixture of both realistic and unrealistic concerns. The latter kept her from dealing effectively with the problems at hand.

Pure fear is often seen in medical practice where patients must face the unknown of diagnostic and treatment procedures. What we regard as standard procedures to many patients are new and fright-provoking. No diagnostic test is "routine" to the patient. If the ECG machine and x-ray instill fear, what then of radioactive counters and cardiac catheterization? Patients' reactions reflect their concern about the possibility of positive findings and, in some situations, fear of harm from the procedure itself. Treatment procedures, such as radiotherapy and chemotherapy, can produce similar effects. A good bit of the patient's uneasiness can be relieved if he or she is given a simple explanation and an opportunity to have any questions answered. The facts are usually less frightening than the patient's fantasies.[1] Unfortunately, many patients don't want to "waste your time with foolish questions." We must then take the initiative and make it clear that we *have* the time and want the questions asked. In the hospital setting, it helps to sit down at the bedside. It says to the patient, "I have time to listen to you." Your 10 minutes, seated, may seem longer to the patient than would twice that time, standing.

Short-term use of a minor tranquilizer (see the section on antianxiety agents) can be of major benefit in helping a patient through a particularly stressful period. And, in addition to your prescription of a drug, your acknowledgement that anxiety is a common reaction in these circumstances may allow the patient to express some of his or her concerns. Many patients feel that to admit fear is a sign of weakness. Give them permission to tell you about it. For example, you could say, "Most people are nervous about surgery (or having had a heart attack). What are your worries?" When you get patients to express their fears you relieve them in two ways: (1) you provide reassurance about specific fears, which is more effective than offering global reassurance, and (2) you help the patient to ventilate, a process that itself is therapeutic. (The management of preoperative anxiety is dealt with in detail in Chapter 15.)

Anxiety can also have serious consequences following illness. The post-myocardial infarction patient provides an example of such problems. Fear of a second myocardial infarction can seriously interfere with a patient's return to a reasonable level of functioning. The special meaning of cardiac illness and the intensive treatment given in the early stages can set the stage for post-myocardial infarction invalidism.[2] The patient's fear can combine with an ill-defined statement from his doctor like "take it easy" to produce serious disability. Such vague instructions are inadvisable for any patient. They produce little or no behavioral change in the patient who denies his illness, and they can immobilize the patient with excessive anxiety. Therefore, give your patients instructions or guidelines that are as specific as possible and then allow time for questions.

Serious sexual problems may develop when the patient's or spouse's fear that intercourse will be dangerous are not dealt with by his or her physician. We must be prepared to answer their questions regarding the risks of sexual activity with specific answers and advice. Where there are no questions, we must open the subject for discussion. (See Chapter 9 for details regarding the management of sexual problems.)

The post-myocardial infarction patient will probably also be quite anxious when he or she comes for the first office visit after discharge from the hospital. Such patients may require considerable reassurance regarding their progress and encouragement to begin constructive activity. Exercise and physical conditioning programs, where indicated, can help in relieving anxiety since they constitute one "do" in a long list of "don'ts."[3] Invalidism usually begins early in convalescence; therefore, anxiety and depression should be identified early. Spouses should be included in these discussions so that your reassurances and instructions can be reinforced after patients return home. The overanxious spouse may require special attention so that she or he does not undermine your constructive efforts. Many of these problems can be avoided if the spouse is brought in for discussion while the patient is still in the hospital.[4] The office visit just before return to work also occurs at a time of heightened anxiety. Additional time should be scheduled to deal with the patient's concerns.

For most patients, ventilation of their fears and provision of specific instructions and information should be adequate. However, if explanations, interpretations and support are not completely effective, then drugs should be used. They can relieve unnecessary suffering and minimize the physiological concomitants of anxiety that can introduce unnecessary physiological complications. For example, the use of a benzodiazepine in the coronary care unit after a myocardial infarction can reduce the incidence of arrythmias by reducing the production of catecholamines.[5] When the acute situation is resolved, the medication should be stopped. Its prolonged use can produce lethargy and weakness that patients will assume is related to their illness. This in turn can create unnecessary anxiety.

Should your efforts fail and the patient remain disabled by anxiety, he or she should be referred for psychotherapy. This referral should be presented positively; that is, patients should be told that it is their anxiety, not the physical effect of the illness, that is preventing them from functioning. The referral for psychiatric help, therefore, can serve as another bit of reassurance regarding the patient's health status.

PHYSICIAN-INDUCED ANXIETY

It has been said, nervous doctors have nervous patients. Of course that is true; it has even been documented. One study of cardiac patients found that 22 percent were considered to have been made unnecessarily anxious by what their doctors said, or failed to say.[6]

Anxious, perfectionistic doctors, fearful of making a mistake, allow their own anxiety to influence what they say, or do not say; what they do or do not do. They have to do every conceivable test to be absolutely certain that they have not missed something. They find it difficult to give their patients unqualified reassurance about anything. They must, therefore, always qualify their remarks and give the more guarded prognosis. (They tell themselves, "We can't be absolutely sure we got all the nodes, can we?") After all, if their patients do well, there can be no recriminations. However, what if they should make a rosy prediction and then things go sour? Then they have made a mistake, and they assume patients and their families will remind them of it. In fact, it is the doctor's own unconscious that he or she fears. It causes the doctor to voice the more guarded prognosis, to avoid making a "public" error. As a consequence, his or her patients live with unneeded anxiety.

Some doctors try to deal with this problem indirectly. They give the patient an optimistic prognosis but then share their concerns with the family. The average spouse cannot cover up distress for very long and so the patient senses the more guarded prognosis and loses faith in the doctor for not being honest. In most situations patient and spouse should be given the same information. If the patient will benefit from a more optimistic prognosis so will the spouse.

Such doctors will feel free of anxiety for a while if they use these self-protective techniques. However, their patients and patients' families are burdened with unnecessary concerns, and their own anxiety will return with the next comparable situation.

This type of behavior is most common in the inexperienced house officer. When it persists beyond training into practice, consultation with a psychiatric colleague may provide an understanding of its source and thus allow some control over it.

A word about the role of doctor-anxiety in informed consent. Many physicians allow their fears of a malpractice suit to influence their judgment in determining what information they provide to their patients prior to procedures. The laws of most states do not require that we burden our patients with a catalogue of every possible complication for each procedure. We are required only to share with them that which is a commonly accepted risk. To do otherwise can only produce unneeded fear or even panic. This can force patients to avoid or cancel necessary procedures. That probably *is* malpractice.

PHOBIAS

A *phobia* is an unreasonable fear associated with some situation or object. It usually results from an unconscious conflict in which the patient detaches the emotion from the conflict and displaces it onto some exterior source. The acute anxiety associated with the feared object or situation is thus actually derived from another source of which the patient is unaware.

In some cases the fear may be an "understandable" one, such as fear of flying or heights; however, for the phobic patient the severity of the response outweighs the actual risk involved. Obviously, many air travel passengers are "nervous" but are able to control their fear with conscious intellectual reassurance regarding the actual risks involved. The phobic patient knows the same facts but still cannot control his or her emotional response. However, these patients do not experience anxiety unless confronted by the phobic situation or phobic object.

Patients may experience a return of phobic anxiety when a change in a stable life situation occurs, upsetting a carefully worked out balance. For example, a patient with a fear of driving did quite well while living in a major city where she could use mass transit. When she moved to the suburbs, where she had to drive, her anxiety reappeared.

A good complete medical history should include an inquiry regarding "fears of certain places or activities, for example, elevators or flying." Some patients are careful to avoid discussing their phobias, out of embarrassment. It is important to help patients overcome embarrassment so that they can obtain appropriate treatment. In many cases, specific phobias can be easily treated by a variety of behavioral techniques such as *desensitization,* in which the patient is led to imagine progressively more frightening situations while he or she maintains a relaxed state.[7] Referral to a psychiatrist or a psychologist may be required for this kind of treatment.

Agoraphobia (fear of public spaces—e.g., streets, shops, crowds) is one of the more common disabling phobias. Patients with this type of phobia usually require that someone accompany them when they go out. The patient who never appears alone in your office, no matter how minor the complaint, may be agoraphobic. Major problems arise when the companion can no longer accompany the patient. Agoraphobia may be a complication of panic disorder (discussed next) as well as the result of unconscious conflicts. Desensitization alone is less successful in the treatment of agoraphobia than in the treatment of more specific, circumscribed phobias.

PANIC DISORDER

Panic disorder was first delineated by Roth in 1960.[8] Patients describe the sudden onset of tachycardia, shortness of breath, choking sensations, dizziness, weakness, and sweating accompanied by fear of impending doom, going crazy, or dying. The attacks are spontaneous and can occur in any situation. Patients often mistakenly restrict their activities, assuming the attacks are related to the particular situation in which they have occurred.

Frequently, when the syndrome first begins, patients go to an emergency room, thinking they are having a "heart attack." This is usually ruled out by electrocardiographic findings. Reassurance that "there's nothing wrong," is only temporarily helpful. With the next attack, which is very likely to occur, patients develop a secondary component of anticipatory anxiety and live in fear of subsequent attacks. They desperately attempt to attribute the reaction to a given place or activity, and thus the phobic cycle begins. Unfortunately, the syndrome is often misdiagnosed as common anxiety, hypoglycemia, or hyperventilation. Patients are placed on benzodiazepines or barbiturates, or they place themselves on alcohol. All of these are ineffective treatments for panic attacks and carry a risk of addiction.[9]

Tricyclic antidepressants have been shown to be remarkably effective in the treatment of panic disorder. Klein has shown that approximately 90 percent of patients obtain marked improvement.[10,11] The drug blocks panic attacks, but many patients require further treatment for the anticipatory anxiety and phobic symptoms.

> A 27-year-old woman was referred for consultation by an internist. She had presented with a two-month history of intermittent episodes of palpitations, and the fear that she was going to die. The first episode occurred in a bus terminal while she was waiting to leave on a visit to her mother. An extensive medical work-up revealed no abnormalities. Two days prior to the consultation she had another severe episode. She called her internist and told him that she could no longer tolerate the situation and that she would be better off dead than living with the symptoms. He placed her on haloperidol, 5 mg bid, and called the psychiatrist, quite concerned that this young woman might be psychotic. He also noted that a significant romantic involvement of hers was about to end, and that she had had several job changes over the past few months.
>
> When interviewed, the patient showed no evidence of psychosis or depression and gave a history compatible with panic disorder. She was started on imipramine, 25 mg po hs, which was raised over a period of ten days to 100 mg po bid (she had never taken the haloperidol). By the end of a month her symptoms had ceased. During this period she terminated her romantic involvement. She continued in psychotherapy in order to understand the difficulty she had had in that relationship.

In the treatment of panic attacks, the usual contraindications for tricyclic antidepressants must be observed (see Chapter 6). The common side effects of dry mouth, constipation, blurred vision, and orthostatic hypotension with rapid changes of position are dose related and should not be a major interference in continuing treatment. Imipramine (Tofranil, Presamine) may be started in doses of 10–25 mg po hs and raised by 10–25 mg each day, dividing the total dosage between the morning and evening, until the patient reaches a daily dose of 150 or 200 mg. There are occasional patients who require up to 300 mg of imipramine a day. If there are no electrocardiographic abnormalities at 200 mg a day, there is no reason not to increase the dose slowly until the patient's symptoms disappear. Sensitivity to side effects may make a slower rate of increase necessary. Some patients may become asymptomatic at doses much lower than those used in the treatment of depression, but this is uncommon.

After several weeks of treatment with the antidepressant the patient will no longer have spontaneous panic attacks but may still have a large component of anticipatory anxiety. At this point the patient still fears that the panics could return, especially in the phobic situation. A benzodiazepine may be helpful in reducing this anticipatory anxiety enough so that the patient will enter into those situations and find out that the panic attacks are now blocked. Behavioral desensitization may also be needed to alleviate this anticipatory anxiety.[7] Where the condition has existed for several years, the treatment may take months or even a year. In situations where the condition has existed only for a few months the treatment can be expected to be quite rapidly effective.

Medication should be continued for six months to a year after which it can be slowly tapered and then stopped. Most patients continue panic free after successful treatment, but approximately 20 percent will experience a recurrence of the disorder within a year of discontinuation of medication. These patients should be placed back on the medication. Another trial off medication can be instituted in 6 to 12 months. Should this fail, the patient may need to be maintained on the drug indefinitely.

Psychotherapy to explore possible underlying conflict as a cause of the initial panic attacks may be helpful to the patient and may increase the likelihood that the patient will tolerate the discontinuation of medication.

A 6′5″, 250 lb executive had become increasingly disabled by his fear of panic attacks. His internist reported that he had treated the patient with diazepam without success. The patient was unable to cross the George Washington Bridge, or use the tunnels into New York City. This posed serious problems, since his company's home office was located in the city and he was required occasionally to come into the city, from his home in New Jersey, for meetings. When he ran out of excuses, his wife would drive him to meetings.

The first panic attack had occurred some years ago. The patient had been called into the office of his superior and criticized for an alleged job failure. He was not responsible for the deficiency, but the senior man would not listen and insisted the failure was the patient's fault. On his way to work the next morning, the patient experienced his first panic attack as he crossed the bridge.

This giant of a man had lived in fear since childhood that he would lose his temper and hurt someone. He remembered vividly the few occasions when, as a teenager, he had used his full strength on the football field, with devastating consequences. Therefore, he would not allow himself to get angry. This was the conflict that was aroused in his supervisor's office that day. The panic attack occurred the next day as he drove to work and unconsciously contemplated the possible consequences of another confrontation—either humiliation or an outburst of murderous rage. Being unaware of the unconscious internal conflict, the patient assumed the anxiety problems were related to the external situation—crossing the bridge. Eliciting the history and airing the conflict provided some, but not complete, relief. The patient was then placed on imipramine, 25 mg hs, which made him feel "jumpy." It was found that 10 mg were sufficient to control the panic attacks. The patient eventually decided to leave his position and became quite successful in a business of his own.

There are some cases in which it is difficult to tell whether medication or psychotherapy plays the major role in treating a disorder. Since medications should not be used without concomitant psychotherapy, this is not an issue in providing appropriate treatment. As the two cases described here demonstrate, individual dose requirement can vary widely. Most patients, however, require doses in the range used in treating depression. A more complete discussion of panic disorder will be found in a recent paper by Muskin and Fyer.[12]

HYPERVENTILATION

The *hyperventilation* syndrome is another commonly seen manifestation of anxiety.[13] Patients experience faintness, visual disturbance, numbness and tingling in the extremities and around the mouth, headaches, sensations of breathlessness or frank chest pains. Occasionally symptoms are unilateral.[14] All of these symptoms are the result of the physiological changes produced by overbreathing. Some patients with panic disorder may have hyperventilation as their primary manifestation of that disorder. The diagnosis can be easily confirmed in the office by having patients breathe deeply and rapidly for a minute or more. This should reproduce their symptoms. Holding their breath will provide rapid relief.

The patient should be instructed to use the breath-holding technique to abort future attacks. This advice is obviously more practical than the suggestion to breathe into a paper bag. (It is also less potentially embarrassing.) Giving the patient some control over his or her symptoms should have a very salutory effect. Many of these patients are inappropriately treated with benzodiazepines. The use of drugs alone is usually not effective, and it prevents the patient from getting help for the underlying problem.

Once the patient has been shown that his or her symptoms can be controlled, inquiries should be made into the possible precipitants of these symptoms. It is usually not very difficult for patients to identify the circumstances in their lives that triggered the first attack.

A 32-year old married woman presented in her internist's office with complaints of lightheadedness, tingling, shortness of breath, and fear of fainting. These symptoms had first appeared during a summer vacation trip but the patient noted them subsequently while shopping and while driving her automobile. The symptoms had made it necessary for her to significantly limit her activities.

The patient was thoroughly worked up and found to have no physical abnormalities. It was clear to the clinician that the symptoms were the product of hyperventilation. He had her hyperventilate for about a minute or so, and was able to reproduce her symptoms in the office. He showed her that by holding her breath she could control the symptoms. He also began to explore with her the possible basis for the episodes.

It soon became clear that these were the product of her inability to say no to any request that was made of her. It also became apparent that she was becoming increasingly frustrated with her husband whose drinking on social occasions was becoming a major source of embarrassment to her. He had resisted any suggestion to seek help with this problem, and she did not know how to deal with her rage in this regard.

The patient's physical symptoms quickly subsided when she was able to identify the emotional source of her symptoms and to understand the basis for the underlying feelings. She was then referred to a psychiatrist to deal with the underlying character problem and conflict with her husband.

TRAUMATIC ANXIETY

This syndrome is seen in victims of such things as automobile and industrial accidents, shootings, stabbings, or disasters such as floods and fires. The individual usually comes away from the situation feeling a sense of heightened vulnerability.

A 25-year-old man was admitted to the hospital following a motorcycle accident during which he suffered a traumatic amputation of the right leg. Several days later the nurses reported that he was not sleeping well and seemed agitated. He readily spoke of his fear that he was "losing his mind" because of the recurrent dreams of the accident. His feeling of helplessness during the episodes was obvious. He was reassured that he was not psychotic but was trying to find a way to get back the control which he felt he had lost in the accident. He was encouraged to talk about the accident and his feelings. Diazepam, 5 mg po qid, was ordered and, after a few days, was switched to 10 mg po hs. After a week, the patient's acute symptoms subsided. He began to talk about rehabilitation and his hopes that he would be able to get a prosthetic device. After two weeks the diazepam was discontinued, with no recurrence of the agitated behavior.

An early clue to this syndrome is a report that the patient is not sleeping. Patients frequently have nightmares, sometimes nightly, which recapitulate the traumatic event and wake them. During the day patients are often irritable and restless and may startle easily, withdrawing from others. Often patients are afraid they are "going crazy" because of their need to relive the experience over and over again. It is beneficial to reassure them that this is a normal reaction to trauma and an attempt by the ego to master the unpleasant experience.

Treatment with a benzodiazepine is most helpful and should be instituted unless there is diagnostic uncertainty about possible head trauma or lethargy. Once such complications are ruled out, the temporary use of anxiolytic medications and the ventilation of feelings about the experience should provide rapid relief of the symptoms. Should the benzodiazepines not provide relief of the nightmares, the tricyclic antidepressant imipramine (Tofranil) may be tried. Imipramine has been reported to reduce the affective component of the nightmares[15,16], that is, dreams may continue to occur but without the very frightening feelings. This action of imipramine may be similar to its effect in blocking panic attacks.

PSYCHOSIS

In the early stages of psychosis the patient may merely appear restless, irritable, easily distracted, and withdrawn. On exploration, the patient may be found to be grossly disorganized, terrified, delusional, and possibly hallucinating. A psychotic patient who is terrified responds poorly to minor tranquilizers such as chlordiazepoxide (Librium) and diazepam (Valium), and appropriate treatment with antipsychotic agents should be instituted as soon as possible. Intramuscular haloperidol, in dosages of 0.5 mg–1.0 mg/hr until the patient is quiet, carries with it few adverse side effects. Intramuscular chlorpromazine in dosages of 10–25 mg/hr is more sedating than haloperidol, but carries the risk of orthostatic hypotension, especially in debilitated and elderly patients. However, for the extremely agitated patient, chlorpromazine, because of its potent sedating effects, is helpful in rapid control of the behavior. Keeping patients flat in bed prevents the hypotensive complication.

Chapter 7 discusses the management of psychosis in greater detail.

DEPRESSION

Patients with clinically significant depression may present as slowed in thought and speech, apathetic, and retarded. However, they may also appear anxious, tense, and agitated. In some cases, the anxiety and agitation may be so overwhelming that the diagnosis of depression is missed, a common and unfortunate error. Remember that the depressed patient, in addition to his anxiety, experiences (1) a loss of capacity to obtain pleasure, or a loss of interest in activities, hobbies, work, and sex; (2) feelings of guilt and worthlessness; (3) a low mood in the morning, with improvement towards the evening; and (4) insomnia characterized by early morning awakening. In both anxiety and depression, patients may have loss of appetite with weight loss and may complain of fatigue or a variety of somatic difficulties.

Tricyclic antidepressants are the appropriate treatment for anxious depression. Patients often find relief from the more sedating tricyclic antidepressants such as amitriptyline (Elavil). A more anxious or agitated depression can also be treated with the simultaneous use of a benzodiazepine and a nonsedating antidepressant such as imipramine. The benzodiazepine will give early relief of the anxiety and insomnia. The drug can be discontinued as soon as the trycyclics become effective, usually in two to three weeks. When, in error, such patients are treated with a benzodiazepine only they rapidly become depressed. The drug is then thought to have "caused" the depression. Actually the benzodiazepine has reduced the agitated component sufficiently to make the depressed mood more obvious. It is therefore important to think about the possibility of depression each time you prescribe a benzodiazepine.[17]

SPECIFIC ANTIANXIETY AGENTS

There are several agents commonly in use today for the treatment of anxiety. These include the barbiturates and the propanediols, the beta-adrenergic blocking agents, the antipsychotics, and the benzodiazepines.[18,19,20]

Barbiturates

The barbiturates are still commonly used as antianxiety agents. However, their primary action is to produce sedation with no specific antianxiety effect, and the dangers of physiological addiction are ever present. In addition, when barbiturates are used for intentional overdosage, the outcome (unlike that associated with the benzodiazepines) is frequently fatal. The barbiturates also stimulate hepatic microsomal enzymes, thus altering the metabolism of other medications such as digoxin, oral inticoagulants, steroids, tricyclic antidepressants, chlorpromazine, and phenytoin. For these reasons, barbiturates are now seldom indicated in the treatment of anxiety.

Propanediols

Meprobamate (Miltown) was popular as an oral treatment for anxiety in the 1950s and 1960s, but controlled studies did not substantiate its use as an antianxiety agent. The propanediols, like the barbiturates, stimulate hepatic microsomal enzymes. Physiological addiction and tolerance develop sooner and at lower doses than with benzodiazepines. Many patients are still receiving these agents. If possible, they should be switched to more effective medication.

Neuroleptics

In those instances where anxiety is accompanied by disorganized thoughts, violent outbursts, inappropriate or bizarre behavior, hallucinations, or delusions, the antianxiety agents are not the drugs of choice and serve only to delay appropriate treatment with antipsychotics.

The antipsychotic agents are the appropriate drugs for patients who are psychotic and who manifest anxiety secondary to their psychosis. Chlorpromazine is an effective treatment both orally and intramuscularly. Its powerful sedating effects are often beneficial in cases of extreme anxiety and agitation. Orthostatic hypotension is an unwanted side effect, and the drug must be used with some caution in the elderly or those at risk; however, precautions can be taken to minimize the side effects. Haloperidol, though less sedating, is an extremely potent and effective antipsychotic agent that is effective both orally and parenterally. The incidence of orthostatic hypotension is much lower than with chlorpromazine but extrapyramidal side effects are much more common.

Beta-Adrenergic Blocking Agents

Many of the peripheral manifestations of anxiety, such as tachycardia, tremors, and hyperventilation respond well to beta-adrenergic blocking agents like propranolol.[21] However the subjective feeling of anxiety is not affected. Propranolol has been used in the treatment of severe stage fright where the cardiovascular symptoms are disabling. [22] Doses of 10 mg po qid may be used following the usual precautions with beta-blockers. Patients with coexisting congestive heart failure or asthma should be excluded from treatment. In those specific conditions where beta-adrenergic blockade is indicated to block cardio-vascular symptoms, the underlying anxiety should be treated with psychotherapy and benzodiazepines.

Benzodiazepines

The benzodiazepines are the most frequently prescribed drugs in the United States today.[20] In the treatment of anxiety, they are the most effective. In comparison with the barbiturates they do not stimulate hepatic microsomal enzymes and they have a more favorable outcome from intentional overdosage. [18,19,20] According to Castillo-Ferrando, however, diazepam can cause changes in digoxin blood levels: in a recent letter to the editor of the *Lancet* (2:368, 1980), he reported a moderate increase in 5 out of 7 subjects taking both drugs. This is thought to be caused by increased protein binding of the digoxin with resultant diminished renal excretion. Whether other benzodiazepine interactions will be reported remains to be seen.

While physiological dependence has been observed, it is uncommon at usual therapeutic dosages. Anyone may become psychologically dependent upon any medication without physical dependence. (The latter implies that an actual withdrawal syndrome will appear when the drug is stopped.) Physical dependence can be developed to many drugs but usually is not seen with doses less than 50 mg/day of diazepam, or an equivalent dose of other benzodiazepines, for less than a month. There is some recent evidence, however, that long-term administration of even moderate doses of diazepam (25 mg/day) may carry a risk of withdrawal reactions.[23] Although this evidence derives from a single case report, it points up the necessity of careful consideration of long-term use of this class of medication. In cases where the dose is greater than 50 mg/day or the equivalent, with prolonged administration, patients are at risk for withdrawal reactions and the benzodiazepines must be tapered slowly. The withdrawal reaction may be delayed for several days, even as long as a week, when the half-life of the drug is very long. This should be kept in mind for drugs like diazepam and chlordiazepoxide especially. The elderly are more sensitive to these drugs, and smaller doses of short-acting forms (oxazepam, lorazepam) should be used to avoid neurological and psychiatric complications from drug buildup leading to ataxia, somnolence, delirium, and what may appear to be a depression.

Recent evidence indicates that there are specific receptors for the benzodiazepines in the brain. [24,25] The barbiturates, ethanol, and meprobanate do not bind to these sites. Frontal and occipital cortex showed the highest affinity for labeled diazepam. In addition, endogenous substances that have benzodiazepine-like activity have been identified. Inosine and hypozathine have been isolated from the brain and are competitive inhibitors of diazepam binding, with similar pharmacologic properties.[26]

Like the barbiturates, the propanediols, and the neuroleptics, the benzodiazepines act synergistically with other central nervous system depressants. This is of particular importance to patients using both benzodiazepines and alcohol, who are often unaware of their level of impairment. [27,28] Patients must be warned of this effect of the medication and cautioned against the concomitant use of tranquilizers and alcohol. The potential health hazard of alcohol–benzodiazepine interactions is considerable. The most serious hazard is to the driver who has consumed alcohol while taking a benzodiazepine, barbiturate, or propanediol. Physicians should caution their patients to abstain completely from alcohol during the period of treatment. Cimetidine (Tagamet) has also been found to elevate benzodiazepine blood levels significantly.[29] The effects of the benzodiazepines on fetal development are not clearly delineated. There is some animal evidence which suggests that prenatal administration of diazepam may slow normal development in the newborn long after the drug can no longer be detected in the body.[30] Pregnant women, therefore, should not be given these drugs unless the anxiety is so overwhelming that the pregnancy cannot continue to term. In these cases a psychiatric consultation may be helpful to explore and treat the source of the anxiety.

Diazepam (Valium)

Diazepam is well absorbed from the gastrointestinal tract but poorly and erratically absorbed intramuscularly. Intravenous administration has a rapid anxiolytic effect that rapidly fades away, most likely related to rapid tissue distribution of this relatively lipid-soluble drug. Unless given too fast and in large doses intravenously, diazepam is relatively safe and the risk of respiratory depression and hypotension are low. Diazepam should never be administered intravenously at a rate faster than 5 mg/min. The half-life of diazepam is between 6 and 40 hours. The major metabolic product has considerable pharmacologic activity, with an even longer half-life. For this reason, after 5–10 days of administration, a steady state is reached and multiple daily administration is no longer necessary. After this point, repeated dosage of diazepam (more than once or twice daily) can result in unwanted cumulative clinical effects. The usual dosage is between 2 and 40 mg/day, as there is considerable individual variation in responsivity.

Chlordiazepoxide (Librium)

Like diazepam this drug is well absorbed from the gastrointestinal tract and intravenously but is poorly absorbed intramuscularly. Respiratory arrest and hypotension can result if the intravenous dose is administered too rapidly. The rapid decline of the perceived effect that is seen with diazepam is less of a problem with chlordiazepoxide as it is water soluble and, therefore, less rapidly and extensively distributed in the tissue. The clinical effect is otherwise quite similar. Although the half-life varies between 6 and 30 hours, active metabolites are also found and danger of cumulative effects exist as with diazepam. The usual clinical dose is between 15 and 100 mg/day.

Oxazepam (Serax) and Lorazepam (Ativan)

These benzodiazepines have a shorter half-life, with much less risk of cumulative effects over time than the other drugs in this group incur. Unlike diazepam, oxazepam is directly conjugated as a glucuronide and excreted in the urine with no active metabolites. There is no parenteral preparation available. The half-life of oxazepam varies between 3 and 21 hours, and the dose varies between 30 and 120 mg/day. Because of its shorter half-life and lack of active metabolites, the drug must be administered three or four times daily.

Lorazepam resembles oxazepam in both its pharmacokinetic and its molecular structure.[31] Well absorbed orally, the half-life ranges between 10 and 20 hours. Lorazepam is transformed into inactive glucuronide that is excreted in the urine. With a multiple dosage schedule, steady concentrations are reached within 3 days. Because of the short half-life and lack of active metabolites, cumulative effects are far less of a risk than in the case of other benzodiazepines. The usual dose is between 2 and 10 mg daily, in divided doses. The parenteral form of lorazepam possesses several clinical advantages over the other benzodiazepines. After intravenous administration, its clinical effects have longer duration than those of diazepam because of less rapid and extensive tissue distribution. More important, it is the only benzodiazepine reliably absorbed intramuscularly.

Flurazepam (Dalmane)

This drug is commonly used as a hypnotic. It is absorbed after oral administration but barely detectable in the blood; however, its major metabolite undergoes a slow biotransformation, with a half-life between 50 and 100 hours. Commonly used in doses between 15 and 30 mg/day, if used on a long-term basis it can result in cumulative effects. A more detailed discussion of hypnotic use can be found in Chapter 14, on sleep disorders.

In summary, benzodiazepines appear to be the best available agents for treating anxiety. However, because of the potential for cumulative effects with long-term usage and because of the potential for physiological dependence, treatment should be both specific and time limited. The occasional use of benzodiazepine prn for anxiety or sleeplessness is harmless, but not if it leads to chronic dependence or the avoidance of a more direct approach to a problem. It is the responsibility of the treating physician to reevaluate a drug's use after 4–6 weeks. If anxiety symptoms persist, the patient should be urged to further explore the source of the anxiety with his physician or he or she should be referred for psychiatric consultation.

RELAXATION THERAPY

This technique has been helpful for some patients with chronic or recurrent anxiety or with stress related illnesses. It is based on techniques such as transcendental meditation which have been used by man for more than a thousand years. Benson has presented these techniques in a non-mystical format that is acceptable to most patients.[32] He believes that the physiological response elicited in this way is similar to the trophotropic response in animals, that is, the opposite of the fight-flight response. The physiological changes are associated with a hypothesized decrease in sympathetic tone, that is, decreased heart and respiration rates and lowered oxygen consumption. It is this "hypometabolic or restful state" that provides the basis for the beneficial effects of relaxation therapy. The relaxation response may have evolved to provide protection from an overresponse to stress while neither fight nor flight is possible.

The relaxation response, done twice a day for 10–20 minutes, has been reported to reduce blood pressure, decrease premature cardiac contractions, and lower blood cholesterol.[33,34] It has also been used, in combination with biofeedback, for the treatment of tension and migraine headaches.

The various techniques used by different cultures to elicit the response have common elements: a quiet environment, a mental device, a passive attitude, and a comfortable position. The patient should, therefore, be given the following instructions:

1. Select a quiet room where you will not be disturbed. If you are at work, be sure no messages are called in for 10–20 minutes.
2. Sit in a comfortable position. Do not lie down since sleep could occur and that is not what is desired. Relax all your muscles.
3. Close your eyes and concentrate on your breathing. Each time you exhale think of the number, "one." When distracting thoughts occur think "Oh, well," and then go back to concentrating on breathing. These distracting thoughts will occur and are just to be ignored.

Patients may wish to select some phrase other than the number "one" to think to themselves. For example, some religious patients may think of a very brief prayer. The content is obviously not what is important. The point is that by means of a repetitive device, they are able to block out stressful thoughts for a given period of time.

The relaxation approach is particularly helpful for patients with more chronic manifestations of anxiety, where drug therapy is not indicated. It can also be used in combination with other forms of psychotherapy, to provide symptomatic relief. For some patients, the reduction in tension can also produce a gratifying sense of control over their bodies.

When used as recommended, twice a day, or occasionally prn, the relaxation response is free of side effects. However, it can produce hypoglycemia in diabetics on insulin and hypotension in patients on beta blockers. If overused by a more disturbed patient, it can also produce an altered state of consciousness.

SUMMARY

A list of the principles we have outlined in this chapter follows. We have emphasized the importance of establishing the basis for anxiety symptoms as a part of the treatment. We appreciate the value of antianxiety drugs but want to emphasize the potential benefit of utilizing the power of the doctor–patient relationship. Even the busiest practitioner who believes he cannot provide the counseling recommended in step 5 should find the time to take his patient through steps 1–4. A failure to do that deprives your patient of an opportunity to be adequately treated. The drug treatment of anxiety without such an exploration is no different from the treatment of fever with aspirin without a physical exam and diagnostic tests.

1. Identify the symptoms as having an emotional basis.
2. Help the patient identify the symptoms as emotionally based.
3. Explore with the patient the possible sources of anxiety or fear.
4. Provide an opportunity for emotional ventilation.
5. Provide counseling.
6. If steps 2, 3, 4, and 5 fail, medicate temporarily with a minor tranquilizer.
7. Treat with specific pharmacologic agents when possible, for example, use a tricyclic antidepressant in panic disorder or anxious depression.
8. If symptoms persist, refer for psychological or psychiatric treatment.

REFERENCES

1. Golden JS, Johnson GD: Problems of distortion in doctor–patient communications. Psychiat in Med 1:127–149, 1970
2. Klein RF, Dean A, Willson M, et al: The physician and post-myocardial infarction invalidism. JAMA 194:123–128, 1965
3. Gulledge AD: The psychological aftermath of a myocardial infarction, in Gentry WD, Williams RB, Jr. (eds): Psychological Aspects of Myocardial Infarction and Coronary Care. St. Louis, Mosby, 1975
4. Hackett TP, Cassem NH: Psychological intervention in myocardial infarction, in Gentry WD, Williams RB, Jr. (eds): Psychological Aspects of Myocardial Infarction and Coronary Care. St. Louis, Mosby, 1975
5. Hackett TP, Cassem NH: Reduction of anxiety in the coronary care unit. Current Ther Res 14:649–656, 1972
6. Wynn A: Unwarranted emotional distress in men with ischemic heart disease. Med J Aust XX:848–850, 1967
7. Wolpe J: Psychotherapy by Reciprocal Intervention. Stanford, Calif, Standord University Press, 1958
8. Roth M: The phobic–anxiety–depersonalization syndrome and some general etiological problems in psychiatry. J Neuropsychiatry 1:293–306,
9. Quitkin FM, Rifkin A, Kaplan J, et al: Phobic anxiety syndrome complicated by drug dependence and addiction. Arch Gen Psychiatry 27:155–162, 1972
10. Klein DF: Delineation of two drug-responsive anxiety syndromes. Psychopharmacologia 5:397–408, 1964
11. Klein DF, Zitrin CM, Woerner M: Anxiety, panic, impramine, and phobias, in Lipton MA, Dimasuo A, Killiam RF (eds): Psychopharmacology: A Generation of Progress. New York, Raven Press, 1978, pp 1401–1410
12. Muskin PR, Fyer A: Treatment of panic disorder. J Clin Psychopharmacol 1:89–90, 1981
13. Pincus JH, Tucker GJ: Behavioral Neurology. New York, Oxford University Press, 1978
14. Tavel ME: Hyperventilation syndrome with unilateral symptoms. JAMA 187: 147–149, 1964
15. Marshall JR: The treatment of night terrors associated with the post-traumatic syndrome. Am J Psychiatry 132:293–295, 1975
16. Logan DG: Antidepressant treatment of recurrent anxiety attacks and night terrors. Ohio State Med J 75:653–655, 1977
17. Murphy G: The physician's responsibility for suicide. I. An error in commission. Ann Intern Med 82:293–295, 1975
18. Greenblatt DJ, Shader RI: Drug therapy: Benzodiazepines, I. New Engl J Med 291:1011–1015, 1974
19. Greenblatt DJ, Shader RI: Drug therapy: Benzodiazepines, II. New Engl J Med 291:1239–1243, 1974
20. Cohen S (ed): Valium—It's use and abuse. Drug Abuse and Alcoholism Newsletter, Vista Health Foundation 5:4, May 1976
21. Imhof P, Brummer H: The treatment of functional heart disorders with beta-adrenergic blocking agents. Postgrad Med 46(suppl):96, 1970
22. James IM, Griffith DWN, Person RM, et al: Effect of oxprenolol on stage-fright in musicians. Lancet 8045:952–954, 1977
23. Winokur A, Rickels K, Greenblatt OJ, et al: Withdrawal reaction from long-term low-dosage administration of diazepam. Arch Gen Psychiatry 37:101–105, 1980

24. Squires R, Braestrup C: Benzodiazepine receptors in rat brain. Nature 266:732–734, 1977
25. Mohler H, Okada T: Benzodiazepine receptor: Demonstration in the central nervous system. Science 198:849–851, 1977
26. Marangos PJ, Clark R, Martino AM, et al: Demonstration of two new endogenous "benzodiazepine-like" compounds. Brain Psych Res 1:121–130, 1979
27. Alcohol-Drug Interactions. FDA Drug Bulletin, 10(2), 1979
28. Prescribing of Minor Tranquilizers. FDA Drug Bulletin, 10(4), 1980
29. Klotz U: Cimetidine/diazepam interaction, letter to the Editor. Lancet 8144:699, 1979
30. Kellogg C, Tervo D, Ison J, et al: Prenatal exposure to diazepam alters behavioral development in rats. Science 207:205–207, 1980
31. Greenblatt DJ, Shader RI: Drug therapy: Prazepam and lorazepam—Two new benzodiazepines. New Engl J Med 299:1342–1344, December 14, 1978
32. Benson H: The Relaxation Response. New York, William Morrow & Co., Inc., 1975
33. Benson H: Systemic hypertension and the relaxation response. New Engl J Med 296:1152–1155, 1977
34. Roskies E, Sperack M, Surkis A, et al: Changing the coronary-prone (Type A) behavior pattern in a non-clinical population. J Behav Med 1:201–217, 1978

Ralph N. Wharton, M.D.
Donald S. Kornfeld, M.D.

6

The Management of Depression

Depressive illnesses are the most common serious psychiatric maladies seen in the physician's office. However, since fluctuations of mood are universal, it is important to distinguish between *unhappiness*, which is in the realm of almost every human being's experience, and *depression,* a true pathological state of mind and body. Not every patient who comes in complaining of "depression" is clinically depressed and in need of treatment for depression. On the other hand, in many situations it requires clinical sensitivity to ascertain that patients may be depressed when they, in fact, deny being depressed.

DIAGNOSTIC CATEGORIES

Since the term "depression" can be used in so many different ways, it is essential that we clarify its use here. The new guidelines and terminology established by the American Psychiatric Association (DSM-III) will be used.[1]

Major Depressive Disorder

This clinical syndrome has, in the past, been called "endogenous depression" or "biological depression," since it is characterized by signs and symptoms that suggest hypothalamic or limbic system dysfunction. This disorder responds very well to antidepressant medication or to electric shock treatments combined with psychotherapy. It is characterized by the following features:

Dysphoric affect. The patient reports he doesn't feel well. He is "sad," "low," "blue," "down in the dumps." He has an ill-defined bad feeling which he may locate in the epigastrium. He feels both helpless and hopeless. His psychic pain is often apparent in his facial expression.

Anhedonia. The patient reports he cannot enjoy any of the activities that previously gave him pleasure. He has lost interest in his job, family, friends, and hobbies. Sexual arousal and performance are diminished.

Psychomotor changes. The patient is slowed down in all psychological and motor activities. He thinks and speaks more slowly. He complains of becoming easily fatigued, of having no energy. He becomes sluggish and clumsy. He complains that his memory is faulty. This *pseudodementia* will disappear when the depression lifts.[2] Some patients become agitated, pace constantly, wring their hands, and are obviously anguished.

Vegetative symptoms. These are the complaints that are thought most likely to reflect hypothalamic dysfunction. Appetite is lost, and there may be profound weight loss. Some patients complain of a nauseous feeling on awakening. There is a characteristic insomnia in which the patient readily falls off to sleep but then awakens early in the morning and cannot fall back to sleep. Some patients are constipated. Diurnal variation is an important diagnostic feature; that is, all symptoms are at their worst in the morning. Patients report they may feel perfectly well late in the evening only to have their symptoms return when they awaken. The loss of interest in sexual pleasure is probably another vegetative symptom. There are often concomitant menstrual irregularities.

Negative state of mind. These patients tend to be quite critical of themselves. They have diminished self-esteem and minimize past achievements ("just luck"). They have no confidence in their ability to accomplish anything in the future. They are often guilt-ridden regarding past errors, or preoccupied with losses. They are indecisive, or when pressed for a decision, may change their mind many times. This may involve major life decisions such as a move or job change, or minor daily decisions about clothing, shopping details, and the like.

Some patients are irritable and occasionally frankly hostile. They may be sensitive about being slighted and demand special reassurance from family or friends that they are still loved.

Suicidal ideation. This is quite common in varying degrees, from the thought, "If this feeling goes on forever, life would not be worth living," to the decision to take one's life, coupled with a specific plan of action. The depressed patient must be asked about suicidal ideation. The inquiry will *not* give him the idea. In fact, most patients are relieved to discuss it, since it is a way of communicating to you how much anguish they feel.

You can say, "Many patients, when they are depressed, can feel life isn't worth living; have you had such thoughts?" If the answer is "yes", ask "Have you thought about how you might take your life?" If the answer is "yes" then you should refer the patient to a psychiatrist for management. The patient should be told that the referral to a specialist is based on your desire to get him or her out of the depression as quickly as possible. If you feel patients are acutely suicidal, keep them in your office until family or friends can accompany them to a hospital.

Reactive versus Endogenous Depression; An Outmoded Concept

The presence or absence of a precipitating event is not a crucial diagnostic issue. The distinction once made between reactive and endogenous depressions is clinically not very helpful and is no longer included in official psychiatric nomenclature. The ability to find a precipitant often depends on your ability to explore in detail the events of the patient's life prior to the onset of the illness and their psychological meaning. This information can be useful in helping the patient understand what triggered the depression and can help in developing a plan to prevent a recurrence; we will discuss the use of this information at greater length later.

Adjustment Disorder with Depressed Mood

This is the technical designation for the difficulty evidenced by patients in whom some life event has produced sadness, demoralization, or transient despondency; for example, the response of a patient to a myocardial infarction or the death of a loved one. The full picture of a major depressive disorder is not present. There are no vegetative signs. Lowered self-esteem and guilt are much less common. Biological treatment is not indicated.

Atypical Depressive Disorder

This category includes patients with a more persistent depression with intermittent periods of normal mood. In addition to the bad mood there may be hypersomnolence instead of the insomnia that is typical of major depressive disorder. These patients are more likely to overeat than to have anorexia. Their mood is not constant and can lift in response to some event. There is no diurnal variation. These patients should be referred to a psychiatrist for treatment.

Manic–Depressive Disorder

This disorder occurs in three forms: It may include both manic and depressive episodes (*bipolar* illness); it may take the form of recurrent mania without episodes of depression; or it may take the form of recurrent depression without mania (*unipolar* illness). The management of mania is discussed in Chapter 7. The depressive episodes are major depressive disorders and are treated accordingly. Treatment to prevent recurrences is discussed later.

ETIOLOGY

No specific etiology for depression has been established. Perhaps no single biological or psychological cause will be found. Instead we may find that there are a variety of paths that lead to these specific symptom clusters. We will briefly review some current hypotheses that do help in our understanding of treatment.

Biogenic Amine Hypothesis

There are data to suggest that drugs that are effective in the treatment of major depressive illness may increase receptor sensitivity or the bioavailability of biogenic amines, primarily norepinephrine or serotonin, at receptor sites in the brain.[3] Similarly, drugs that cause depression or that are effective in the treatment of mania may decrease the activity of these amines at receptor sites. It is likely that future research will delineate a variety of subgroups of depression with neurotransmitter markers for specific drug responsivity. The catecholamine response may be found to be a final common pathway for a variety of metabolic vulnerabilities to depression.

Neuroendocrine Hypothesis

Patients with major depressive disorders secrete adrenal cortical hormones differently when ill.[4] The normal cycle, with a peak in the early morning and a low during the early night hours, is flattened. Blood levels are generally higher during the depressive episode. Although some believe these hypothalamic changes have etiological significance, it is also possible that the disordered circadian rhythm is a secondary phenomenon.

Genetic Factors

Although there does seem to be a tendency for major depressive disorders to run in families, the genetic role is seen clearly only in the manic-depressive variety. A statistically significant increase in illness of approximately 10 to 15 percent is found in first-degree relatives of diagnosed cases.[5]

Psychodynamic and Psychoanalytic Issues

The issues of self-esteem, security, and reaction to loss which have been recurrent themes in the classical psychoanalytic literature are still important in explaining the psychological mechanisms that trigger the physiological changes of depression. Recently, Arieti and Bemporad have contributed an outstanding text on the role of psychotherapy in the treatment of major and minor depressive illness.[6] With the chronically or recurrently depressed individual, those character traits that contribute to the patient's vulnerability can benefit from an analytic approach. Patterns of learned helplessness in the face of early or repeated frustration, exaggerated needs for love, and a defective sense of self-esteem can be modified with long-term psychotherapy.

Iatrogenic (Drug-Induced) Depression

The use of some medications has been found to be associated with a clinical picture of depression. The effects of some drugs (for example, reserpine and methyldopa) on neurotransmitters could account for the production of a depression. With many of the other drugs listed in Table 6-1 the mechanism by which the depression is produced is not clear.

These drug-induced depressions are rare. They are more likely to occur in patients with a prior history of depression. In such individuals, alternative forms of treatment should be used. If the latter is not possible,

Table 6-1
Commonly Used Drugs that May Induce Depression with Chronic Use

L-Dopa	Reserpine	Oral Contraceptives
Methyldopa (Aldomet)	Steroids	Benzodiazepines
Propranolol (Inderal)	ACTH	Glutethimide (Doriden)

the patient should be closely monitored. These drug-induced depressions are sometimes dose related, and may be treated by reducing the dose. In most cases, however, the drug will have to be discontinued.

If a patient with a history of previous depression in association with steroid therapy again requires the drug, a tricyclic antidepressant can be given simultaneously. Lithium carbonate has been successfully used in the prophylaxis of steroid-induced mania,[7] and it can also be tried for the prophylaxis of depression.

The chronic use of diazepam (Valium) on a three- or four-times-a-day basis for a period longer than ten to fourteen days may lead to the development of a clinical picture that resembles major depressive disorder. Such an event may be explained by any or all of the following mechanisms:

- The general "depressing" effects of the accumulation of diazepam and its metabolites on the central nervous system
- The psychomotor slowing effects of the drug and the patient's response with feelings of despair and helplessness
- The worsening of an undiagnosed depression that initially presented with anxiety as a chief complaint

The treatment of choice in such situations is gradual cessation of diazepam and the institution of antidepressant therapy. Murphy suggests that each time you start to write a prescription for a benzodiazepine you should ask yourself, "Are you sure this patient isn't really depressed?"[8,9]

PROBLEMS IN DIFFERENTIAL DIAGNOSIS

The classic picture of major depressive disorders is easy enough to diagnose once you understand the diagnostic criteria. What is necessary is to maintain a high enough index of suspicion for this very common problem.

When the chief complaint is a dysphoric affect—for example, "I feel down in the dumps"—the diagnosis may appear to be obvious. However, a differentiation must be made between an adjustment disorder with depressed mood and a true major depressive disorder. The physician should inquire about a past history of sadness, unhappiness, and depression. Does the patient have a history of cyclical mood swings? Fleeting moods of depression may be promptly reported by some, whereas depression of several months' duration may be tolerated by others. It is also of importance, as with any report of pain, to get explicit information about the onset, duration, and time of day of the depressed mood. It is important to know if the depression occurs only in the morning, lasts all day, or clears at night and whether it goes on primarily at the office, at home or both.

Depressed patients often complain of difficulties with memory and concentration. Such a complaint can suggest the presence of a brain tumor or of dementia. However, the changes in mentation are more likely to be related to the neural synaptic deficit and the patient's preoccupation with his or her depressed thoughts, producing a pseudodementia. Depressed patients are usually more likely to complain themselves of memory loss; the family of the patient with an organic dementia is more likely to note the patient's memory difficulty. The mental status exam may not be too helpful since apparent memory deficiencies can occur with depressed mood; however, most patients with pseudodementia do well on these simple tests. Of course, the presence of focal neurological signs are an indication for neurological consultation. The symptoms of pseudodementia will clear with adequate treatment of the depression.

Patients with brain tumor or dementia can present with a picture that resembles depression. A history of personality changes, sensory or motor changes, or forgetfulness prior to the depressed mood make neurological illness more likely. Accurate information in this regard may be obtained only from the family.

Depression with Bereavement

One of Freud's important papers dealt with the differential diagnosis between mourning and melancholy.[10] Certainly mourning after a loss is a natural and usually self-limited response. However, we must be able to identify those patients in whom mourning becomes melancholy. This is major depressive disorder and is treatable. Those bereaved individuals who begin to experience these symptoms outlined earlier in this chapter, especially the vegetative signs and symptoms, should be treated with antidepressants. The patient will need to be told that your goal is not to make the patient happy, since no medicine can do that in the face of their loss. However, medicine can eliminate the debilitating depressive symptoms, such as early morning awakening and anorexia. The patient must be helped to recognize that while mourning is normal, the clinical symptoms of depression are an unnecessary additional burden.

Depression with Physical Illness

What about the patient with serious physical illness who becomes "depressed?" Is this an "understandable" reaction, to be treated differently from other forms of depression? We must, again, make the important distinction between unhappiness and depression. The former is to be expected and may not be amenable to our intervention. However, depression in these patients, like all others, is an illness and should be treated.

How common is depression in patients with serious medical illness? Surprisingly, not many studies have been done using specific diagnostic criteria. In one study of cancer patients 30 percent were reported to be depressed.[11] In post-myocardial infarction patients, a sense of despondency is often found in patients for 2–3 months after the event, and serious depression after one year has been reported in approximately 10–25 percent.[12] The history of the patient's mood prior to the infarction should be obtained since there are patients in whom depression was present prior to the coronary event. In these patients an additional emotional stress may have precipitated the myocardial infarction, and the depression can worsen as a consequence of the illness.

The management of illness-induced despondency can be considered in two phases: acute and long-term.[13] In the acute phase, for example, immediately after a myocardial infarction, the patient should be encouraged to express his concerns regarding what he believes the illness may mean to his future life. Some realistically based reassurance will help. The patient should be told that the weakness he will feel initially on ambulation is not due to his weakened heart, but is instead related to his long stay in bed or to the tranquilizers he has been given and that it is, therefore, soon reversible.

For some patients, depression will occur on return home, as a reaction to this weakness. Therefore, a specific program of physical rehabilitation is important to counter this effect. Such a program provides the patient with both psychological and physical benefits.[14] Your availability to answer questions, spoken or unspoken, is essential during this phase.

During the early weeks at home most patients have a heightened awareness of physical sensations arising from the area they consider damaged. For the post-myocardial infarction patient, any unexpected sensations in the chest are cause for concern. Some explanation regarding the likelihood of a wide variety of benign chest pains can help. They should also be told that their concern with their bodies is normal and does not reflect a permanent change in their personalities. Otherwise, concern that he or she is becoming a "hypochondriac" can further lower the patient's self-esteem.[15,16] This pattern can be expected to follow a wide variety of physical disorders.

It should also be noted that patients with serious illness who become depressed are often responding to more than the illness per se. We have found that many of these patients have other personal problems that are exacerbated by the illness, triggering the depression. We can too easily assume that a patient is despondent because of the illness alone. It is important, therefore, to explore other areas of the patient's life, since psychotherapeutic intervention can be very effective. For example:

> A 53-year-old widowed mother of three was admitted to a gynecological service for the reassessment of her treatment for endometrial cancer. It was discovered that a recurrence had developed and further radiation treatment and surgery were considered. The patient started on radiation treatment and then refused to continue. She stopped eating and suffered insomnia accompanied by feelings of futility. It was assumed that she was upset by the spread of cancer. Several of the house staff and attending physicans tried unsuccessfully to convince her to continue her treatment. After the psychiatric consultant was called, it was learned that the patient's brother and sole staunch emotional support had died between the initial diagnosis and treatment and the second course of treatment. After exploration of her feelings about the loss of her brother and with continued support from her physicians, she went on with her radiation treatment.

Depression can also occur after viral illness: flu, hepatitis, and infectious mononucleosis. These depressions do not usually meet the criteria for major depressive disorder and respond to reassurance and time. However, the same indications for drug treatment should be applied as outlined above.

When should antidepressant drugs be considered in medically ill patients? The general indications for their use with these patients are the same as with all others. The most important additional consideration is the possibility that there may be specific medical contraindications that limit their use. For example, in the postmyocardial infarction patient, cardiac findings may preclude their use. In such a situation three alternatives are available:

- If the depression is not too severe, one can use psychotherapy alone and allow for time to bring relief.
- Monamine oxidase inhibitors may be used since they have fewer direct cardiac effects than other antidepressants.
- If the depression is itself life-threatening, electric shock treatment can be considered, with close anesthesiology supervision. Treatment should not be given until the myocardial infarction scar has healed adequately.

The use of monamine oxidase inhibitors and electric shock treatment are discussed below.

The "Masked" Depression

Certain individuals use their bodies to express their emotions. These individuals are unable to acknowledge, even to themselves, that they are depressed and focus instead on physical complaints as a way of expressing their suffering.[17]

An attractive 35-year-old woman, mother of five children, was hospitalized on the weekend of Mother's Day for pain in the neck and the assessment of a cervical disc. X-ray examination showed mild osteoarthritis with minimal clinical indications to suggest myelography. When the patient's personal history was being taken, she reported that she had unequivocally not wanted the fifth child, now three years old. She was completely unable at times to resolve the inevitable conflicts between her husband and the four older boys or among the boys themselves. The patient's insomnia, anorexia, pain, and depression were slowly resolved after a series of family conferences combined with a course of antidepressant medication.

A 61-year-old widowed secretary, mother of one, was seen for evaluation of abdominal pain following cholecystectomy and a series of negative gastrointestinal and barium enema studies. As this sad patient told her story she burst into tears, sobbing and complaining of insomnia, anorexia, a 12-pound weight loss, and inability to work. She was unwilling to leave her apartment to visit her only son or grandchildren. Resentment and rage at her son who had not visited her when she was ill and to whom she had loaned considerable sums of money were explored. After six sessions she was able to restructure her financial and emotional relationship with her son and grandchildren. Her abdominal complaints, which had persisted for over a year following her operation, completely subsided after a course of antidepressants and the psychotherapy.

It is important to recognize that the choice of the presenting physical symptom does not usually represent special symbolic significance but may be related to an underlying physical illness. Therefore, the presenting symptoms may be:

- The apparent exacerbation of a physical illness
- Identification with a relative or friend with a physical ailment
- The reappearance of a symptom at a site of previous injury

TREATMENT OF MAJOR DEPRESSIVE DISORDERS

A medical practitioner can treat most depressed patients in his office quite effectively. This can be among the most gratifying of clinical experiences, since these patients, who suffer so deeply, can be completely relieved of the illness that pervades their lives and that of their friends and families. Of course, some patients may require hospitalization or prove resistant to standard treatment regimens, but these events are relatively rare.

Most patients will do best with a combination of psychotherapy and antidepressant medication.[18] The initial therapy should be supportive and should include some further history-taking while allowing time for the drugs to take hold. During this period the patient will require regular, frequent (at least weekly) visits with you. He or she should be reassured that improvement will occur after adequate blood levels of the drug are reached. Adequate treatment may require no more than 15–20 minutes per patient each week for 4–6 weeks, by which time most patients have had significant symptomatic improvement. Failure to respond after 6 weeks indicates the need for psychiatric consultation.

Suicidal Risk

A suicide risk is present when the patient has considered a specific plan and the means are at hand. It is more frequent among the aged, in men, and among the single, divorced or widowed. Alcoholism, a family history of suicide, or a previous suicide attempt are also associated with increased risk. It has been said that patients who talk about suicide will not attempt it. This is true only if those around the patient take his or her statement seriously as a plea for help and institute appropriate action. Depressed patients often have suicidal thoughts. Death appears to be a way out of their suffering. Such a thought does not have to lead to an attempt if we indicate our understanding of the intense suffering that prompts it, and then initiate effective treatment. However, if the patient has formulated a clear plan, psychiatric consultation should be obtained without delay. Hospitalization will probably be indicated. Such patients should not be left alone until definitive treatment has been instituted. The management of the surviving family after a successful suicide is discussed in Chapter 18.

Tricyclic Antidepressants

These drugs have been used for the treatment of depression since the late 1950s. They are antidepressants and not stimulants, like amphetamine. Their effect seems to be mediated through their ability to increase receptor sensitivity or the availability of certain biogenic amines (primarily norepinephrines and/or serotonin) at synapses in the brain. Some tricyclics are said to be more effective in increasing norepinephrine, others, serotonin.[19] The clinical application of this distinction is not yet clear.

The choice of a specific agent will depend on (1) the need for sedation and (2) concern regarding specific side effects, which vary in intensity with different agents (Table 6-2).

Table 6-2
Drugs Useful for Treatment of Major Depressive Disorder

	Sedative Potency	Starting Dose	Therapeutic Dose		Anticholinergic Effects (rated intensity, 1–10)
			Average	High	
Tricyclic antidepressants					
Amitryptyline (Elavil, Endep)	High	10–25 mg/tid	150	250	10
Imipramine (Tofranil, Presamine)	Low	25 mg/tid	200	300	4
Nortriptyline (Pamelor, Aventyl)	Moderate	10–25 mg/tid	100	150	3
Desipramine (Pertofrane, Norpramin)	Low	25 mg/tid	200	300	4
Doxepin (Sinequan)	Moderate	25 mg/tid	150	300	3
MAO inhibitors					
Tranylcypromine (Parnate)	None	10 bid	30	50	
Phenelzine (Nardil)	None	15 bid	60	90	

Amitryptyline (Elavil), the most sedating of this group, is the drug of choice for the agitated patient or the patient with severe insomnia. The larger portion of the dose can be given at bedtime. Doxepin (Sinequan) also has sedating properties.

Imipramine (Tofranil) and desipramine (Norpramin) are relatively less sedating drugs. They should be given to patients who have little anxiety and who show psychomotor retardation. These patients might not respond well to the more sedating effects of amitryptyline.

The anticholinergic side effects (dry mouth, constipation, urinary hesitancy, and blurred vision with accommodation) within this group of drugs vary primarily in degree of severity.[20] Most patients learn to adapt to them. Urinary retention can occur in patients with prostatic enlargement. Narrow-angle glaucoma (not the common form) can be worsened. However, a patient who is receiving appropriate treatment for glaucoma can be treated with these drugs. Hard sour candy can provide some relief from the dry mouth. Laxatives may be needed for the constipation. Urecholine (5–10 mg tid) can help with the urinary hesitancy. In some patients, particularly in the elderly, memory deficits and delirium can occur.

Some male patients report retarded ejaculation or impotence in association with use of these drugs. This problem can sometimes be alleviated by having the patient avoid taking a dose for 6–12 hours before sexual intercourse.

Tricyclics and other neuroleptics have also been reported to produce nightmares and somnambulism in association with single, large, nighttime doses.[21] If this should occur, switch to a divided daily dose schedule.

Cardiovascular Effects

Orthostatic hypotension is quite common. This symptom is of concern in patients with coronary or cerebrovascular disease in whom a sudden large drop in arterial pressure can have serious consequences. It is most likely to occur after a sudden change in position following a prolonged period of sitting or lying down. Patients should be cautioned to rise slowly; for example, to sit on the edge of the bed before arising. Men should be told not to "stand at attention" while shaving. If the effect should occur and persist despite a reduction in the dose, elastic support stockings, or an abdominal binder can be used. Fluorocortisone acetate (Florinef), a salt-retaining steroid can also be used in very small doses (0.05–0.3 mg/day) in the rare cases in which all other measures fail. This drug reduces the hypotensive effect by increasing blood volume. There is a danger of inducing hypertension in the recumbent position.[23]

Cardiac effects can occur by direct or indirect action. The anticholinergic effect of these drugs can indirectly produce a sinus tachycardia. The less anticholinergic compounds such as desipramine can be used should this be a concern. The conduction system can also be affected directly. When this does occur the drug effect resembles the action of quinidine, slowing conduction in the His-Purkinje system.[24] The ECG can show prolongation of PR, QRS, and QT intervals. Both atrial and ventricular depolarization can be slowed. It has even been suggested that these drugs could be used for the treatment of premature ventricular contractions.[25,26] Doxepin (Sinequan) is said to be the only tricyclic that does not show this direct cardiac effect. It also has lower bioavailability than the other tricyclics; therefore, at higher, more effective doses cardiac effects may still occur. In patients without cardiac disease, there need be no concern regarding the use of these agents. In the absence of a conduction defect the tricyclics can also be used safely in cardiac patients, providing weekly ECG's are taken.

In the presence of conduction defects, such as bundle branch block, monamine oxidase inhibitor drugs or electric shock treatment should be considered.

Newer Antidepressants

A number of new antidepressants with modified chemical structure are now being introduced after clinical use in Europe. They are said to have more rapid onset and fewer anticholinergic and cardiovascular side effects than drugs now in use. The ones currently available, maprotiline (Ludiomil) and Amoxapine (Asendin), have not been available in the United States long enough for us to report on the accuracy of these claims.

Drug Interactions

Both the effectiveness of tricyclic antidepressants and their side-effects can be influenced by other medications the patient may be taking (Table 6-3). For example, barbiturates and tobacco stimulate hepatic enzymes; this produces a more rapid metabolism of the drugs and makes larger doses necessary. On the other hand, the simultaneous use of a phenothiazine inhibits tricyclic metabolism; in this case lower doses may be required. Thyroid hormones may also enhance their effectiveness by making receptor sites more responsive. The tricyclics may also have adverse effects on other drugs; for example, they will reduce the hypotensive effect of methyldopa (Aldomet), guanethidine (Ismelin), and clonidine (Catapres).

The effects of alcohol can be potentiated by the tricyclics. The degree of this effect varies widely among people. Patients must therefore be cautioned to avoid alcohol while on treatment, or at least to use it with caution, keeping in mind that their tolerance has probably been lowered.

Table 6-3
Interaction of Drugs and Other Chemical Substances with Antidepressants

Interacting Substances	Effect/Mechanism
Tricyclic antidepressants in general with	
Amphetamine Methylphenidate (Ritalin)	Tricyclic antidepressants can inhibit the metabolism of stimulants and increase their therapeutic and toxic effects. Tricyclic antidepressants increase brain levels of stimulants. Methylphenidate can inhibit tricyclic antidepressant metabolism and increase serum levels. Stimulants may increase the antidepressant effects of tricyclic antidepressants.
Phenothiazines Neuroleptics	Concomitant use may increase serum levels of both; it may also increase the risk of tardive dyskinesia. Phenothiazines can inhibit the metabolism of tricyclic antidepressants.
MAO inhibitors	Fatal reactions may follow concomitant treatment, or treatment courses that are spaced too closely, especially with intramuscular medication.
Anticonvulsants	Anticonvulsants can lower tricyclic antidepressant serum levels by increasing metabolism. Tricyclic antidepressants can lower the seizure threshold. However, this is not a problem in patients who are adequately medicated with anticonvulsants.
Central nervous system depressants: hynotics sedatives benzodiazepines meprobamate barbiturates narcotics general anesthesia	The hypotensive and the central nervous system depressant effects may be additive.
Ethchlorvynol (Placidyl)	Delirium, central nervous system depression
Barbiturates Methaqualone Chloral hydrate Lithium	These drugs can lower tricyclic antidepressant serum levels.

(continued)

Table 6-3 (continued)

Interacting Substances	Effect/Mechanism
Alcohol Glutethimide (Doriden) Diphenhydramine (Benadryl)	
Diuretics	Used together may increase the risk of orthostatic hypotension.
Methyldopa Guanethidine Clonidine	Tricyclic antidepressants may lead to a reduced hypotensive effect.
Reserpine	Tricyclic antidepressants may block or reverse the depressant, as well as the hypotensive, effects of reserpine.
Oral anticoagulants	Tricyclic antidepressants can decrease the metabolism of dicoumarol and thus increase serum levels.
Phenylbutazone	Tricyclic antidepressants can decrease gastrointestinal absorption of phenylbutazone.
Epinephrine Norepinephrine Phenylephrine	Tricyclic antidepressants can enhance the pressor effects.
Antihistamines	Concurrent treatment can lead to mutual potentiation.
Tyramine	Tricyclic antidepressants can diminish the pressor effect.
Alkalinizing agents: acetazolamide bicarbonate	Making the urine alkaline may increase tubular reabsorption. This is important.
Central anticholinergics	The increased anticholinergic effect may have toxic consequences.
Methyltestosterone	A group of depressed men developed a paranoid psychosis after combined therapy.
Antacids	Can interfere with absorption.
While the following interactions have been reported with individual drugs, they probably apply to tricyclic antidepressants in general.	
Imipramine with	
Thyroid hormone	Hypothyroidism may retard response to tricyclic antidepressants. Thyroid hormone (triiodothyronine, 25 μg) may hasten a therapeutic response.* Imipramine may enhance the response to thyroid hormone.

Table 6-3 (continued)

Interacting Substances	Effect/Mechanism
Imipramine with	
Estrogen	An adverse interaction has been described, characterized by lethargy, nausea, headache, coarse tremor, and hypotension. Probably rare.
Amitriptyline with	
Diazepam	Diazepam may increase the half-life of amitriptyline and raise the serum concentration.
Methyldopa	Increased pulse and blood pressure by decreasing effect of methyldopa.

Adapted from Gaultieri CT, Powell SF: Psychoactive drug interactions. J Clin Psychiatry 62:720–729, 1978
*Wilson et al.[37]

Dosage Requirements

The spectrum of dose response is broad and may differ as much as ten-fold from one patient to another; some individuals may respond at 30 mg of imipramine and others at 300 mg. There is great individual variability in absorption, bindings, metabolism, excretion, and central nervous system sensitivity, which influences dosage effectiveness. For the typical adult patient, start Imipramine or Amitriptyline at 25 mg tid and then gradually build up the dose at 25-mg intervals every 48–72 hours, until a daily dose of 150 mg is reached.

Up to 50 percent of the dose can be given at sleep to reduce the discomfort of anticholinergic side effects. When amitryptyline is being used, this can often quickly help with the insomnia. Although the total dose can be given at sleep during the maintenance phase of treatment, we do not recommend it in the earlier phases. A twice- or three-times-a-day schedule will produce more consistent drug blood levels. A very large sleep-time dose can also produce problems with orthostatic hypotension in the elderly patient who awakens during the night to void.

It should be noted that geriatric patients are more sensitive to both the therapeutic effects and the side effects of these drugs. They must, therefore, be treated more cautiously. Start with 10 mg bid and then increase the dose by 10-mg increments. The elderly can respond to one-fourth to one-half of the dose required for younger patients. (The management of depression in the elderly is discussed in more detail in Chapter 12.)

It is essential to check the patient's pulse and blood pressure *both* sitting and standing (upon rising and after one minute) before starting a patient on these drugs. These observations must be repeated before any incremental dose changes are made.

If the patient has a drop in systolic blood pressure of 20-mm Hg or more, associated with symptoms of dizziness, weakness, or lightheadedness, then an incremental dose change should not be made. Most patients can tolerate the 20-mm Hg drop without any difficulty whatsoever, and a dose change can be made until symptoms secondary to postural hypotension occur.

In the absence of symptoms of distress even with measurable postural changes of the order of 20-mm Hg, patients should still be reminded to be careful when standing after prolonged sitting or lying down. They should also be advised not to stand without moving for any prolonged periods.

Usually mild autonomic side effects occur before clinical benefit is felt. If you warn patients in advance, they will rarely discontinue the drug because of side effects. Patients should be told at the start that they will have a dry mouth and may have transient blurring of vision. They should be told that these are signs the medicine is being properly absorbed.

The dose can be left at 150 mg for a week. Should the patient not respond the following week, the dose should be raised to 200 mg. Weekly 25–50-mg increments can then be used, until a maximum dose of 300 mg is achieved. Most patients will respond in the 150–300 mg range over a period of 4–6 weeks. Smoking tobacco and the use of barbiturate drugs enhance hepatic enzyme activity and can thereby increase this dose requirement.

A special word regarding nortriptyline dosage. The drug appears to demonstrate the therapeutic window phenomenon, that is, above drug blood levels of 170–180 ng/ml the treatment response drops off.[27] This makes dosage adjustment difficult in the patient who is not responding and therefore makes this a less desirable agent.

Blood levels of tricyclics are becoming more readily available from hospital and commercial laboratories. They are not needed in most clinical situations; however, they can be helpful when a patient is not responding to a reasonable therapeutic dose. Occasionally, because of problems with absorption or metabolism, patients on usual drug doses still do not attain what is considered a therapeutic blood level (therapeutic levels differ for each of these drugs.) In these situations larger doses can then be used, with subsequent blood level monitoring.

It is helpful to clarify to the patient how you expect his or her symptoms to respond to the medications. Most patients expect to feel better shortly after taking a pill. Explain that this medicine requires about 2 weeks before it starts to work. It begins by gradually reducing the intensity of symptoms, and does not abruptly eliminate them all (for example, initally insomnia will improve, then appetite, etc.). The biological symptoms usually respond before mood and thinking improve. Mood improvement will usually occur first at the end of the day. Thus the patient should be told not to be discouraged when the low mood reappears the next morning. The morning mood is the last to improve. It is important to offer the patient hope but to make it clear that the drugs are very slow acting and that relief may take a few weeks.

The depressed patient may be so despondent that he will feel that you cannot help him. It is therefore important to state at the onset something like, "In your depressed state you may not believe that medicine or anyone can help you. . . . That pessimism is a symptom of your illness. Try to remember that so that you do take your medicine." The family will have to be told the same thing since they will soon become frustrated at their inability to get the patient to accept the good prognosis. Depression is a self-limited illness. Without drugs, the average depression in an outpatient will end in 6 months; with drugs, it should lift in 3–6 weeks.

A 66-year-old businessman from New York had been anticipating his retirement with great pleasure for some time. He had many intellectual interests that he had not had time to pursue, and he expected that retirement would allow him the time he needed to study and even to do some writing. He expected that the Florida climate would be good for his health and would allow him to golf year round.

However, within two months after his arrival in Florida his mood shifted. He had lost interest in everything, was unable to concentrate, and complained of a failing memory. He had enrolled in two college courses but had to drop out. He could not develop any enthusiasm for golf or music. He became preoccupied with what he considered to be early failures in his life. He lived with a nameless fear that was particularly severe early in the morning. He had lost his appetite and was having trouble sleeping, often awakening at 4 A.M. unable to return to sleep. He found that 2–3 oz. of alcohol before dinner gave him temporary relief. Diazepam also helped relieve his tension, but his sad mood persisted.

The patient was started on amitryptyline 25 mg bid. Three days later, it was increased to 25 mg in the morning and 50 mg at sleep. The next week the patient reported that he was sleeping better and his mood was somewhat improved in the evening. The dose was raised in 25-mg increments over the next 3 weeks, to a total dose of 125 mg/ day. At that level he reported he was feeling significantly better with improvement in mood, appetite, and sleep.

He then began to discuss the factors that contributed to his depression. Since the death of his father when he was 14, he had been forced to be self-sufficient. There was a constant need to prove himself, probably related to the need to demonstrate he could adequately substitute for his father. However, oedipal guilt made it necessary for him to diminish his successes since he had, in fact, replaced his father. He was therefore never satisfied with his performance no matter how successful a venture might have been. He was thus able to understand that retirement left him with no way to prove himself and therefore, his self-esteem had no immediate support.

Over the next few months, the patient found that he was able, on occasion, to enjoy his successes without having to subsequently diminish them. He found that with his improvement in mood, his interests in music and reading returned, and these activities began to give him real pleasure. He began to think of himself as entitled to this free time after almost 50 years of devotion to work. The amitryptyline dose was reduced over a 6-month period. His mood has remained satisfactory since.

Monoamine Oxidase Inhibitors

Monoamine oxidase (MAO) inhibitors block the enzyme system that metabolizes catecholamines, thereby increasing the quantity of catecholamines available for neurotransmission. Over a decade ago, there was a brief recall of all of these medications because of reports of severe hypertensive episodes. However, at that time the need for dietary control was not understood. Now it is known that the hypertension is easily avoided by certain dietary and drug restrictions. The toxic foods that must be avoided are those containing tyramine: pickled herring, chicken livers, most wines and beer, broad beans, chocolate, soy sauce, any aged cheeses, and drugs containing phenolethylamine compounds. The common stimulants—amphetamines and cold remedies that contain ephedrine—must be avoided. MAO inhibitors should also not be used in association with alcohol and narcotics. Hypoglycemia can occur if these drugs are given to patients on insulin. (The manufacturer will supply you with a printed list of food and drug incompatibilities for your patients to carry with them.)

Tranylcypromine (Parnate) 20–50 mg/day and phenelzine (Nardil) 30–75 mg/day are the most common drugs in this group. The onset of action of these two drugs is somewhat more rapid than that of the tricyclics, but they must be used with cooperative patients. Two to four weeks of treatment are usually required to achieve an effect. These drugs, like the tricyclics, can produce orthostatic hypotension, however with MAO inhibitors it may develop insidiously over a period of weeks. This class of drugs has fewer anticholinergic or direct cardiac effects. Like the tricyclics these drugs can produce memory deficits and delirium. They can also produce cardiovascular problems should the patient require vasocontrictor drugs. Therefore a 10–14 day washing-out period is required before surgery. These drugs are not for use in an actively suicidal individual since by describing the hazards of certain food–drug interactions, we may be giving the patient a way to kill himself.

MAO inhibitors are most often used after a trial of tricyclics fails to achieve effects. A 10-day drug-free period is required before starting MAOI treatment.

Electric Shock Treatment

Electric shock treatment (EST)[28] was the first definitive treatment for depression. It remains the most rapid and most effective treatment for major depressive disorder. It might more properly be called *electric-stimulating treatment,* since this more accurately reflects its mode of action. The "shock" has been taken out of electric shock treatment by the concomitant use of the muscle relaxants succinylcholine or curare and the hypnotic sodium pentothal. The only motor signs of such a treatment may be a few small twitches of the eyelids.

EST is now used when a rapid treatment response is needed, for example, with the acutely suicidal or mute patient, or if drug treatment fails. Treatments are generally given three times a week for 2 weeks. The average course of treatment for depression is six treatments in a 2–3 week period. Treatments are usually given on an in-patient basis. Outpatient treatment can be given if there are no potentially complicating medical problems and the necessary resuscitative equipment and trained staff are available.

EST is safe except in the presence of recent myocardial infarction or intercurrent infection. It has been given successfully to patients with a clipped cerebral aneurysm, a history of cerebrovascular accident, and an implanted cardiac pacemaker. There need be no fears about permanent brain injury, persistent amnesia, and/or fracture. The temporary amnesia for recent events produced by a brief course of treatment may be minimized by the use of unilateral treatment to the non-dominant hemisphere. This transient amnesia must be differentiated from any persistent memory disturbance that many patients and physicians still fear. Objective evidence of persistent difficulty with memory has been found only in patients who have received multiple prolonged or intensive courses of treatment (40 treatments or more). No such data have been demonstrated with the usual brief course of 6–8 treatments given for depression. Newer methods of delivering the electrical current unilaterally, with better current control, have reduced the risk of memory loss still further. Maintenance EST may be necessary in some patients. Maintenance anti-depressant medication should be given post-EST in all patients.

Use of Maintenance Drugs

It is judicious to keep an individual on antidepressant medication for a minimum of 6 months following a single episode of severe depression; however, the patient should be seen and followed through the anniversary of the illness. Once the therapeutic level of the drug has been reached, with good clinical response, it is essential to maintain that dose level for approximately 6 weeks to 2 months. Following remission for 2 months, the dose level can be gradually reduced by one-third, one month at a time. For example, if a patient responds to 225 mg of imipramine, we will reduce the medication to 150 mg after 2 symptom-free months. Over the next 3 months, the dose can be reduced to 75 mg hs and kept there, if necessary, as a maintenance dose for at least 6 months. It can then be reduced at the rate of 25 mg every 2 weeks. When there is a history of recurrent depression (three or more episodes), the patient should be kept on treatment for a longer period of time, perhaps 5 or more years. This sort of patient is relatively rare, however, and decisions about long-term maintenance should be made with the assistance of psychiatric consultants. Some may consider lithium preferable for prophylaxis.

Some patients on maintenance tricyclics will note a weight gain that is usually associated with an increased craving for sweets. This is probably a direct effect of the drug, but the mechanism of action is unclear. The symptom is dose related and will also diminish somewhat with time.

With certain manic-depressives or unipolar depressives, relapse seems to occur without any obvious precipitants. However, on closer examination it will often be found to have occurred on the anniversary of some important event in the patient's life, for example, the death of a close family member. Where such anniversary reactions are likely, the drug dose should be increased from maintenance to therapeutic levels, in advance of such dates. Discussing the impending anniversary may also help avoid a recurrence.

There is often significant resistance to drug maintenance. Most people resent the dependence implied in having to take drugs every day for long periods of time. Medication also serves as a reminder of the illness and their vulnerability. It is, therefore, necessary to understand and deal with the meaning of taking the medicine to the individual patient. For example, where there are preadolescent or adolescent children in the family, the patient–parent may be uncomfortable taking drugs at home in front of children, or even "behind their backs." If a concerned spouse pressures the patient about taking the medicine, the pills can become a source of resentment in the relationship. If the patient is a nurse or a physician, the significance of taking medicine over a long period may be especially difficult, since it represents a role change. Where such psychological reactions are anticipated, discussing them early on may help make these issues conscious and avoid the problem.

When a decision is made to take a patient off maintenance tricyclic treatment, taper the medicine quite slowly, for example, by 25 mg reductions every two weeks. An abrupt discontinuation of the drug can produce withdrawal symptoms; most commonly, these are gastrointestinal. Although the half-life of the drug is approximately 24 hours, its effect on catecholamine uptake persists for days.

After the mutual agreement to stop medication, follow-up visits are essential. The telephone may also be used, but calls should be planned at a specific time of the month. It is unwise, especially at times of weaning from medicine, to consult exclusively over the phone. Usually it is better to schedule brief follow-up visits, without writing a prescription, as a way of validating the patient's ultimate capacity to function without medicine and yet maintain contact with you. Patients should be taught the early signals of relapse—for example, loss of appetite or early morning awakening—and they should be encouraged to contact you as soon as early symptoms appear. They must be kept from feeling that a recurrence of the depression is a sign of weakness.

Psychotherapy

Ongoing psychological support may include a variety of techniques: attentive listening to patient's global as well as specific concerns; intervention to enlist the support of other family members; practical suggestions or guidance, and/or providing patients with opportunities to ventilate pent-up feelings. In the course of such support, certain therapeutic themes should be emphasized. For example, the overly perfectionistic patient can be reminded of how this attitude makes him more vulnerable to depression. The long-suffering patient can be urged to take time off "on doctor's orders" (since he wouldn't do it on his own initiative). You should emphasize the need for some patients to learn to think and feel about themselves in new ways. For example, some patients will require encouragement to express hostile or assertive feelings appropriately. These patients often do not understand the difference between reasonable, self-assertion and a truly angry outburst or temper tantrum. As a result, they will inhibit any expression of their own needs and produce a self-imposed passivity. Certain patients need to develop social networks rather than dependence on a single central figure in their lives. Others may need to develop a specific hobby interest outside of a work compulsion. Some patients may require a referral for psychotherapy to modify such established patterns of behavior.

The Management of Tricyclic Overdose

More commonly, tricyclics are being used in intentional overdose. In toxic doses these drugs are respiratory depressants; however, their effects on the cardiovascular system are the most distinctive and potentially lethal.

If the patient is treated soon after drug ingestion, treatment with gastric lavage and activated charcoal via nasogastric tube is important, since dialysis is ineffective. These procedures are worth doing regardless of the apparent time interval since ingestion of the drug.

The cardiovascular complications are so severe and prolonged that these patients should be hospitalized in a cardiac intensive care unit. The manifestations of cardiovascular toxicity include cardiac arrhythmias and conduction defects as well as hypotension.[29] The conduction defect may present as an atrioventricular (AV) block or as an intraventricular conduction disturbance. The AV block occurs in the ventricular portion of the conducting system. Neither atropine nor catecholamines are helpful in treating the AV block.

Management, therefore, requires placement of a catheter electrode in the right ventricle to provide pacing of the heart below the block. The intraventricular conduction defects usually do not require specific therapy. However, if the QRS widening is marked and thought to contribute significantly to ventricular arrhythmias it should be treated as is the intraventricular conduction disturbance of quinidine toxicity—with molar sodium lactate. If this is unsuccessful, the use of catecholamines, such as isoproterenol, should be considered. However, these drugs must be used with extreme caution since the uptake of catecholamines by sympathetic nerve terminals is blocked by tricyclic drugs.

The ventricular arrhythmias may occur as an isolated manifestation of cardiac toxicity or in the setting of the conduction disturbances. If heart block is present, ventricular pacing should be assured before attempting suppression of the ventricular arrhythmias. Ventricular pacing alone may be successful in terminating the ventricular arrhythmias in the presence of heart block.

The choice of the appropriate anti-arrhythmic drug for suppression of the ventricular arrhythmias remains controversial. Theoretical concerns make Type I anti-arrhythmic drugs such as procainamide (Pronestyl) undesirable since their effects on cardiac conduction resemble those of the tricyclics. Propranolol (Inderal) may be useful, but its depressant effect on myocardial contractility may outweigh its benefit as an anti-arrhythmic. The use of lidocaine is fraught with risk since it has a significant slowing effect on conduction and can worsen the conduction block produced by the tricyclic drug.

Hypotension is a common complication of tricyclic toxicity. Volume replacement should be initiated, and if hypotension is severe or persistent, early monitoring is necessary. Placement of a pulmonary artery catheter with measurement of pulmonary artery systolic, diastolic, and wedge pressures as well as cardiac output will permit more intelligent management. If the pulmonary artery wedge pressure is low, reflecting a low atrial pressure, fluid should be administered to expand volume. If the pulmonary artery wedge pressure is above 15–18 mm Hg and the cardiac output and peripheral vascular resistance are low, an agent like dopamine or dobutamine should be used, albeit with caution, to increase cardiac contractility. Catecholamines such as norepinephrine are relatively contraindicated.

The respiratory depression may require intubation and mechanical ventilatory support. Close monitoring of arterial blood gases is necessary. Intubation may also be necessary to protect the patient's airway during treatment with gastric lavage.

The central anticholinergic effects of tricyclic overdose can produce a picture of agitation and toxic delirium that is associated with peripheral signs of cholinergic blockade: Fever, flushing, sweating, dilated pupils, increased salivation, and bronchial secretion, urinary retention, and decreased bowel mobility. Myoclonic jerks and choriathetoid movements are also common and can be misdiagnosed as seizures. An EEG should show no seizure activity. It is important that this distinction be made, since the unnecessary use of central nervous system depressants, such as barbiturates or diazepam, can depress respiration.

The pseudoconvulsion and other central and peripheral anticholinergic effects can be reversed with physostigmine, an anticholinesterase drug, which does cross the blood–brain barrier. However, it is short acting (it has a half-life of half an hour), and potentially hazardous. It can produce nausea and vomiting, and can provoke a seizure, an asthmatic attack, or a heart block. Physostigmine can slow a sinus tachycardia but has no proven benefit in the management of ventricular arrhythmias.

Physostigmine should, therefore, be reserved for use as a test agent where the diagnosis of anticholinergic toxicity is unclear.[30,31] If used, 2 mg should be given intramuscularly, or 1–2 mg should be given very slowly intravenously (no faster than 1 mg/min), with ECG monitoring. Should serious bradycardia occur, atropine at one-half the physostigmine dose should be administered.

The myocardial effects can persist beyond the period of coma; therefore, monitoring should be continued until the QRS returns to normal. The QRS is the best variable to follow serially. Transient agitation, hypomania, or paranoid ideation can occur when consciousness is regained. Diazepam is the drug of choice for control of these symptoms since the phenothiazines can produce cardiovascular effects.

Lithium Salts

Lithium salts are effective in the treatment of mania and in the management of manic-depressive episodes. Their effectiveness as antidepressants has not been established.

Manic-depressive illness is the primary indication for lithium. It is a relatively rare disease and often difficult to diagnose in late adolescence or early adulthood, especially when initial attacks are not classical. In the late 30s or early 40s the diagnosis is often clearer.

Some believe that lithium should be used immediately after the first attack of bipolar illness—especially late in life—and then for the rest of the patient's lifetime. However, there are a number of manic-depressives who have only one attack and others who may have one attack at twenty and may not have another until eighty. There is agreement that the frequency of manic-depressive attacks, generally, increases with age and that therefore, late-onset illness is more likely to be repetitive. We recommend that a patient who may possibly be manic-depressive be referred to a psychiatrist for confirmation of the diagnosis and a decision regarding treatment. The consultant can start treatment, establish an appropriate blood level, and then send the patient back to the referring physician for maintenance treatment.

The usual maintenance dose ranges between 600 and 1800 mg/day. For the first year, monthly blood levels should be taken and the drug maintained at 0.6–1.0 mg. After the anniversary of the initial attack has passed, the need for continued treatment can be discussed with the psychiatric consultant. If the patient is then placed on maintenance therapy, blood level checks of lithium can be done 4–6 times a year. Should the patient gain a significant amount of weight, the dose may have to be increased.

Lithium can be easily tolerated by most patients if blood levels are properly monitored and certain specific laboratory examinations are periodically carried out. Diarrhea and nausea do occasionally occur early in treatment but can usually be controlled by temporarily lowering the dose. Heart failure, salt-restricted diets, decreased glomerular filtration, or the use of diuretics can increase the likelihood of toxicity. If lithium must be used in these circumstances, much more frequent blood levels should be taken.

Blood pressure measurements, thyroid studies, and urine analysis should be done. A small but significant incidence of hypothyroidisms and thryoiditis and an occasional case of hyperthyroidism have been reported. Polyuria and increased thirst are fairly common. There may be a transient loss of ability to concentrate urine. Kidney changes of uncertain clinical significance have also been reported.[32] Serum creatinine levels can be monitored, and a 50 percent increase over baseline should prompt further investigation.

Lithium can produce reversible T wave changes on ECG (flattening or rarely, inversion). This may reflect intracellular myocardial potassium depletion by lithium;[33] sinus node dysfunction has also been reported.[34]

Serial ECG's are therefore recommended more frequently in patients with known cardiac arrhythmias.

Lithium can have a wide range of central nervous system effects that are dose related. At therapeutic levels, patients can experience some slight hand tremor and mild diminishing of coordination—for example, in hand writing. These symptoms may gradually disappear without any changes in dosage. More severe symptoms, such as somnolence, tinnitus, muscle twitching, dysarthria, confusion, vertigo, and seizures, are clear evidence of drug toxicity. There have been reports that some patients on long-term lithium maintenance develop cogwheeling.[35,36] However, there is no convincing evidence to date that long-term use of lithium produces any central nervous system damage.

COMMON ERRORS IN THE TREATMENT OF DEPRESSION

- *Misuse of minor tranquilizers.* Physicians may be misled by a patient's emphasis on the tension or irritability that often accompanies depression. A medication like chloridazepoxide (Librium) or diazepam (Valium) may, therefore, give a few days' relief, only to have the depression appear more obvious as the anxiety diminishes.
- *Underdosage of tricyclic medications.* Some individuals may need doses up to 300 mg/day to insure an adequate trial of treatment.
- *Inadequate time allowed for drug effect.* Weeks, not days, of treatment are needed. At least three weeks are required at a therapeutic level, which may be 300 mg/day for some patients.
- *Inappropriate use of lithium carbonate.* Lithium carbonate is an effective drug for the management of bipolar manic-depressive illness. It is not an antidepressant for acute episodes.
- *Difficulty in diagnosing the occult depression.* Masked depression comes in many disguises, which the clinician must learn to identify.
- *Reluctance to refer patients for psychotherapy.* Some physicians rely too much on drugs, while others rely too much on talking treatment. For most patients there is an optimal blend of both.
- *Underutilization of the doctor–patient relationship.* The use of mood-altering medications in no way lessens the need for support of the physician's presence during the patient's depressive episodes. Your emotional support of the patient during the acute phase will do much to relieve suffering and to provide hope until the illness begins to respond to specific treatments.

REFERENCES

1. Diagnostic and Statistical Manual, ed. 3. Washington, D.C, American Psychiatric Association, 1980
2. Wells CE: Pseudodementia. Am J Psychiatry 136: 895–900, 1979
3. Schildkraut JJ: Depression and biogenic amines, in Hamburg D, Brodie K (eds): American Handbook of Psychiatry, Vol 4. Philadelphia, WB Saunders, 1979
4. Sachar EJ: in Krieger, DT (ed): Neuroendocrinology. Sunderland, Mass, Sinauer and Associates, 1980, pp 177–183
5. Mendelowicz J, Fieve RR, Rainer J: Manic-depressive illness: A comparative study of patients with and without family history. Br J Psychiatry 120: 523–530, 1972
6. Arieti S, Bemporad J: Severe and Mild Depression. New York, Basic Books, 1978
7. Falk WE, Mahnke MW, Poskanzer DC: Lithium prophylaxis of corticotropin induced psychosis. JAMA 241:1011–1012, 1979
8. Murphy GE: The physician's responsibility for suicide. I. An error of commission. Ann Intern Med 82:301–304, 1975
9. Murphy GE: The physician's responsibility for suicide. II. Errors of omission. Ann Intern Med 82:305–309, 1975
10. Freud S: Mourning and melancholia, in Collected Papers, Vol. 4, Rivere J (ed). New York, Basic Books, 1959, pp 152–170
11. Plumb MM, Holland J, Park SK, Dyksira LJ, Holmes J: Depressive symptoms in patients with advanced cancer: A controlled assessment, abstracted. Psychosom Med, 1974
12. Stern MJ, Pascale, L, McLoone JB: Psychosocial adaptation following an acute myocardial infarction. J Chronic Dis 29:513–526, 1976
13. Cassem NH: in Massachusetts General Hospital: Handbook of General Hospital Psychiatry St. Louis, CV Mosby, 1978, pp 210–216
14. Hackett TP, Cassem NH: Psychological intervention in myocardial infarction, in Gentry MD, Williams RB (eds): Psychological Aspects of Myocardial Infarction and Coronary Care, St. Louis, CV Mosby, 1975
15. Wynn A: Unwarranted emotional distress in men with ischemic heart disease. Med J Aus 2:847–851, 1967
16. Klein RF, Dean A, Willson LM et al: The physician and postmyocardial infarction invalidism. JAMA 194:143–148, 1965
17. Lesse S: Masked Depression. New York, Jason Aronson, 1974
18. Dimascio A, Weissman MM, Prusoff BA, et al: Differential symptom reduction by drugs and psychotherapy in acute depression. Arch Gen Psychiatry 36:1450–1456, 1979
19. Maas JW: Biogenic amines and depression: Biochemical and pharmacological separation of two types. Arch Gen Psychiatry 32:1357–1361, 1975
20. Snyder SH, Yamamura HI: Anti-depressants and the muscarinic acetylcholine receptor. Arch Gen Psychiatry 34:236–238, 1977
21. Flemenbaum A: Pavor nocturnus: A complication of single daily tricyclic or neuroleptic dosage. Am J Psychiatry 133:570–572, 1976
22. Gaultieri CT, Powell SF: Psychoactive drug interactions. J Clin Psychiatry 62: 720–729, 1978
23. Chobanian AV, Volicer L, Tifft CP, et al: Mineral corticoid-induced hypertension in patients with orthostatic hypotension. N Engl J Med 301:68–73, 1979
24. Kantor SJ, Bigger TJ, Glassman AH, Macken DC, Perel J: Imipramine-induced heart block. JAMA 231:1364–1366, 1975
25. Giardina EA: The electrocardiographic anti-arrhythmic effects of imipramine hydrochloride. Circulation 60:1045–1052, 1979

26. Bigger TJ, Giardina EA, Perel J, et al: Cardiac anti-arrhythmic effects of imipramine hydrochloride. N Engl J Med 296:206–207, 1977
27. Kragh-Soresnen P, Hansen C, Gaastrup T, et al: Self-inhibiting action of nortripyline to anti-depressant effects at high plasma levels. Psychopharmacologica 45:305–312, 1976
28. Weiner RD: The Psychiatric Use of Electrically Induced Seizures. Am J Psychiatry 136:1507–1517, 1979
29. Bigger TJ, Kantor SJ, Glassman AH, Perel JM: Cardiovascular effects of tricyclic anti-depressant drugs, in Lipton MA, Dimascio A, Killiam RF (eds): Psychopharmacology: A Generation of Progress New York, Raven Press, 1978
30. Gramacher RP, Baldessarini RS: Physostigmine, its use in acute anticholinergic syndrome with antidepressant and anti-Parkinson drugs. Arch Gen Psychiatry 32: 375–380, 1975
31. Bigger T, Kantor SJ, Glassman AJ: Is physostiomine effective for cardiac toxicity of tricyclic antidepressant drugs? JAMA 237:1311, 1977
32. Hestbech J, Hansen IT, Amdisen A, et al: Chronic renal lesions following long term treatment with lithium. Kidney Int 12:205–213, 1977
33. Tilian AG, Schroeder J, Kao J, et al: The cardiovascular effects of lithium in man. Am J Med 16:665–670, 1976
34. Roose SP, Nurnberger JI, Dunner DL, et al: Cardiac sinus node dysfunction during lithium treatment. Am J Psychiatry 130:804–806, 1978
35. Shopsin B, Johnson G, Gershon S: Neurotoxicity with lithium: Differential drug responsiveness. Int. Pharmacol Psychiatrics 5:170, 1970
36. Kane J, Rifkin A, Quiktin F, et al: Extrapyramidal side effects with lithium treatment. Am J Psychiatry 135:851–853, 1978
37. Wilson IC, Prange AJ, McGlane T, et al: Thyroid hormone enhancement of imipramine in non-retarded depression. N Eng J Med 282:1063–1067, 1970

Stuart Yudofsky, M.D.

7

The Management of Psychosis

Psychosis is an impairment of thinking or mood in which the patient's interpretation of reality of his or her daily functioning is grossly compromised. Like pain or fever, the presence of psychosis in no way points to a specific etiology, nor does it discriminate between organic or functional illness. Psychosis is a final common pathway for a disordered brain. Although psychological factors probably contribute to the complex etiology of psychosis, there is enough evidence to suggest that psychosis associated with affective illness or schizophrenia may be a manifestation of a neurochemical disorder of cerebral function; therefore, schizophrenic psychosis may be as "organic" as the psychosis associated with delirium tremens. For clinical purposes, however, it has been useful to make a distinction between psychosis associated with schizophrenia and affective illness and the so-called organic psychoses associated with known physical factors.

CHARACTERISTICS OF PSYCHOSIS

The psychotic patient, regardless of etiology, may exhibit one or more of the following characteristics or features:

Disorder of thinking. The most common thought disorder is delusional thought. A *delusion* is defined as a false belief that is not attributable to the patient's culture and that cannot be refuted by the use of logic or rational persuasion.

A patient complained to an internist of difficulty in sleeping and of lethargy. On physical examination, the patient was found to be in a normal state of health although markedly dehydrated. Even though the patient did not appear to be depressed, the physician gently questioned her about her relationships, her work, and her thoughts. To his surprise, she eventually told him of a conviction that her next door neighbor had poisoned her dog (which had died two years earlier). The patient now firmly believed that her neighbor was poisoning the local water supply as well as all bottled fluids.

Somatic delusions can assume a variety of forms—from the preoccupation with bodily odors of a patient who is psychotically depressed to the schizophrenic patient's request of a plastic surgeon that he "redo my nose so it doesn't look like a penis."

Disorder of perception. *Illusions* are misperceptions of sensory input; for example, the rustle of the wind in the trees can sound like someone calling your name. This is not necessarily pathological. *Hallucinations* are the most common disorder of perception found in the psychotic patient. Here there is no external sensory input. Hallucinations can include voices or such sounds as buzzing, ringing, or music. Although auditory hallucinations are more often seen in depression and schizophrenia and visual hallucinations in organic psychosis that is secondary to toxins, brain lesions, and so on, both types may be present in either organic or functional disease.

Disorder of language. *Circumstantiality,* the elaboration of topics with extraneous detail, is a common trait and not diagnostic. *Tangential thinking* is characterized by associations that are coherently linked but stray from any central idea. The patient with tangential thought appears incapable of answering a direct question or staying with the point. In *loosening of associations,* unrelated thoughts are juxtaposed so that communication is impaired. Initially, the physician will have trouble understanding the patient and may feel that he has not been listening closely. However, when he stops concentrating on content and studies the thinking process itself, he will discover that the patient's thoughts are not logically related. *Blocking* is an abrupt, involuntary, and usually brief cessation of speech. The patient appears unaware of such interruptions, which are often followed by a total shift in the train of thought. *Concreteness* is a disorder of thought in which there is excessively literal thinking. When asked by the physician, "What is on your mind?" the patient said, "My skull."

Disturbance of affect. *Affect* is the emotional feeling tone attached to an object, idea, or thought. *Mood* is a prolonged emotion that colors the entire psychic life of the individual. Inappropriate affect refers to an emotional feeling tone that is not consistent with the patient's thoughts. Labile affect is an emotional feeling tone that is unstable and fluctuates more rapidly than is normal. This is often found in patients with brain damage. A patient who laughs, cries, and is angry all within the course of a few moments is exhibiting labile affect. A reduced emotional response may also be present in the psychotic patient. Such words as dull, blunted, apathetic, and shallow are frequently used to describe the emotionality of certain chronically psychotic patients. *Mania* is a state of excessive euphoria, excitability, agitation, activity, and energy that is most commonly associated with a decreased need for sleep and uncharacteristically poor judgment.

PSYCHOTIC SYNDROMES

Organic Brain Syndromes

An organic mental disorder is a transient or permanent dysfunction of the brain that is attributed to a specific nonpsychological factor. Any disorder of memory, orientation, attention, or comprehension; any visual, tactile, or olfactory hallucinations, and any neurological signs or symptoms suggest a possible organic component to a psychosis. Medical laboratory evidence, positive findings on physical examination, or a history of specific etiologic factors are necessary before a diagnosis can be made.

Delirium is an organic brain syndrome with a rapid onset of a fluctuating clinical picture that involves disturbance of attention, memory, and orientation. In addition, reduced wakefulness, insomnia, perceptual disturbances, and impaired motor activity are also commonly seen. Disturbances of attention are manifested by impairment of the abilities to sustain attention to environmental stimuli and to sustain goal-directed thinking, as well as goal-directed behavior. The memory impairment in delirium often involves impaired recall of memories formed prior to the onset of delirium, that is, *retrograde* memory impairment. *Anterograde* memory impairment, which is failure to retain information received following the onset of the delirium, is also common. In the delirious patient thinking is often fragmented and disjointed. Speech may fluctuate from incoherence to lucidity for minutes or hours at a time. Patients with delirium are characteristically disoriented to time and place, and they may have difficulty recognizing the roles and identities of other individuals. Perceptual disturbances in the delirious patient are common. Although all varieties of hallucinations may occur, visual hallucinations and illusions are the most frequent disorders of perception. In the past the term *delirium* has suggested the potential for reversibility. Since such a prognostic statement is often impossible to make, it is no longer considered a necessary criterion.[1] Table 7-1 summarizes etiological factors to be considered in delirium.

Table 7-1
Causal Factors in Delirium

- I. Intrinsic central nervous system (CNS) disease
  - A. Tumor
    - 1. Primary
    - 2. Secondary
  - B. Infections
    - 1. Encephalitis
    - 2. Abscess
    - 3. Meningitis
    - 4. Neurosyphillis
    - 5. Fungus and protozoa
  - C. Epilepsy
  - D. Ischemia
    - 1. Diffuse or multifocal blood vessel obstruction
    - 2. Large-vessel disease
      - a. Thrombosis
      - b. Embolism
    - 3. Intravascular coagulation
      - a. Collagen disease
      - b. Subacute bacterial endocarditis (SBE)
  - E. Hypertensive encephalopathy
  - F. CNS bleeding
    - 1. Subarachnoid
    - 2. Subdural hematoma
    - 3. Bleeding diathesis
      - a. Purpura
      - b. Clotting disturbance
      - c. Leukemia
  - G. Degenerative diseases
    - 1. Senility
    - 2. Presenility
    - 3. Metabolic errors
    - 4. Demyelination
- II. Non-CNS vascular disorders
  - A. Hypoxia due to pulmonary disease
  - B. Hypoxia due to cardiac disease
    - 1. Congestive heart failure
    - 2. Arrhythmia, including cardiac arrest and Stokes-Adams syndrome
    - 3. Shock, as with myocardial infarction
    - 4. Valvular disease, as with aortic stenosis
  - C. Reduced peripheral resistance
  - D. Disorders of blood volume and viscosity
    - 1. Polycythemia
    - 2. Cryoglobulinemia and macroglobulimemia
  - E. Anemias and hemoglobinopathies
    - 1. Pernicious anemia
    - 2. Carbon monoxide poisoning
    - 3. Methemoglobinemia
- III. Non-CNS organic disease
  - A. Liver
  - B. Kidney
  - C. Lung
- IV. Endocrine hypo- or hyperfunction
  - A. Thyroid-myxedema, thyrotoxicosis
  - B. Parathyroid: hypo- and hyperfunction
  - C. Adrenal: Addison's and Cushing's diseases pheochromocytoma
  - D. Pancreas: diabetes, hypoglycemia
  - E. Pituitary hypofunction

V. Ionic or acid-base imbalance
   A. Water intoxication or dehydration
   B. Hyper- and hyponatremia
   C. Hyper- and hypokalemia
   D. Hyper- and hypocalcemia
   E. Hyper- and hypomagnesemia
   F. Acidosis, metabolic or respiratory
VI. Infections
   A. Acute, such as: pneumonia, typhoid, malaria, acute rheumatic fever
   B. Chronic
VII. Environment
   A. Low-oxygen hypoxia
   B. Starvation hypoglycemia
   C. Vitamin deficiencies: thiamin, niacin, pyridoxine, B_{12}, folic acid
   D. Heat and electricity
   E. Radiation
   F. Sensory monotony
VIII. Exogenous poisons
   A. Medications
      1. Sedatives, barbiturates, and other hyponotics
      2. Minor tranquilizers: diazepam, chlordiazepoxide
      3. Phenothiazines
      4. Opiates
      5. Anticholinergics
      6. Tricyclic antidepressants

From Heller SS, Kornfeld DS: Delirium and related problems in Relser M (ed): American Handbook of Psychiatry, vol 4. New York, Basic Books, 1975

Psychosis in the Intensive Care Unit

The Intensive Care Unit (ICU) probably has the highest prevalence of delirium in the general hospital. This is due to the severity of the illnesses found there and the special environment of the units.[2] The psychoses associated with these environmental factors have been referred to as *ICU psychoses*. However, every psychosis in the ICU is not an ICU psychosis. In fact, the psychiatric symptoms found in the ICU are much more likely to be associated with the serious medical-surgical illnesses and their treatment that bring the patient to the ICU. The major problem, delirium, when accompanied by anxiety or agitation, can pose a threat to the life of a critically ill patient. The treating physician who mistakes these symptoms for a purely psychological reaction to the environment may delay the diagnosis and treatment of a serious underlying medical problem. When in doubt, an underlying organic basis should be sought.

There are psychiatric problems that appear to be related to the unique environment of the ICU itself. The nature and extent of these problems can vary. This variation may reflect differences in the construction and atmosphere of the individual ICUs. Some ICUs comprise a small facility in which patients, separated only by curtains, are surrounded by monitoring equipment and are all within the sight and hearing of each other. On the other hand, the ICU may be constructed with patients in individual sound-proof cubicles where monitoring equipment is judiciously concealed. Obviously, the environment in each of these ICUs is quite different, and the psychological reactions to each vary accordingly.

The concept of the ICU syndrome developed out of reports of the high incidence of delirium following open heart surgery. Typically, this delirium developed in the open heart surgery recovery room, after a lucid postoperative interval. Although a variety of operative factors and preexisting organic factors could contribute to the delirium, the environment of these rooms played a major role. Patients were often anxious and severely sleep deprived. The inadequate discrimination between days and nights added to the confusion. The ideal way of treating delirium related to the ICU environment is to transfer the patient to a standard hospital setting. When this is not medically possible, every effort must be made to provide the patient with adequate sleep. An hypnotic dose of a sedative should be given. Should these measures fail, the delirium should be treated as outlined in the next section.

It is possible to reduce certain stressful aspects of the ICU environment. The lighting on the unit can be varied according to day–night cycles. The ICU can be designed with windows visible to the patients to help orient them to time of day. If a stay in the ICU is anticipated for a surgical patient, the staff can describe the setting in advance. During the patient's stay, efforts should be made to orient the patient to time and place. Nursing procedures should be scheduled to avoid waking the patient. Try to avoid exposing patients to the emergency resuscitation procedures that may be required for other patients.

Treatment of Delirium

The patient's physical status must first be carefully reviewed. The physician should ask such questions as, Are there any neurological signs? Is the electroencephalograph abnormal? What new drugs have been given? How are the electrolytes, blood urea nitrogen, and hemoglobin? How well is the patient oxygenated? Prior to hospitalization, had the patient been drinking alcohol or taking some sleeping pill or tranquilizer from which he has abruptly been withdrawn?

While this diagnostic workup is in progress, symptomatic treatment can begin. Antipsychotic medications are beneficial in treating the agitation, the confusion, and the delusions and hallucinations. These patients often respond to smaller doses than would be required for the treatment of psychosis with schizophrenia. They may also be more sensitive to the drug side effects.

The drug of choice is a phenothiazine or haloperidol. The fear of cardiovascular complications has caused some physicians to refrain from using phenothiazines. When judiciously used, there is no significant danger, especially in the setting of the intensive care unit where the patient's vital functions can be monitored. In many cases the patient's agitation is a more serious threat to his or her well-being than are the drug side effects.

It is our policy to begin treating the agitated patient with chlorpromazine, 25 mg IM. Larger single doses should not be used initially. An elderly or debilitated patient might first be given a test dose of 12.5 mg IM. A regimen of repeated doses, such as 25 mg IM qid, while awake, is then established for each patient. This regular dosage schedule, based on the patient's physical status and response, is used until the psychosis is cleared. This is preferable to the exclusive use of PRN doses which often results in a more labile and extended course of the delirium. Vital signs must be monitored frequently, even though hypotension is less problematic in the recumbent patient. Should hypotension or oversedation occur, lowering the dose is usually adequate treatment. Additional 25-mg doses, when needed, can be used to supplement the basic regimen during the initial acute phase. As soon as possible, the patient should be shifted to an oral dose of approximately double the intramuscular dose.

If fear of cardiovascular side effects preclude the use of phenothiazines or if a less sedating agent is needed, haloperidol (Haldol) can be used. One-half to two milligrams can be given intramuscularly or orally. Doses must be determined on the basis of the patient's age, weight, and general medical condition. If the drug is well tolerated, the dose may be increased gradually. Daily doses of more than 10 mg/day of haloperidol are rarely required or tolerated in the patient with organic brain disease. Minor tranquilizers should not be used to treat the anxiety or agitation of patients with organic psychoses. Such medications often overly sedate these patients without affecting the psychotic symptoms and may even aggravate their agitation and confusion.

In addition to the drug treatment, patients with delirium require special treatment by the staff. If possible, a private duty nurse or aide should be utilized. One person whom the patient can learn to recognize and trust is preferable. If family members or friends are available and cooperative, they should be asked to spend time at the bedside. The patient's bed should be in a room with a safely secured window to assist with orientation to time and place.

Psychosis Related to Substance Abuse

The psychoses associated with substance abuse are among the most common organic psychoses. Acute alcohol intoxication and alcoholic withdrawal delirium (delirium tremens, or the DTs) are the most common. Details regarding their management can be found in Chapter 13. Other commonly abused substances include cannabis, opiates, barbiturates, cocaine, and amphetamines. Without the benefit of historical or laboratory information, the psychosis brought about by chronic amphetamine abuse is indistinguishable from acute schizophrenic psychosis. Of special significance to the primary care physician are the psychoses that are associated with prescribed medication; Table 7-1 also lists the categories of drugs that are most likely to produce psychosis.

Sedative and hypnotic ingestion is usually associated with labile mood swings, release of sexual and aggressive impulses, hostility and combative behavior, and even paranoid thought processes. Psychosis is much more common following precipitous discontinuation or withdrawal from these drugs. These acute withdrawal states are often produced inadvertently when patients are admitted to the hospital on an emergency basis and their supply of drugs or alcohol is cut off. With barbiturates withdrawal, tremor, weakness, sleep disturbances and irritability may develop within 24 hours of discontinuation. Depression, confusion, and irritability are also common in the second 24 hours after withdrawal. If untreated, grand mal seizures, delirium, and hallucinations may emerge, and withdrawal is potentially fatal. The hallucinations are most frequently visual, with vivid, bizarre, and terrifying imagery. The patient is usually agitated, and delusions may also develop. Tactile and auditory hallucinations may also be present. This state, occasionally accompanied by fever, develops 36 to 72 hours after precipitous withdrawal from barbiturates. Treatment requires establishing the diagnosis from history or blood and urine analyses and establishing, as accurately as possible, the dosage, duration, and pattern of barbiturate ingestion. A patient experiencing delirium with withdrawal has probably been taking at least 800 mg of barbiturate daily. Slower-acting barbiturates such as phenobarbital are more safely utilized to withdraw patients from barbiturates because of their more stable blood levels. An adequate initial substitution dosage is 30 mg of phenobarbital for every 100 mg of drug consumed daily.

Withdrawal from glutethimide (Doriden), methaqualone (Quaalude), and ethchlorvynol (Placidyl), produces a similar picture to withdrawal from barbiturates. Phenobarbital can also be used for ethchlorvynol and glutethimide withdrawal. The basic principle of the phenobarbital-withdrawal method is to substitute one sedative dose of phenobarbital (30 mg) for each hypnotic dose of the short-acting sedative or hypnotic.[3] Methaqualone must be used for the treatment of methaqualone withdrawal.

Glutethimide remains in the stomach longer than barbiturates; gastric reabsorption and blood levels are therefore, unpredictable. The variable absorption of glutethimide from the stomach can result in a patient going into coma, even after having begun to recover from an overdose. It is therefore essential that gastric lavage should be undertaken up to 24 hours subsequent to an overdose of glutethimide.

The benzodiazepines may, on rare occasions, be associated with paradoxical agitation and confusion—particularly in elderly patients or those with preexisting neurological lesions. The combination of benzodiazepines and alcohol potentiate the central nervous system depressant effects of both drugs. Withdrawal symptoms similar to barbiturate withdrawal can occur, although the most common reaction is anxiety, tremor, and insomnia. It is important to note that because of diazepam's (Valium's) long half-life, withdrawal symptoms are often minimal for the first 5 days after discontinuation of the drug, but emerge and peak between days 5 and 9. Thus detoxification from high doses of diazepam requires tapering the drug for at least 10 days beyond the date of the last high-dose use.

Psychosis Associated with Hallucinogens[4]

Acute dysphoric psychotic reactions to such hallucinogens as LSD (lysergic acid diethylamide), mescaline, psilocybin, THC (tetrahydrocannibinol, the active element in marihuana and hashish) and PCP (phencyclidine, also commonly called "angel dust") often occur shortly after the ingestion of the drug. Panic, anxiety and fear of loss of mental control are common. In addition, patients may express fearful disorientation, delusions, illusions, and hallucinations with concomitant agitation or bellicose behavior. Chronic PCP users may manifest unprovoked violent outbursts.

Physical examination of such patients will often reveal evidence of sympathetic hyperactivity, tachycardia, tremulousness, diaphoresis, and hyperreflexia. The clinical history and presence of neurological signs such as nystagmus, ataxia, or fluctuating levels of consciousness help in the differential diagnosis from acute schizophrenic psychosis.

These patients are best treated in a quiet environment with someone in attendance to provide reassurance. The patient should be told that the effects of the drug will "wear off in time," that he or she is not "going crazy," and that no permanent damage will occur. Sedatives and other tranquilizers should be avoided if possible, since they may act synergistically with some of these drugs, producing respiratory or cardiovascular depression. If agitation is so severe that a benzodiazepine must be used, remember that diazepam is poorly absorbed when given intramuscularly. Lorazepam (Ativan) is more reliable given this way. Should psychotic symptoms persist, an antipsychotic agent can be used. Haloperidol (Haldol) is preferable to the phenothiazines since it has less severe anticholinergic effects.

Psychosis Associated with Anticholinergic Drugs

Anticholinergic psychosis can be produced by toxic doses of a wide variety of substances. For example, many of the over-the-counter sleep medications contain scopolamine or methapyrilene. The antihistamines as a group have anticholinergic effects. Antiparkinsonian medications and many antipsychotic and antidepressant drugs are anticholinergic. Therefore, the syndrome is often found in association with overdoses of these drugs.

The physical manifestations of anticholinergic crisis are distinctive. Tachycardia, mydriasis that is unresponsive to light, dry skin and mucous membranes, urinary retention, decreased or absent bowel sounds, hyperreflexia, flushing, and fever. Paralysis of visual accommodation may also be present.

Patients are usually hyperactive and agitated and are plagued with visual and tactile hallucinations. They often swing at imaginary objects in the air or pick imagined creatures off their skin and clothing. Fluctuations in the mental status are common, and the patient often moves quickly from central nervous system excitement to central nervous system depression.

The diagnosis may be corroborated by the slow (no more than 1mg/min) intravenous injection of 1–2 mg of physostigmine. The comatose patient may become more alert. Psychotic symptoms will cease, and somatic anticholinergic symptoms will diminish. Physostigmine, however, is a potentially toxic drug and can produce tachycardia and seizures. Therefore, the usual treatment of anticholinergic or antihistaminic psychosis is reassurance and passive protection of the patient. Only in the cases of uncontrollable agitation or hyperpyrexia should physostigmine, 1–3 mg IV or IM, be used. This is a short-acting drug, and doses may have to be repeated in 1–2 hours. An electrocardiogram should be monitored as the drug is given. Should serious bradycardia occur, the physostigmine effect can be reversed by administering atropine, at half the dose of physostigmine given.[5] It is important to note that phenothiazines are contraindicated since they will add to the anticholinergic effect.

Psychosis Associated with Amphetamine and Cocaine

Amphetamine psychosis is clinically indistinguishable from many functional psychoses. The reaction, which most often occurs after prolonged amphetamine use and high doses of the drug, is characterized by restlessness, hyperactivity, anorexia, sleeplessness, pressured speech, and characteristically paranoid delusions. The paranoia may be simple suspiciousness and jealousy or it may involve elaborate, systematized delusions. Auditory and visual hallucinations are often present. Physical examination can reveal a restless, agitated patient with wet skin, dilated pupils, tachycardia, increased blood pressure, and, occasionally, hyperreflexia and hyperpyrexia. Toxic drug screens reveal amphetamine in the serum or urine. Phenothiazines or haloperidol are specific antidotes for amphetamine psychosis but should be reserved for use only when the diagnosis is certain and when the patient's physical state is jeopardized by agitation, hypertension, or hyperrexia. A sedating phenothiazine such as chlorpromazine in dosages from 25 to 50 mgs IM is the most commonly utilized agent. However, in view of the alpha-adrenergic blocking effects of phenothiazines, they must be used cautiously to avoid hypotension. Amphetamine excretion can be increased by acidification of the urine with 1–2 g of oral ammonium chloride every four hours. Intravenous phentolamine (Regitine) may be used to treat severe hypertensive crises.

Cocaine is used for its euphoriant and stimulant effects much as amphetamine has been used. Its central stimulant and sympathomimetic effects also resemble those of amphetamines, but are shorter acting. It can produce an acute anxiety reaction, with elevated blood pressure, tachycardia and paranoia. Hallucinations are less common. The psychosis is more common in those who take the drug intravenously rather than the more common nasal route. The pyschosis resembles the syndrome found with amphetamines but is not likely to last as long.

Severe anxiety reactions can be treated with intravenous diazepam (10-mg doses), administered very slowly. An alternative treatment is the use of propanalol (Inderal) which blocks cocaine's sympathomimetic effects.[4]

Toxic Psychosis Associated with Adrenal Corticosteroids

Psychosis may result from protracted use, high levels, or withdrawal of steroids. The incidence and severity of these reactions is unpredictable. Although a previous history of psychosis or of high doses or prolonged use of steroids increase the likelihood of steroid psychosis, the psychosis can occur in patients who were previously treated with steroids without psychological incident. Symptoms of the psychosis include any or all of the following: insomnia, agitation, irritability, euphoria, increased energy levels, grandiosity, auditory hallucinations, visual hallucinations, pressured speech, hyper-sexuality, flight of ideas, impaired social judgment, and affective lability. The symptoms are clearly distinct from the commonly observed euphoria of patients on corticotrophin and steroid treatment.

Treatment of toxic psychosis associated with adrenal corticosteroids includes reduction or discontinuation of the steroid (where safe to do so) and the treatment of manic and psychotic symptoms with major tranquilizers in dosages dictated by the patient's clinical condition. Where it is not possible to lower the steroid dose, antipsychotic medication can be helpful in controlling the psychotic symptoms. The dose required for control of psychotic symptoms may be much less than required for a schizophrenic psychosis.

Patients may show depressive symptomatology on being withdrawn from steroids or they may develop depression while on the drug. Symptoms include irritability, tearfulness, affective lability, pessimism, sadness, decrease of interest, decrease of appetite, and insomnia. Such symptoms may develop into full-blown psychotic depressions with hallucinations, delusions, and high suicide risk. Treatment involves protecting the patient from suicidal behavior and standard antidepressant medication. Such patients often require lower doses of antidepressants to achieve therapeutic benefit.

Recent studies have shown that patients on adrenocorticotropin (ACTH) who are treated simultaneously with lithium (with serum levels in the range of 0.8–1.2 mEq/l) have a significantly lower incidence of toxic psychosis.[6] Although it is possible that ACTH may have a direct effect on the central nervous system it is more likely that increased steroid levels play a role in these psychiatric disturbances.

Dementia

The management of psychosis associated with dementia is discussed in Chapter 12.

SCHIZOPHRENIC DISORDERS

Schizophrenic disorders occur in 1 percent of most populations. They occur equally in males and females, are present in every culture, and have been shown by epidemiological investigation to have higher prevalence among biologically related family members. It is likely that future investigators will prove the schizophrenias to comprise several separate disorders, each with a specific neurobiological defect. For the purposes of this chapter we shall focus on two common forms of the illness. The first type has an insidious onset, a chronic course, and a poor prognosis. The second variety occurs later in life, has a more abrupt onset, and is more responsive to treatment.

The essential feature of all schizophrenias is the disorganization of a previous level of higher social and psychological functioning. In the chronic variety the first symptoms often appear just after puberty. At this time the patient becomes less involved in social activities with peers and increasingly idiosyncratic. Thereafter, the patient becomes progressively eccentric in his interpersonal relationships, may neglect his personal hygiene, and ignore other social niceties. These initial changes mark the prodromal phase and comprise the hallmark of the chronic, more disabling type of schizophrenia. Soon the characteristic disturbances of language, thought, perception, and affect appear and mark the acute phase of the illness.

The chronically disabling form of schizophrenia is marked by exacerbations and remissions. Residual symptoms, which often accompany the remissions from the more acute episodes, include the following:

- Social isolation or withdrawal.
- Marked impairment of role functioning in work, school, or home
- Eccentric behavior
- Impairment of personal hygiene or grooming
- Blunted or flattened affect
- Tangential, circumstantial, or overly metaphoric speech
- Bizarre ideation or magical thinking

A second variety of schizophrenic illness characteristically appears in the late twenties or early thirties and does not have a prodromal phase of social isolation and deterioration of role functioning. The onset of language, thought, perceptual, and affective disorders is rapid. Often there are clear precipitating stresses. The symptoms are highly responsive to antipsychotic medications, and, in the residual phases, the patient may be asymptomatic.

TREATMENT OF THE PSYCHOTIC SCHIZOPHRENIC PATIENT

General Principles

Differential Diagnosis

Antipsychotics are usually effective in the treatment of the symptoms of all forms of psychosis, so care must be taken that these drugs do not mask symptoms that give clues to other potentially dangerous or reversible organic diseases. As with other medical symptoms, the differential diagnosis of psychosis is best made on the basis of a meticulous and thorough history. Since the psychosis may impede the securing of an accurate history, information from family members, previous physicians, and medical records should be vigorously sought. A primary care physician who is familiar with the responses of his or her patients to previous life stresses has an advantage in making a differential diagnosis. For example, if a middle aged patient without previous psychiatric history presents with the acute onset of paranoid fears, visual hallucinations and agitation, it is not likely to be schizophrenia, and organic etiologies must be vigorously investigated.

Histories should not only focus on the psychiatric symptoms but should include (1) a thorough family history of genetically related illnesses such as schizophrenia, bipolar affective illness, Huntington's disease, and senile dementia; (2) a careful history of past medical illnesses, including such categories as amnesias, metabolic disorders, previously treated neoplasias, trauma, infectious diseases, and vascular disorders; (3) inquiries concerning alcoholism, drug abuse, or exposure to toxic substances; and (4) a careful review of all medications the patient is currently taking or has recently taken.

Occasionally, the emergence of organic psychotic symptoms in patients with previous functional psychosis is not detected by the family or the clinician. The following should be the minimal medical evaluation in all patients with acute psychotic episodes: (1) A complete physical and neurological examination; (2) A thorough evaluation of the neurological mental status, including attention, orientation, alertness, speech, comprehension, memory, naming, repetition, reading, writing, and calculations; (3) laboratory screening, including complete blood count, erythrocyte sedimentation rate, serum electrolytes, glucose, blood urea nitrogen, serum creatinine, serum calcium, serum phosphate, liver function tests, serum vitamin B_{12}, T_3, T_4, VDRL, and toxic screen of urine or blood. Neuropsychological testing and an eletroencephalograph are also helpful in making a differential diagnosis.

Where the clinical findings suggest a possible neurological etiology, in a noncommunicative patient, the use of intravenous amobarbital (Amytal) can be helpful.[7] The Amytal is given by way of an intravenous line kept open with a dextrose solution. It is injected into the vein slowly at approximately 25 mg/min or in such amounts as to render the patient groggy but not somnolent. The patient with an underlying functional psychosis or catatonic state will become agitated and loquacious and will reveal characteristic paranoid or other psychotic fears. Therefore, you must be prepared to deal with a more acute agitated patient before you begin the test. The organic patient will become more confused and disoriented or will fall off to sleep with minimal amounts of the barbiturate.[7]

Hospitalization

The decision to hospitalize is based on an evaluation of the following possibilities:

- The patient is suicidal or otherwise self-destructive.
- The patient's psychological state renders him or her potentially dangerous to others.
- The patient's thinking, perception, memory, or intellectual functions are impaired to the degree that everyday activities are risky for him or her. The manic patient on a spending spree, the demented patient who is indifferent to traffic, and the patient who is toxic on phenocyclidine and who jumps from a window "to experience a feeling of flying," are examples.
- A thorough, rapid workup of the etiology of the psychosis requires the technology and concentrated coordinated efforts of a hospital service.
- The patient's present or projected physical state requires medical care; Examples are the delirious patient withdrawing from alcohol and the dehydrated and emaciated patient with a psychotic depression.
- Treatment of the patient's psychosis may be more safely and effectively managed in a hospital. Examples are the elderly, depressed patient whose cardiovascular status should be monitored while being placed on tricyclic antidepressants; the patient who requires electro convulsive therapy or the confused and agitated schizophrenic patient who could benefit from the support and protection of a therapeutic milieu.

Although psychotic patients are not commonly violent or self-destructive, the primary care physician should have preestablished office procedures that are designed to protect the patient as well as the physician and his or her office staff. Once patients are determined to be a danger to themselves or others, the physician should ensure that they are protected from the moment of that determination until they are safely secured on the requisite hospital unit. It is not uncommon for a suicidal patient to jump from the moving car that is transporting the patient from the physician's office to the hospital facility. Family or friends can be helpful, but for some patients the local police may be needed. Obviously, no one relishes the need to use coercive force. However, most patients are ultimately grateful for your forceful constructive action.

Somatic Treatment of Schizophrenia

A group of drugs are available that are quite effective in the treatment of the symptoms of psychosis. The principle action of these drugs is not sedation, so the term tranquilizer is a misnomer. Although some can produce sedation, they all can reduce or abolish psychotic symptoms. They all have the capacity to block central dopamine receptors, and this observation has been the basis of much research on the underlying mechanisms of psychosis. The phenothiazines, butyrophenones, and thioxanthenes are all equally effective when used in appropriate doses. Their differences lie in their individual side effects. Some, for example, are more sedating than others; some have more extrapyramidal side effects than others. The practitioner can, therefore, successfully treat the symptoms of most acute psychoses if he is familiar with as few as two agents, a sedating phenothiazine such as chlorpromazine (Thorazine) and a nonsedating agent such as the butyrophenone, haloperidol (Haldol). Table 7-2 lists the more common antipsychotic agents and compares them with respect to dosage and intensity of side effects. Of course, any of these drugs can be selected for your personal armamentarium. It is unnecessary to become familiar with a host of agents; instead, master the use of two or three. Occasionally, a patient will fail to respond to one agent but will respond to another.

Dosage

The required dose of an antipsychotic agent will vary with the individual patient. The patient's size and age are factors to consider. Table 7-2 includes information on dose equivalencies among six such agents. There is a wide therapeutic range between effective dose and toxic dose, so the physician can feel free to raise the medication level should the patient not respond to treatment.

Unlike psychotic patients with organic mental illness, patients with acute symptomatology of schizophrenia can often tolerate inordinately high doses of major tranquilizers. When initiating an antipsychotic medication, a small test dose is indicated: an equivalent of 50 mg PO or 25 mg IM of chlorpromazine. Haloperidol can be used in relatively higher doses (5–10 mg PO, 2–5 mg IM) since it does not have the cardiovascular side effects of the other drugs. If the medication is tolerated, it may be rapidly increased to effective therapeutic ranges in order to develop an adequate blood level quickly. Initially the medication should be given four times a day, for example, chlorpromazine, 100 mg PO qid, or haloperidol, 5 mg PO qid. During the first day, however, the agitated patient may require more frequent doses, which may have to be given intramuscularly. Half the oral dose should be used. Multiple small doses are

Table 7-2
Drugs Used in Treatment of Psychosis

	Single Dose (mg)	Usual Therapeutic Daily Dose (mg)	Sedative Effects	Extra Pyramidal Effect	Hypotensive Effects[a]	Anticholinergic Effects
Chlorpromazine (Thorazine)	25–50	200–800	***	**	**	***
Thioridazine (Mellaril)	25–50	100–600	***	*	**	****
Perphenazine (Trilafon)	4–8	8–32	**	***	*	**
Fluphenazine[b] (Prolixin, Permitil)	1.25–4	2–10	*	***	*	**
Trifluoperazine (Stelazine)	1–2	4–15	*	***	*	**
Haloperidol (Haldol)	1–5	2–20	*	***	*	*

Symbols: *, minimal or minor; **, moderate; ***, major.
[a] More severe when given intramuscularly.
[b] Available as a depo-preparation

preferable to larger single doses. Individual intramuscular chlorpromazine doses should be limited to 25 mg; individual haloperidol doses to 5 mg.

A recent study found that there was no advantage to rapidly increasing haloperidol dosage.[8] Patients given 10 mg PO/day did as well after 10 days as patients in whom the dose was increased up to as much as 100 mg in 5 or 10 days. Of course, those patients who do not appear to respond to the lower dose should have the dose increased. Some patients respond slowly to these drugs, and the duration of treatment may be more important than the dosage, once an adequate dose is achieved. Therapeutic daily doses for acute schizophrenic symptoms can range from 100 mg to 2 g of chlorpromazine or an equivalent antipsychotic medication. The average antipsychotic dose is approximately 600–700 mg of chorpromazine or approximately 15 mg of haloperidol (Haldol). The lowest dose that achieves symptom control is recommended.

Side Effects

The antipsychotic drugs are potent and, perhaps as a consequence, have a wide variety of often serious side effects. However, the average patient is readily treated without untoward incident or discomfort. Of course, a good working knowledge of these side effects is essential to assure optimal use and minimal difficulty.

Anticholinergic effects. A dry mouth is a very common early effect. The intensity diminishes with time, and patients usually tolerate it. Constipation and reduced bladder contractility can also occur. Laxatives for the former and urecholine (10 mg tid) for the latter are sometimes needed. Blurred vision, with accomodation, can also occur. Although anticholinergic agents produce mydriasis and, therefore, can worsen glaucoma, the patient adequately treated for the illness with miotics can be treated with antipyschotic agents. Inhibition of ejaculation can also occur, especially with thioridazine. Having the patient withhold his dose for 6–12 hours before sexual relations may help.

The intensity of these symptoms varies within this group of drugs. Table 7-2 indicates the relative intensity of each drug's anticholinergic potential.

Cardiovascular effects. Orthostatic hypotension is a common problem. It occurs early in treatment and often will gradually disappear. It is most marked in the morning after a prolonged period horizontal in bed. Patients should be alerted to this effect and trained to get up in stages, sitting for a minute on the side of the bed before standing. Support hose can also be helpful. The patient's blood pressures should be taken sitting and standing while the drug regimen is being established. Haloperidol is less likely to produce the effect than are the phenothiazines.

A severe episode of orthostatic hypotension should be treated by having the patient lie down with his legs elevated. This is usually adequate; however, if necessary, levarternol (Levophed) can be given. Phenothiazines produce relative alpha-adrenergic blockade; therefore, epinephrine should not be given since it can produce a paradoxical hypotension. Psychotic asthmatic patients who may require epinephrine should, therefore, be treated with haloperidol, which produces relatively little alpha-adrenergic blockade.

Electrocardiographic changes do occur with the phenothiazines. The usual such changes are an increased QR interval and flattening of the T-wave, and they are most likely to occur with thioridazine in doses above 300 mg. They are thought to have no clinical significance and will respond to lowering of the dose. The anticholinergic properties of the drugs can also produce a relative tachycardia that is dose related.

Central nervous system effects. The antipsychotic drugs vary in their ability to produce sedation. This effect appears to be independent of their ability to reduce psychotic symptoms. Relative sedative potentials are indicated in Table 7-2. The sedative effect often disappears in a few days or weeks. If this becomes a problem, the bulk of the dose can be given at sleep since the antipsychotic effect is a long-lasting one (days) whereas the sedative effect is much shorter (hours). The single bedtime dose is also much cheaper; for example, one 200-mg tablet of chlorpromazine is approximately one-third the cost of four 50-mg tablets.

Since all antipsychotic agents block dopamine receptors, it is not surprising that these drugs affect the extrapyramidal system. They produce three types of symptoms: a parkinsonian syndrome; dyskinesia; and akathisia.

The parkinsonian syndrome includes the usual elements of that disorder, including mask-like facies, tremor, stiffness, bradykinesia, and rigidity. The dyskinesias include a variety of peculiar movements of the neck and head—for example, torticollis—and buccofacial or lingual movements. The akathisia refers to a restlessness, especially in the lower extremities. This latter syndrome can be misdiagnosed as agitation and the drug dose mistakenly increased rather than reduced or neutralized with an antiparkinsonian agent.

Although all current antipsychotic drugs can produce parkinsonian effects, they do vary in their ability to do so, as Table 7-2 indicates. The more sedating, high-dose drugs such as chlorpromazine and thioridazine are less likely to produce these effects than are the low-dose drugs such as fluphenazine or haloperidol. These extrapyramidal effects can be readily treated by reducing the dose or by administering antiparkinsonian medication. For example, benzotropine (Cogentin), 2–4 mg/day, or trihexyphenidyl (Artane), 4–8 mg/day, are usually effective. The acutely disabling dyskinesias can be treated with intravenous diphenhydramine (Benadryl), 50 mg, or with intramuscular benzotropine (Cogentin), 1–2 mg, which is rapidly absorbed and can be repeated in 15 minutes if there is no response.

While the antipsychotic drugs can lower the seizure threshold, they can be safely used in patients with a seizure disorder if these patients are adequately covered with antiseizure medication. Untreated psychiatric symptoms are more likely to contribute to an increase in seizure frequency than the drugs used to treat them.

Tardive dyskinesia. Tardive dyskinesia[9] is the potentially most serious of the side effects, since no satisfactory treatment for all cases is available. The syndrome is characterized by abnormal movements of the face and tongue, such as sucking movements of the lips, tongue protrusion, and facial grimacing. It usually occurs after prolonged use (more than a year) of relatively large doses, or occasionally, after discontinuation of the drug. The elderly may be more prone to develop it. The overall incidence of tardive dyskinesia associated with the prolonged use of antipsychotic drugs is 10–20 percent of patients at risk.

Tardive dyskinesia is not likely to occur in association with the treatment of an acute episode. However, there should always be good indication for the use of antipsychotic agents. Some patients require the continued use of these drugs to avoid recurrence of psychotic episodes, and the risk of tardive dyskinesia must be measured against the disability and the social destructiveness of the psychotic symptoms.

Should tardive dyskinesia develop while the patient is on the drug, the medication should be discontinued. If the medication is discontinued shortly after the appearance of a dyskinesia, the symptoms are likely to disappear in weeks to several months. New antipsychotic agents that do not cause extra-pyramidal effects are currently being developed and tested. A psychiatric consultant should be aware of the latest developments in this area.

Skin and ocular effects. The phenothiazine agents can sensitize some patients to the dermatologic effects of sunlight. Chlorpromazine is especially prone to do this. Sunscreen lotions and appropriate clothing and the avoidance of direct sunlight can prevent this from becoming a problem. Some patients on chronic drug use can develop pigment deposits in areas exposed to sun.

The phenothiazines have also been found to produce ocular pigmentary deposits when used in larger doses for long periods of time. Chlorpromazine in doses exceeding 300 mg, taken for more than 2 years can produce deposits in or near the lens and cornea. These do not appear to have clinical significance. Thioridazine above 800 mg./day has produced retinal deposits that are harmful (retinitis pigmentation) and, therefore, doses should not exceed that level.

Antipsychotic Drug Interactions

The physician prescribing the antipsychotic drugs should be aware of how they interact with other classes of agents. For example, they can potentiate the CNS depressant effects of the opiates. They may diminish slightly the hypoglycemic effects of insulin and oral hypoglycemics. They may block the antihypertensive effects of guanthidine. Especially important is the interaction between the phenothiazines and epinephrine. Since the phenothiazines are alpha blockers, using epinephrine for the treatment of hypotension will usually worsen the problem, because the beta-adrenergic, vasodilating effect of epinephrine goes unopposed. Should a patient on a phenothiazine develop hypotension that does not respond to being placed in a horizontal position with legs elevated, than levarternol (Levophed) or phenylephrine (Neo-synephrine) can be used. Table 7-3 lists many of these drug interactions.

The Office Management of Schizophrenia and Other Psychoses

Patients who suffer acute psychotic episodes as well as chronic schizophrenic patients with recurrent psychotic breaks can often be managed as outpatients. In both conditions antipsychotic agents and the patients' trusting relationship with the medical practitioner play key roles. The non-chronic patient who recovers from an acute psychotic episode often returns to a reasonably normal state of social adjustment and mental functioning. Studies have shown that such a patient does not benefit from indefinite maintenance on antipsychotic medications.[10] As a result, they are usually tapered off medication by 6 months after the psychosis has been reversed. During this 6-month period the psychiatrist will have worked with the patient to identify and ameliorate the stresses that precipitated the pyschotic episode. To follow such a patient in an optimally effective manner, the medical practitioner should then pay careful attention to the following factors: (1) the patient's "normal" or baseline functioning; (2) the stresses that were thought to have precipitated the psychosis; (3) the "early" changes in the patient's behavior that occured *prior* to the emergence of the frank psychosis; (4) the specific medications and doses that ultimately reversed the psychosis; and (5) the psychotherapeutic, social, and behavioral interactions that the psychiatrist felt were useful in the treatment of psychosis.

Table 7-3
Interaction of Drugs and Other Chemical Substances with Antipsychotic Agents

Interacting substances	Effect/Mechanism
Antipsychotic drugs with	
Amphetamine Methylphenidate (Ritalin)	Neuroleptics in low doses may inhibit the metabolism of amphetamine and thus increase effects. In higher doses phenothiazines may antagonize the amphetamine effect on catecholamine systems. Methylphenidate may aggravate the symptoms of schizophrenia in certain patients. Long-term neuroleptic therapy can enhance amphetamine-induced stereotypy, presumably by increasing dopamine receptor sensitivity. Chlorpromazine can prolong amphetamine-induced hypermotility by increasing brain levels.
Tricyclic antidepressants	Concomitant use may increase serum levels of both; it may also increase the risk of tardive dyskinesia. Phenothiazine can inhibit the metabolism of tricyclic antidepressants.
Monoamine oxidase inhibitors	Monoamine oxidase inhibitors may inhibit the metabolism of phenothiazines, thus increasing serum levels. The combination may have an additive hypotensive effect.
Lithium	Possibly an additive hyperglycemic effect. Phenothiazines may increase lithium excretion.
	Combined use, especially with haloperidol, may lead to severe extrapyramidal reactions and hyperpyrexia.
Phenytoin Phenobarbital	Phenothiazines may inhibit phenytoin metabolism. Prolonged therapy with phenobarbital may increase chlorpromazine metabolism, increase urinary excretion and diminish clinical effects. Chlorpromazine and thioridazine may lower the seizure threshold.
Opiates Sedatives Hypnotics Barbiturates Antihistamines	Central nervous system depressant effects (and hypotensive effects) may be additive.
L-Dopa	Probably a mutually antagonistic interaction.
Hydroxyzine	Hydroxyzine may decrease the clinical effects of phenothiazines. Hydroxyzine may potentiate the cardiac effects of thioridazine.

Interacting substances	Effect/Mechanism
Centrally-acting anticholinergics, e.g. benztropine	Concomitant long-term use may increase the risk of tardive dyskinesia. Anticholinergics may decrease the risk of tardive dyskinesia. Anti-cholinergics may decrease absorption of phenothiazine, lowering serum levels. The combination may interfere with the thermoregulatory system, resulting in hyperpyrexia.
Oral anticoagulants	Concomitant use can lead to an increased hypoprothrombinemic effect.
Oral anticoagulants	Haloperidol may lower the anticoagulant effect through enzyme induction.
Halogenated anesthetics Enflurane Isoflurane	Profound hypotension may ensue.
Succinylcholine	Phenothiazines may lower anticholinesterase levels, prolonging neuromuscular blockade.
Thiazide diuretics	Hypotension
Acetaminophen	Acetaminophen derivatives may inhibit chlorpromazine metabolism and increase effects.
Insulin Oral hypoglycemics	Phenothiazines may decrease the hypoglycemic effect.
Digoxin Steroids	Phenothiazines may increase absorption of these substances by decreasing gastric motility.
Estrogens	Estrogens (e.g. oral contraceptives) may increase phenothiazine blood levels.
Diuretics Corticosteroids	Hypokalemia may enhance thioridazine-induced cardiac toxicity.
Gel antacids Aluminum and magnesium ions	Simultaneous intake will compromise gastro-intestinal absorption of chlorpromazine
Cholestyramine Activated charcoal	Simultaneous intake will compromise gastrointestinal absorption of phenothiazines.
Fruit juice, milk, tea, coffee	Phenothiazine elixirs mixed in these beverages will form an unpalatable mess; a complex that is insoluble even in hydrochloric acid.
Thyroxine	Thyroxine may increase the likelihood of haloperidol toxicity.
Cigarette smoking	Smoking may increase the metabolism of chlorpromazine.
Chloroquin	Chloroquin may increase the likelihood and/or severity of extrapyramidal symptoms.
Quinidine	Thiordazine has quinidine-like effects on the myocardium. Avoid simultaneous administration.

(continued)

Table 7-3 (continued)

Interacting substances	Effect/Mechanism
Guanethidine	Phenothiazines may block the antihypertensive effect of guanethidine and related compounds by blocking neuronal uptake.
Methyldopa	The hypotensive effects may be addictive. Methyldopa may potentiate the effects of haloperidol.
Epinephrine	The phenothiazines are alpha-blockers. Using epinephrine to treat phenothiazine-induced hypotension may compound the problem, perhaps because the beta-adrenergic (vasodilating) effects of epinephrine go unopposed.

Adapted from Gaultieri CT, Powell SF: Psychoactive drug interactions, J Clin Psychiatry 62:720–729, 1978.

It is essential that patients feel that their doctors have not lost respect for them because of their psychosis. Psychosis can be thought of as an aberrant neurochemical response to stress over which the patient has no control. Physicians should communicate to their patients their belief that this response should be considered no more embarrassing than such psychophysiologic reactions to stress as a duodenal ulcer, asthma, or colitis.

The following case example describes a patient whose first acute psychotic episode was treated on an inpatient basis and whose second psychotic episode was handled on an outpatient basis by her primary care physician.

> Mrs. A, was a 37-year old, married mother of three children with no previous psychiatric treatment. During a time when her husband, a successful novelist, was away for a month on business, the patient began to act peculiarly. She began to be fearful for the safety of her youngest child—an 8-year-old girl. She would not allow her daughter to go to school in the usual car pool and later began to keep the child at home "to protect her from the germs." In addition, the patient began to arrange her furniture in a cross-like formation, "to prevent the Andromeda strain from breaking into our house." The patient heard voices that told her to bury the family photo albums as well as her husband's clothing in the backyard. The voices also called her disparaging names, and warned her that harm would come to the children. She was hospitalized after she burst into her daughter's principal's office and screamed incomprehensible warnings about the safety of the students.
>
> At the time of her psychiatric hospitalization the patient was agitated, fearful, and somewhat oppositional. Her associations were loosened, and she spoke openly of her fears of infection from the Andromeda strain as well as of the threatening voices. Prior to this psychotic episode, the patient had no history of psychosis. She had many friends, highly developed intellectual interests, and adult activities. Since the patient was in excellent physical condition she was placed on liquid chlorpromazine 25 mgs/hr while

she was awake, and this dose was raised over the next week to 200 mg PO qid plus 400 mgs PO hs. Within one week the patient was no longer agitated, was not hearing voices, and displayed no thought disorder; she was still mildly fearful of contamination from germs.

Daily inpatient psychotherapy revealed that the patient had learned, 1 month prior to the onset of her symptoms, of the marital infidelity of her husband. The husband joined his wife in inpatient family psychotherapy, where this and other issues were discussed and resolved. The medication was changed from liquid to tablets and tapered to 50 mg PO qid, the patient's dose at discharge, after 3 weeks of hospitalization. She was seen by her psychiatrist weekly for 6 months after discharge, and her medications were tapered and then discontinued. The patient's primary care physician, whom she trusted, was apprised of all of the details of this psychotic episode, and she was discharged from psychotherapy to his care.

Two years after the patient had terminated her psychiatric treatment, a classmate of one of her children was seriously injured in an automobile accident. The patient again became fearful, restless, and overprotective of her children. Thereafter she began to hear voices and to behave in a paranoid fashion. She refused to see the psychiatrist but did accept chlorpromazine from her primary care physician, who saw her daily as an outpatient. Her practitioner placed her on increasing doses of chlorpromazine until she received a total of 1 g/day. The patient was cared for at home by her husband and her mother; under this regimen, the psychosis, which was not allowed to achieve its previous level of severity, resolved within 1 week.

Patients with chronic schizophrenic illness often have recurrent psychotic episodes as well as moderate social and behavioral impairments during the residual phase of their illnesses. Such patients are usually followed on a continuing basis in psychiatric outpatient groups, medication clinics, or sheltered workshops. Some of these patients may become acutely psychotic with each attempt to reduce or discontinue their antipsychotic medications. Such patients may require continuous maintenance on antipsychotic agents, in consultation with a psychiatrist.

These patients often have frightening somatic fears that can be mitigated by a trusting and understanding primary care physician. When the practitioner becomes comfortable and familiar with the highly symbolic and idiosyncratic communication of schizophrenic patients, he or she can find these people fascinating and highly rewarding to treat. An established relationship between the primary care physician and the schizophrenic patient becomes particularly important at times when the patient is medically ill or requires surgery. Such occasions are often highly stressful to this patient, who can misinterpret the meaning of his or her symptoms or the medical procedures. The familiar and trusted primary care physician is in the best position to understand and interpret the patient's fears and concerns.[11]

MANIC ILLNESS

Manic episodes include several of the following characteristics:

- Mood elevation, feelings of euphoria, excessive optimism, expansiveness, and inflated self-esteem
- Increased activity, in which the patient has unusual energy and may be restless or have an unusually increased work capacity
- Decreased need for sleep
- Increased sexual activity
- Increased alcohol or drug intake
- Talkativeness, often with very rapid, "pressured" speech
- Flights of ideas in which rapid successions of thought are often without logical connection
- Distractability, in which attention is too easily diverted by irrelevant, external stimuli
- Poor judgment, in which the patient may go on buying sprees, engage in grandiose business endeavors, make reckless investments, or show sexual indiscretions
- Irritability: occasionally the manic phase has a dysphoric cast, in which the excessively active patient may be loud, socially intrusive, quarrelsome, and even violent

Patients who have had one or more manic episodes and, in addition, have had one or more serious depressions are said to have *manic depressive illness,* now called *bipolar affective disorder.*[1] The onset of bipolar illness typically occurs before age 30; the illness is thought to be transmitted on the X chromosome. Manic episodes are prototypically well demarcated: They begin suddenly, escalate rapidly, and may persist for several days to several months; they may terminate abruptly, or they may be closely followed by a depressive episode.

The antipsychotic agents are beneficial in controlling the symptoms associated with mania. Because of its sedative properties, chlorpromazine—often administed in a liquid oral form in doses ranging from 300 mg/day to 1 g/day—is especially effective in treating acute manic episodes. Lithium carbonate is less effective than antipsychotic agents in treating *acute* manic episodes, since it is not fully active until 7 to 10 days after initiation of treatment. In well-established bipolar patients, however, lithium has been proved to be highly effective in the prophylaxis of recurrent manic episodes. In addition, there is excellent evidence that lithium also reduces the number and the intensity of recurrent depressive episodes associated with bipolar illness. Therefore, in a patient with bipolar illness who presents with acute mania, major tranquilizers should be initiated immediately for the treatment of the acute manic symptoms, and lithium should be simultaneously introduced to begin the prophylaxis.

It should be noted that there have been case reports of an acute severe neuroleptic syndrome characterized by hyperpyrexia, rigidity, mutism, and irreversible dyskinesia, which have been attributed to the combined use of haloperidol (Haldol) and lithium. Some investigators have questioned whether it is the combination of these drugs which has caused the syndrome, since it has also been reported with high doses of haloperidol and other neuroleptics alone. The combination of lithium with a phenothiazine such as chlorpromazine (Thorazine) can also increase the likelihood of lithium toxicity.[12] While these complications are rare, it does seem advisable when trying to control acute severe mania with a combination of lithium and a neuroleptic to use chlorpromazine, monitor lithium blood levels carefully, watch for evidence of lithium toxicity and discontinue the chlorpromazine as soon as possible. Where there is a specific contraindication to the use of the phenothiazines, haloperidol can be used but in relatively smaller doses (5–30 mg/day). Electroconvulsive therapy is also a very effective treatment for an acute manic episode.

Prior to the administration of lithium carbonate, the following baseline studies should be taken: thyrotropin, T_4, T_3. Baseline renal function should be assessed with serum blood urea nitrogen and creatinine. Where renal function is impaired, 24-hour creatinine clearance should also be done. Because lithium may cause reversible flattening, isoelectricity, or inversion of T-waves, an electrocardiogram should be taken prior to the administration of lithium. Certain sinoatrial node-induced arrhythmias have also been attributed to lithium.[13]

Lithium carbonate should be initiated at 300 mg PO and increased by approximately 300 mg/day. Serium lithium concentrations should be drawn every other day, 12 hours after the last oral dose of the drug. Once a serum level of 0.8–1.2 mEq/L is reached, therapeutic ranges have been achieved. Most patients achieve this level with doses in the 900–1800 mg/day range. At this point, the oral dose should be made constant.

Serum levels should be maintained higher (in the 1.2 mEq/L range) for the treatment of acute mania, and then reduced to between 0.6 and 1.0 mEq/L for prophylaxis. This level can usually be maintained with the patient on 600–900 mg/day. Major tranquilizers should be gradually reduced and then discontinued once manic symptoms have abated. Prominent side-effects of lithium include thirst, tremor, dryness of the mouth, nausea, and polyuria. At toxic levels, (above 1.5 mEq/L), lethargy, muscle fasciculations, ataxia, hyperactive deep tendon reflexes, dysarthria, confusion and, occasionally, convulsions and coma can occur. In addition, euthyroid goiters and interstitial changes in the kidney of uncertain clinical significance have been detected in certain patients on maintenance lithium levels. Following serum creatinine levels is a reasonable way of monitoring possible renal involvement. A 50 percent increase over baseline or early treatment levels warrants further renal evaluation.[14,15]

In some patients on prophylactic lithium maintenance, manic episodes may "break through." Often these episodes can be managed on an outpatient basis by medicating the patient with major tranquilizers in the aforementioned doses. The serum lithium level should be adjusted to between 1.0 and 1.2 mEq/L during the manic phase. After the patient has been euthymic for three weeks, the major tranquilizers should be gradually reduced until discontinued and the serum lithium level returned to the 0.6–1.0 mEq/L range.

RAGE REACTIONS

Rage and violence occurs occasionally in psychotic patients. The problem is rarely found in depressed patients, but may be a concomitant of manic, schizophrenic, or organic psychoses. Treating the patient's underlying psychosis with major tranquilizers, with reassurance, and with a safe nonthreatening milieu usually reduces the dangers of violence. Very recent research has shown that propranolol in very high doses (600–2000 mg/day) may be effective in treating agitation in schizophrenic patients as well as disinhibited rage and violence in patients with acute and chronic organic brain syndromes when other forms of treatment have failed.[16,17]

REFERENCES

1. Diagnostic and Statistical Manual, ed 3 (DSM III). Washington, DC, American Psychiatric Association, 1980.
2. Kornfeld DS: Psychiatric problems of an intensive care unit. Med Clin North Am 55:1353–1364, 1971
3. Khantzian EJ, McKenna GJ: Acute toxic and withdrawal reactions associated with drug use and abuse. Ann Intern Med 90:361–372, 1979
4. Grinspoon L, Bakalar JB: Drug dependence: Non-narcotic agents, in Kaplan HI, Friedman AM, Sadock BJ (eds): Comprehensive Textbook of Psychiatry, ed 3, vol 2. Baltimore, Williams & Wilkins, 1980, pp 1614–1628
5. Gramacher RP, Baldessarini RS: Physostigmine, its use in acute anticholinergic syndrome with anti-depressant and anti-parkinsonian drugs. Arch Gen Psychiatry 32:375–380, 1975
6. Falk WE, Mahnke MW, Poskanzer DC: Lithium prophylaxis of corticotropin-induced psychosis, JAMA 241:1011–1072, 1979
7. Weinstein R, Kahn R, Sugarman L, and Malitz, S: Serial administration of the amytal test for brain disease (its diagnostic and prognostic value) AMA Arch Neurology 71:217, 1954
8. Donlon PT, Hopkin JP, Tupin JP, et al: Haloperidol for acute schizophrenic patients: An evaluation of three oral regimens. Arch Gen Psychiatry 37:691–695, 1980
9. Tardive Dyskinesia: Summary of Task Force Report of the American Psychiatric Association. Amer J Psychiatry 137:1163–1172, 1980

10. Greenblatt AJ, Shader RI: Antipsychotic agents, in Meiller RR, Greenblatt DJ (eds): Handbook of Drug Therapy. New York, Elsevier, 1979, pp 546–559
11. Brody EB: Factors in the recognition and management of the non-hospitalized schizophrenic medical patient. Mod Treatment 6:695–703, 1969
12. Spring G, Frankel F: New data on lithium and haloperidol incompatibility. Am J Psychiatry 136:818–821, 1981
13. Roose, SP, Nurnberger JI, Dunner DL, et al: Cardiac sinus node dysfunction during lithium treatment. Am J Psychiatry 136:804–806, 1979
14. Cole J: Lithium and the kidney. Psychiatric Opinion, pp 40–41, October 1978
15. Jefferson JW, Greist JH: Lithium and the kidney. Semin Psychiatry pp 81–104, 1979
16. Yudofsky SC, Williams D, Gorman J: Propanolol in the treatment of rage and violent behavior in patients with chronic brain syndromes. Am J Psychiatry 134:218–220, 1981
17. Yorkston N, Grugelier J, Zaki S, et al: Propranolol as an adjunct to the treatment of schizophrenia. Lancet 2:575–578, 1977

Michael R. Milano, M.D.

8

The Management of Family and Marital Problems

Family therapy began in the 1940s as a new development in psychotherapy and in the study of human behavior. Contributions from pediatrics, child and adult psychiatry, and social systems theory were used to conceptualize emotional problems and/or deviant behavior in the context of faulty interactions of the patient's family. Traditional emphasis on traumatic individual development or characterological flaws reflecting intrapsychic conflicts was given less importance. In short, for the family therapist, there is no distinction between psychiatric patient, whether child or adult, and the patient's family. The family, and the interaction within that family, is the patient.

Before exploring the many practical applications of family and marital therapy for the family practitioner, we must first consider the physician's usual experience with families. Although family medical practitioners are involved with the health of the entire family they treat, their physical ministrations typically involve treating a sequence of individuals over time. Preventive medical care, treatment of pneumonias, fractures, allergies, and the like primarily involve interactions between doctor and individual patient. Family practitioners have considerable data about the social, economic, and interpersonal progress of their patients' families, but they treat patients as individuals and not as members of a special group, the family.

As a result, the practitioner tends to view each family member as a distinct psychological entity with his or her own strengths and weaknesses with each operating independently of the others. The doctor who sees an alcoholic husband, a depressed wife, a truant son, and an obedient daughter in the Jones family treats each separately and hears quite a few complaints about what the others are doing. The doctor may use individual treatment modalities for each: disulfiram (Antabuse) or Alcoholics Anonymous for the husband, antidepressants and Alanon for the wife, a school conference for the son, and social advice and congratulations for the good daughter. The doctor rarely sees the entire family for ninety minutes while they grapple with an issue and affect each other in stereotyped ways that provoke each individual's problems.

Basic family therapy technique can illuminate the ways in which the feelings—healthy or unhealthy—of each family member are interdependent. It can expose the family practitioner to new types of data, and it requires rethinking concepts of emotional health. For example, Mrs. Jones interacts with the doctor in a healthy, trusting fashion, but is intimidated and tentative in her dealings with her son. This child responds intensely but very differently to his mother and his father, and his sister seems to respond very little to either parent. Where then is the psychopathology? Does it reside in the individual or in the interaction?

If we were to observe some of these interactions, expanded over the 90 minutes of a family session, we would probably conclude that family therapy was indicated. But to undertake such treatment would place unrealistic demands on the time of the medical practitioner and would require special training. It is preferable that the family practitioner use selected techniques from family therapy, tailoring them to the practical necessities of medical practice and to the problems of each family. Before considering specific issues of therapeutic intervention, the family practitioner must learn to think of his or her patient and family as constituting a "system." This system is little more than a habitual pattern of response to a problem, which involves predictable responses by all family members. As these patterns deepen, each member becomes "enmeshed" in a limited pattern of response, and is trapped in his or her own ways and the ways of the family. No one person "causes" the other to be a certain way. Rather, each elicits from the other a characteristic type of statement, feeling, or response that become codified into family members' "roles." Each role reinforces the other, and the whole reinforces each role.

The more rigid and predictable the roles, the more dysfunctional the family (and vice versa). Dysfunctional families can be identified as either *enmeshed* or *disengaged*. The enmeshed family follows rigid patterns, as described above. The disengaged family has no established channels of communication or fixed and reliable roles. It is essentially a "free for all," with each member disconnected from each other (and frequently overconnected with street life, work, or other issues outside the family).

Merely observing family members interacting wtih one another allows a descriptive understanding of whether this "system" operates in an enmeshed or disengaged fashion. A hypothetical example of enmeshment follows.

> Mrs. A discusses with her physician the poor school performance of her 11-year-old son, John. It is immediately apparent that Mrs. A fears both John and Mr. A. She constantly intervenes to ask the school for "special treatment" for John. And she asks the other, healthy family members (two academically oriented older daughters) for "special understanding" about Mr. A's temper. These kinds of patterns become fixed and repetitive and each member becomes "enmeshed," seeing no other way to be.
>
> If the physician were to spend several hours with this family he or she would see a programmed set of interactions each morning. Mrs. A awakens feeling tense about whether John will go to school. Mr. A snaps at her and criticizes her for being so helpless. The daughters then tease John a bit. He becomes angry and cuts school. Mrs. A's role then is to define who was sick, that is, John, and to seek help from her physician, who hears only about John's school failure and defiance—not about the roles all the family members play in John's difficulties. The goal is to get John well without offending anyone else in the family (except Mrs. A) and without stirring any of the other latent conflicts. Everyone is trapped and repeats the cycle of behavior in a systematic, that is, habitual way.

The family practitioner with an orientation toward family interaction will be led by his basic knowledge of the family and his experience to ask several questions of Mrs. A. How does Mr. A feel about John's school refusal? Does Mr. A help with the problem? How do the children relate to one another? At this point the family practitioner will try to comprehend how the A family operates systematically around the issue of John's school attendance.

Planning a strategy of intervention will aim at changing the entire pattern of interaction. First, however, the practitioner must come to understand this entire pattern and not just the part played by John or Mrs. A. He may do this in one of several ways. He may already be able to piece together much information from his individual contacts. He may ask Mrs. A if he can call Mr. A and arrange an appointment with *both* of them. This will relieve Mrs. A of the burden of prodding Mr. A with her fearfulness and guilt. (This procedure virtually ensures that a reluctant husband or wife will eventually appear for help.) Finally, the physician may ask for a "family conference" in which everyone is asked to discuss the issue. His observation of the discussions will provide him with an "instant replay" of the family interaction around this issue.

WHEN IS FAMILY OR MARITAL THERAPY APPROPRIATE?

Most family practitioners will hear numerous descriptions of marital difficulty, usually from only one partner. The practitioner should be prepared to respond with an intervention and/or referral. Common overt problems focus on money, sex, lack of communication, and the interference of "outside" forces (in-laws, affairs, drinking, friends, etc.). Marital intervention is clearly indicated where the marriage itself is presented as the problem by both partners. A major problem arises when only one partner describes the difficulty. Rather than respond directly to the issue, the practitioner should first attempt to ensure that both partners will address the problem from the outset. A direct call to the absent spouse, or an invitation for him or her to call you, will lay the groundwork for talking to both members about the situation.

Many psychotherapists have applied family therapy to the entire gamut of adult and childhood syndromes, but it is rare for a family to request therapy or family intervention directly. Family intervention should be considered for families in which (1) there are multiple problems with several members; (2) adolescent behavior problems (rebelliousness, drug use, school avoidance) focused on a child reluctant to acknowledge the need for help directly; (3) the presenting patient is reluctant to enter therapy alone; (4) family members constantly blame one another; and (5) the parents disagree about how to solve the problems of their children. These are the kinds of problems with which individual referrals are least often successful. The practitioner should be most alert to the need for family or marital therapy in two additional circumstances:

- *When an adequate trial of individually directed interventions has failed.* This circumstance may indicate a problem so deeply embedded in the patient's family structure that no amount of pharmacotherapy, brief dynamic intervention, or even prolonged individual psychotherapy will succeed. Many chronic psychological problems involve the development of caretaker relationships, in which a marriage or a family becomes organized around attending to a "sick" individual. The sickness may be physical or psychological, but it comes to dominate and define the entire relationship. Both the sick patient and the caretaker cease to have a relationship apart from the illness. Other marriages may have rigidified into patterns such as those in which one partner is cold, ungiving, and dominating while the other is needy, emotionally unstable, and dependent, or in which one spouse is suspicious, controlling, and paranoid and the other is depressed, masochistic, and long-suffering. In these chronic situations, there may be many complaints of psychological distress, but well planned individual interventions will have yielded little gain or only transient improvement. The family practitioner should consider working with or referring both partners.

- *When the presenting difficulty is a complaint about someone else.* Individual therapy is designed to ameliorate complaints about the self, and about one's own personality structure. Commonly, however, a patient will see a problem in a spouse or child and describe his or her own situation as helpless frustration. "If only I could change my daughter's promiscuity or bad friends, but she refuses to listen to reason," might be a typical complaint about someone else. Trying to force someone else to behave or feel properly usually fails, and helplessness and/or angry complaints follow. The family practitioner, knowing the stubbornness of each family member and their frustration with one another, is ideally positioned to suggest that they "work this problem out together."

WHAT ARE THE GOALS OF FAMILY THERAPY?

In the natural practice of their art, family practitioners are in the enviable position of being able to view the developmental sequences of both the individuals and families they treat. They are not usually limited to the sickness-healer model that dominates the practice of most medical specialists. In helping families to work on family psychological issues the broader model of involvement is useful. For a depressed individual, pharmacologic involvement may produce a cure. However, the goal of helping a family is less focused on cure and more geared to restoring the normal developmental flow of the family by altering a specific disturbance of communication. The initial problem or symptom will change if the therapeutic intervention succeeds, but neither the family practitioner nor an experienced family therapist need grapple with the desire to produce the "ideal family."

In confronting decisions about which families need intervention and in setting goals for intervention, the family practitioner needs to be alert to his own needs and limitations. Some of these will be reflections of the exigencies of his practice, such as managing office hours and fees. However, it is usually possible to schedule an hour every week or every other week for five sessions to work with a couple or a family. Most families recognize the need for an hourly fee for counseling and are appreciative of efforts to "help them get started on the right road." Don't allow your reservations about charging a reasonable fee for "just talking" deprive your patients of this very important help. If you do not take the initiative, they may never get the treatment they need.

Family therapy, like other psychotherapeutic interventions, requires a great measure of honesty, openness, and common sense on the part of the family practitioner. The practitioner usually has a limited fund of personal experience on which to base an understanding of the many types of interactions and differing values espoused by the families he or she treats. Probably a majority of physicians have experienced only one set of parents and siblings, and their values are indelibly marked by that experience. What have been their experiences as husbands or wives? Can they be open and nonjudgmental in helping a couple with values and problems different from their own? Can they accept the fact that other parents may choose an approach to children with which they would not be personally comfortable?

The guidelines for a healthy, normal, or ideal individual are unclear, and the definition of a healthy, or normal, family is even more nebulous. Family practitioners working psychologically with families will feel personally buffeted by cross currents of conflicts about how a family and an individual should be. In order to work successfully practitioners must be flexible, tolerant of diversity, and able to suggest change without being critical. These are qualities of effective therapists who work with individuals or families. It is hoped that the information in this and other chapters of this book will deepen family physicians' understanding of the healthy and troubled families they see. It is then a matter of their wisdom and judgment in deciding when help is needed, and when they themselves can provide that help.

TECHNIQUES OF MARITAL THERAPY FOR THE FAMILY PRACTITIONER

Several concepts are helpful in diagnosing and understanding marriages and in attempting marital therapy. To make these concepts useful and practical, family practitioners are encouraged to employ them in examining their own marriages and those of friends and patients. In doing a descriptive analysis, the goal is to look for patterns of complementarity and of symmetry. *Complementarity* is best exemplified by the phrase, "opposites attract"; it refers to the fact that each partner brings special skills to a relationship. This division of skills and responsibilities may be highly practical ("I earn the money and my wife takes care of the bills"), or it may be emotional ("Fathers do the discipline when the kids get home . . . mothers are to heal your hurts").

The degree of complementarity, or specialization, may vary from issue to issue. When the complementarity is cooperative, couples speak of "meeting one another's needs." Over the course of a fundamentally cooperative marriage, spouses may adopt one another's strengths. Father becomes a little softer, and mother a little tougher (or vice versa). They speak of having "a nice blend." Such patterns are easily observed or described by the couples themselves.

However, not all individuals are basically cooperative. Where complementarity becomes competitive, admiration is replaced by criticism, and couples become expert at pointing out shortcomings in one another. This is the commonest malfunction of complementarity. Working on an individual level, the family practitioner will try to get each partner to accept his own shortcomings and, if possible, to make an effort to make changes ("If you're not perfect, why should your spouse be?"). Working on a marital level affords family practitioners additional leverage. They can point out that the atmosphere of criticism and competition ("I'm okay and you're not") makes any change impossible. They should insist that the first and the most important step is for both partners to change this atmosphere.

Where antagonistic complementarity reaches sufficient intensity, marital partners no longer see themselves as pursuing common goals and begin to focus on each other's shortcomings. Individuals in such a relationship can no longer acknowledge certain psychological traits or needs in themselves. The husband who fears "weakness" in himself projects this trait onto his wife. By constantly attacking his wife as "weak," or "fickle-minded" he can defend himself against feeling weak, vulnerable, or needy. Marital roles harden, and his wife, fearing her own capacity for anger or vindictiveness, may attack her husband as "the beast." He can present himself as if he had no vulnerability or needs, and she can present herself as if she had no anger or grudge except as a response to her husband's behavior. Both partners can remain "stuck together," each representing part of a whole human being. In this situation there is no sharing. The intense conflict in such marriages makes the average person quail, and divorce seems, to many, the only solution. In fact, such relationships are frequently quite stable, and the partners are highly interdependent.

The family practitioner working with marriages that involve intense strife and competitive complementarity may accomplish a great deal if he or she is able to involve both partners and avoids taking sides. Frequently, intense marital battles may be short-lived and related to a particular issue, rather than chronic and a way of life. Under these circumstances, "clearing the air" in a focused, less critical atmosphere may restore the status quo. If the couple is then able to repeat healthier interactions, deeper changes in the marriage will ensue. However, the family practitioner should not be surprised or disappointed if little progress is obtained. Such couples may have adopted chronic differences as a way of life and may be willing to do no more than use the family practitioner as a spectator while each member competes against the partner for the physician's approval and support. Under such circumstances, a graceful withdrawal and/or referral is appropriate.

Violence may be a feature of such a relationship. The violence may be part of an uncontrolled competition, or it may be an effort by one partner to stifle the mate. Frequently violence is used to silence and subjugate a dissatisfied partner. Communication is seen as a danger. Family practitioners must emphasize to each patient that they cannot condone violence, but that they cannot stop it either. As in child abuse, the victim may have to draw in appropriate social agencies (including the police) if talking, "cooling off," and attempts to foster communication are not voluntarily initiated and accepted by both partners. If the couple is able to accept the family practitioner's offer to serve as a bridge of communication, this may provide an alternative to violence.

Many of the dynamics of competitive complementarity and fixed blaming may be seen when a couple is in conflict about divorce. Here the family practitioner may again be able to reopen communication and enable both parties to find a path of mutual benefit. He or she should avoid taking sides about whether divorce is justified. Frequently, a young couple will want to discuss divorce with the family practitioner in an effort to "try everything" and thus prove to one another that there really is no hope. Both partners may be seeking permission to give up the struggle. They will appreciate the family practitioner's providing a neutral listening ear before they proceed with separation and divorce. The therapist may then be able to help both partners accept their feelings of failure.

Contrasting with complementary patterns of marital relatedness, the family practitioner will be able to observe patterns described as those of symmetry. Healthy symmetrical patterns involve an equal sharing of talent in the same area, either practical or emotional. Here the theme is, "We can both do it well separately, but it's best doing it together." Many current social forces, from women's liberation movements to the need to share household, child raising and breadwinning duties, are also attempts to develop marriages with less specialized roles. Here both partners share all tasks more equally. Observing life teaches us that each marriage is an individual blend of complementary and symmetrical functioning.

Whereas complementary patterns most often go awry in competition, antagonism, and struggles for power, the unhealthy aspect of symmetry produces stagnation. Excessive symmetry may occur where both partners are prone to be overly sensitive to their own hurts and those of others and overly needful of approval and sanction for their feelings and actions. Afraid of hurting themselves or their partners, such couples cannot discuss difficult issues and finally end up with no communication at all.

Symmetrical relationships commonly lead to timidity and avoidance and are prone to generate a fearful attitude affecting parents and children. The most frequent area of marital disturbance is likely to be sexual. With partners eager to "do the right thing for one another" and "perform well," the stage is set for many of the sexual disorders described in Chapter 9. Sexuality is best gratified with two partners symmetrical in approach, but it is necessary for each to be able to pursue his or her own feelings and pleasures, as well as those of the partner. Many of the sexual disturbances most easily helped by the family practitioner will grow out of disturbances in this area. If both partners are more occupied with "doing the right thing" than with the experience of sexual pleasure, they will develop disturbances of sexual arousal. In the absence of deeper marital strife, rapid improvement, with the help of therapy, is the rule.

Before we consider clinical examples of marital intervention, it should be emphasized that the goal of marital interventions is to alter and enhance communication between partners. The ability of the family practitioner to produce an observable change in the communication occuring in his office is a good index of how well his patients can address their marital problems at home. To this end, the following steps are suggested as guidelines for how to intervene.

1. Start with both partners. If the complaint is marital, ask the absent partner to contact you and arrange for both to start together. The only way you can study their communication is to have both partners present.
2. Be a good model of communication. Be cool with angry competitive couples and encourage them to try your approach. Push the timid partner a bit. Be a little daring in questioning the inhibited.
3. Establish a positive, supportive link with both partners. If you have talked in an understanding fashion about the feelings of Mr. B, talk in the same way with Mrs. B. Then pull back and see if they can do it with one another.
4. Try to develop a task for Mr. and Mrs. B to pursue at home that will parallel the change in communication produced in the office. This "homework" is designed to promote a change in roles. Sharing household duties, having someone different do the bills or make the sexual advances, and so on offers couples opportunities to "do it on their own."
5. Build on your successful interventions. Get the timid partner to be a bit more assertive in the session. If this works, then give a homework task that will reinforce the observed change. If an angry demanding father can be corralled into listening to his children during the office session, then he can be given the homework task of visiting each child at bedtime. This will reinforce newly developed behaviors.

6. After a few sessions, explore with the couple whether they are progressing. They may be satisfied with limited gains already achieved. If you feel they need more work, or if you all agree that a different approach is needed, do not hesitate to refer them for further marital counselling.

The following examples describe marital interventions that illustrate some of the foregoing principles.

Mr. and Mrs. C, recently divorced, sought marital help from their family practitioner in deciding whether to remarry each other. Mr. C. had always felt confused and overwhelmed by his wife's emotional capriciousness and had been angered by her complaints that he never talked. Mrs. C had felt blamed for all the problems in the relationship, had never been able to get a verbal response from her husband, and always felt like a burden. Despite all of these difficulties, the C's had a good sexual relationship, enjoyed the same things, and were similar in their approach to raising their children. They divorced after Mrs. C had an affair with someone who "understood her better."

In many ways Mr. and Mrs. C were more alike than different, and they were both frightened by their desire to remarry. They were unable to discuss what had happened in their marriage and feared a repetition. But both were eager to talk and respected one another's feelings. The family practitioner needed only to approach the problem in a straightforward way. Mr. C's mother (also a patient of the physician) was a disagreeable hypochondriacal person, and Mr. C was aware that he had learned long ago to tune out anything said by women. Mrs. C was reminded that her father had died during her adolescence. When asked whether this might have made have made her reluctant to trust men, she cried and described her sadness at that loss.

Both Mr. and Mrs. C were trusting of their doctor and of the process. It was immediately apparent that this time Mr. C, rather than Mrs. C, was the pursuer. He wanted to know more about why their relationship had failed, and why Mrs. C had chosen a lover. The pattern was a reversal of the previous marital structure where Mr. C had avoided his wife's desires for communication. Because this was a healthy change, the physician had little restructuring of communication roles to accomplish. After five sessions, Mr. and Mrs. C were satisfied that they had worked out their problem. No further therapy was needed, and their remarriage was successful.

Mr. and Mrs. D fought about everything. In the course of treating them as medical patients, their family practitioner was able to recognize deeply ingrained patterns of antagonism and competition. Mr. D criticized his wife as demanding and overemotional but sexually cold. Mrs. D described her husband as buried in his work, rather dull, and "weak" toward his children. Both children had had difficulties and it was after they found marijuana in their 23-year-old son's room that Mr. and Mrs. D called their physician. They were threatening divorce over a disagreement about whether to eject the son from the house.

The family practitioner knew that Mr. and Mrs. D were highly complementary and fit one another's needs despite intense friction. He saw them together with the limited goal of tiding them over the immediate crisis. No attempt was made to restructure the marriage. Mr. and Mrs. D were told to refrain from sacrifices "for their children" for two months and to take better care of one another. A referral was provided for the son. There was little mention of divorce during three thirty-minute sessions two weeks apart. By then the crisis had passed and no further intervention was necessary.

Mr. and Mrs. E had a highly complementary relationship in which Mr. E was the caretaker for Mrs. E's chronic psychological difficulty. This difficulty was expressed in complaints of insomnia and in rapidly escalating barbiturate use. Mr. and Mrs. E were in their mid 50s but had had a chronic marital problem of poor communication and absent or infrequent sex for 20 years. Mr. E, a workaholic, had a prior myocardial infarction. He had used his passion for work to avoid much marital contact. As their only two children were leaving home simultaneously, Mrs. E began escalating barbiturate use for insomnia. She was resistant to seeing her personal crisis as related to any psychological problems within herself.

The family practitioner was encouraged, through psychiatric supervision, to use routine medical visits to do covert marital therapy. He recognized the need to reinforce the "caretaker" link that made Mr. E the "strong, capable person" able to be attached in such a fashion to a dependent wife. Mr. E was allowed to dole out the medication on a supervised, gradually diminishing schedule; this tactic reinforced his role as the strong caretaker. The E's were seen for 20 minutes every other week for 6 months, and the physician made "casual" inquiries about their marriage, stimulating communication and getting them to resume a limited sex life.

The family practitioner, operated as a "go-between" in developing marital tasks that included Mrs. E's successful withdrawal from barbiturates. The latter would not have been possible without both the direction of their physician and Mr. and Mrs. E's willingness to reengage one another. Many recalcitrant psychological problems embedded in marital relationships can be best treated by the family practitioner who is aware that these problems may present themselves in the form of medical symptoms.

TECHNIQUES OF WORKING WITH THE FAMILY AS A SYSTEM

We have discussed the importance of understanding families as systems. Within the family as a whole there exist important subsystems. The most obvious are the marital and sibling systems. Sibling systems resemble marriages. In some families siblings are symmetrical. Other families contain specialists—for example, an athlete, a scholar, a black sheep. The marriage itself should have an area of distinctness within the family, and it should have its own set of rules. The children should have "lives of their own." Each system should be separate from the other, each should have strong inner generational loyalties, and each system should have clearly demarcated boundaries. In addition, there are boundaries that separate the family from the families of origin of each parent, and spouses should have loyalties to each other deeper than those toward parents. Finally, the family has a psychological boundary that differentiates it from the outside world. Each of these boundaries can be thought of as semi-permeable membranes, allowing interchange without loss of identity. The establishment, maintenance, and periodic revision of boundaries are the crucial tasks of all developing families. For example, it is across the outer boundary of the family that members interact with work, school, and friends. The boundary of the family changes when children go to school or when they enter adolescence and friends become more important. It is helpful in conceptualizing our patients' families, or our own, to think of the various ways in which boundaries can be used to explain strengths and disturbances. Common experience will tell us the following:

- Some parents, out of fear or ambition, cannot tolerate the viscissitudes of their children's development and, as a result, intervene too deeply and too often in an attempt to govern their children's lives. They never allow the essential generational boundary between parent and child to develop naturally and clearly.
- Some parents, either overworked or disorganized, provide little guidance or relatedness. Their children become swamped by street life or friends. Such parents are never able to establish a boundary between the family and the outside world, and little sense of family develops.
- Some parents have never lost their primary loyalty to their family of origin and are always on the phone with their parents or comparing their spouse to their siblings. There is no boundary between them and their family of origin, frequently at the expense of the marital system.
- Some marital partners form extramarital liaisons (e.g., barroom or coffee klatch friends, lovers) that overwhelm marital loyalties, breaching the boundary of both family and marital system. Frequently children in these families will have "bad friends," who recapitulate breaches of marital boundaries.
- Some children never interact with their siblings, always looking upward to parents or outward to friends for approval. Such "parentalized children" have been removed from sibling status and promoted to parental roles. This often interferes with their own acquisition of friends.
- Some families (especially those with schizophrenic members or the very rich) are aware of their peculiarity or uniqueness and defend

themselves with a fortress mentality that excludes any meaningful contact with the outside world. This too-rigid and exclusive boundary impairs development of friendships.

The classical conduct of family therapy involves gathering all available family members (including members labeled "healthy" or not part of the problem). Therapists then work to help change balances within the systems. They may, by requiring that both change, try to diminish the gap between the black sheep and the angelic children. They will try to sharpen or loosen boundaries. They may insist that parents spend time alone together to intensify their marital bond in a way that does not involve the children. This develops marital boundaries.

In addition to an awareness of boundaries within the family, the family practitioner will develop a sensitivity to the existence of triangles within the families he or she treats. The concept of *triangulation* was introduced by Murray Bowen to describe typical emotional interactions within families (see Guerin, 1976). In an emotional triangle, two family members, or two individuals, "gang up" to attack, avoid, or exclude a third person. Triangles may exist within a subsystem, when two children gang up on a sibling, or they may exist across boundaries, when a husband and his mother agree that the spouse is defective in some way. The excluded member of a triangle usually then finds a partner of his or her own. For example, the spouse may form an unconscious pact with her son that daddy is impossible. This sets up a complex system of balanced triangles that stabilizes the family but prevents the solution of problems.

In working therapeutically with families, the family practitioner will be particularly alert for triangles that involve the presenting problem patient. Most therapists pay special attention to triangles or partnerships that cross the boundary between parents and children. Suppose, for example, that a hardworking, distant father is cut off from contact with a lonely wife and a daughter with a school phobia. Here the women will cling together while the man goes off to do business with the world. This triangle disrupts both marital boundaries and sibling boundaries, creating a special place for the entangled child and separating her from her siblings. Having all family members present makes it easier to diagnose triangles. In this family, father and the other children would sit separately while mother and the phobic daughter would sit close to one another and communicate constantly. The family practitioner who has diagnosed such a triangle will plan his intervention to restore normal boundaries and return the family to its on-going developmental processes.

The following series of steps is similar to those followed in doing marital intervention.

1. Communicate directly with all of the involved members, to arrange an initial meeting. If, for example, the index problem is a reluctant

or rebellious adolescent, it is better to speak to him or her directly rather than through the parents. If you need to use a parent as a messenger, use the parent who seems least involved and least interested in getting help.

2. Define the problem in terms of family systems, at least in your own mind. Explore everyone's side of the problem, and see what happens when they try to find a solution by themselves. Does mother worry too much and start to take over? Then make father the helper to the child and ask mother to be a truly supportive wife. Does father try to dominate with threats? Help him to take a back seat while others suggest new ideas. Give the "irresponsible" child some responsibility in a nonconflicted area to "prove she can do it." But keep your attention on the ways they communicate, and have the family focus on "getting along better" rather than devoting all of their attention to curing the identified patient.
3. Develop a specific problem for them to work on at home. Again, this should parallel the problems in communication. Know everyone individually if possible. Since the therapeutic contract will probably be brief, it is essential to focus on one or two key problems.
4. Observe the results of initial interventions and recalibrate tasks and strategies as necessary.
5. Disengage when your major objective has been achieved.

The following examples illustrate some of the principles of doing family evaluations and family therapy.

The F family. Therapeutic intervention in this family in many respects resembles the advice-giving typical of pediatrics practice. The family practitioner in this case focused on strengthening the marital subsystem and detriangulating a child:

> Mrs. F, a 27-year-old housewife, spoke to her family practitioner about her two-year-old daughter's "insomnia" and constant visits to the parental bedroom throughout the night. Some further exploration revealed that Mrs. F was very unhappy about her marital communication and that sexual interaction had virtually disappeared. The physician asked Mr. F to appear for a second discussion. Six sessions focused on tasks designed to correct structural abnormalities growing in the family. Mr. F was asked to tend to all of his daughter's nocturnal needs, strengthening his relationship with both his daughter and wife and freeing Mrs. F from setting limits at that time. The family practitioner helped Mrs. F, a rather perfectionistic mother, to verbalize her fears of being a "bad mother," which had been stirred by her inability to control her daughter. Mr. F was less conflicted and able to let his daughter "cry it out." This blend of child guidance techniques with structural moves is typical of working with child-oriented families.

In addition, Mr. and Mrs. F had developed two nocturnal marital disturbances. They had little sex, and Mr. F, an isolated person, tended to roam the house alone after his wife had gone to bed. Both Mr. and Mrs. F were able to talk openly of the distance that had grown between them, and after two sessions, they resumed "dating" and going to bed together. Ultimately, feelings of closeness and a sexual life returned. They were able to maintain a normal bedtime cycle for three more sessions and continued in an improved state while the daughter learned to sleep without parental presence. It is notable that these family dynamics, and this therapeutic approach, have been useful in relieving many early school phobias, where mother and child share separation anxiety and father excludes himself from parenting interactions.

The G family. The G family struggled with adolescent individuation, a typical indication for family intervention. Structurally, there was disruption of marital and sibling systems, with constant triangulation across generational boundaries.

Mr. G called to say that his 16-year-old daughter had pummelled Mrs. G and threatened to poison the family. Mr G was a fortyish workaholic with a wife who gained his attention only when he was called upon to intervene in family fights. He blustered and threatened and sometimes hit, legitimizing violence. Mrs. G cried and complained. An older daughter had left home after much unsuccessful individual therapy. The sixteen-year-old daughter was bright, ambitious, and a good student but she was fresh, bossy, and physically dominated her mother, and her father hit her. A younger son was invited for the first and subsequent sessions. He was a silent, uninvolved "good boy" who was an academic underachiever.

Wading through a welter of complaints, a number of structural moves were planned. Mr. G triangulated himself in as Mrs. G's rescuer, usually hitting his daughter. Mrs. G snooped on her daughter to find out about marijuana use, thus stirring overt anxiety attacks in the daughter. Mrs. G and her daughter were willing to restore generational boundaries by refraining from snooping and from hitting. Both were asked to write out their feelings for discussion in the family session rather than hitting. Their problem were redefined as "fears of being overwhelmed." The youngest son was promoted to an unaccustomed position of family prominence, and Mr. and Mrs. G began to push him to study harder. As he began to argue and refute them several changes occurred. He allied himself more with his sister, and relieved her of the burden of being "the family problem." His grades improved as he became more verbal and less inhibited. His sister acknowledged she no longer wanted to destroy her family, and began helping him with homework. Mr. and Mrs. G became aware that they had abandoned their own friendship. They were, therefore, asked to spend two brief periods of time together each week in which they could talk about anything but their children.

As marital and sibling boundaries coalesced, the family, over about 10 sessions of 30 minutes each, talked about working too much (Mr. G), about adolescent freedom, and about Mrs. G's unhappiness over the illness of her parents. Nothing was solved in the sense that the individuals became "perfect," but they began to appreciate the positive ambitions of each. Subsequently, they continued with the "normal" problems and conflicts of a developing family.

The H family. Both the F and G families demonstrated *enmeshment*. They repeated the same conflicts with one another with great regularity and were developing faulty, fixed roles. The H family represents *disengagement*. Theirs was a multiproblem free-for-all with no consistent shape or structure. Instead, each member found his or her support outside the family.

Mr. and Mrs. H called about their 15-year-old son, who was involved in heavy drug use. An older son had run away and two younger children battled each other with great vigor, failed in school, and had "bad friends." Mrs. H had resisted many referrals to Alcoholics Anonymous and was actively alcoholic. Mr. H had recently started an affair and was thinking of leaving the family (this only became known a year later). Both Mr. and Mrs. H had been good medical patients on an individual basis, though they spent much time berating one another. Three attempts to bring Mr. and Mrs. H together with the three children failed for one reason or another. At this point the family practitioner decided, with supervision, that "discretion is the better part of valor." Recognizing the absence of stable family structures with which to work, he referred the 15-year-old son to an adolescent drug program, and the family was referred for more extensive counseling with an agency.

These clinical examples are necessarily brief, but they represent interventions well within the capacity of an active medical practice. In no case were ordinary office routines interrupted, and the family practitioners involved set reasonable limits on their time in advance. The couples and families paid an hourly, or half-hourly fee in each circumstance. Ultimately, all were appreciative of the interventions, though not all interventions were "successful."

GUIDELINES FOR FAMILY INTERVENTIONS

It is hoped that the family practitioner will be alert to the emotional well-being of the families he treats and will experiment with some of the techniques suggested. Merely to treat the emotional and physical symptoms of each individual overlooks the opportunities to help relationships within the families. The following checklist reviews a few principles important in guiding interventions.

- *Set limited goals.* Most of the examples discussed here involved interventions to solve a discrete problem. If normal development can be restored, or a single fixed pattern altered, later gains will come automatically.
- *Stick to the point.* Families always present a multitude of problems, and family members may shift the issue defensively to avoid trying something new. Restrictions of available time and clarity of purpose will lead the family practitioner to limit his or her intervention to a specific issue and this is good practice.
- *Be a good go-between; do not choose sides.* Where family members have sharply conflicting roles or divergent, complementary positions, usually one will appeal to the family practitioner more than the other. The goal of facilitating communication is met only when the family practitioner "understands" and separately supports the healthy aspects of all protagonists (not necessarily simultaneously). The physician can then back away and see if he or she has been successful in helping them to bridge the gap.
- *Always watch for triangles, especially when you are invited to be a member in one.* When Mrs. J describes her marital problems and states that Mr. J "doesn't believe in getting help," you are being invited into a triangle. Sympathize with Mrs. J's real dissatisfactions and, at the earliest opportunity, ask Mr. J to describe his marital dissatisfactions, thus "detriangulating" and forming an equal relationship with both partners. After two or three go-rounds, Mr. J will usually be happy to instigate marital therapy.
- *Look for structural situations; avoid fixing upon the specific complaint.* Families can present a bewildering prolixity of complaints, problems, and personalities. However, only a limited number of structural distortions can occur, and these appear regularly. Attention to triangles, boundaries, roles, and so on will simplify planning interventions.
- *Try to give individual family members tasks that challenge deeply entrenched family roles.* Have the ogre or the workaholic put the children to bed before talking with his wife. Have the mournful, critical wife of an alcoholic patient prepare a special "fun" meal before discussing the fact that she talked with you about his drinking. Along the way, try to be a model of clear, honest communication.
- *Do not get into deep discussions of a contested divorce, especially with one member absent.* Facilitate communication between the partners and be supportive if they both decide to separate or divorce. Do not take sides in an attempt to justify the divorce or in attempts to argue against it. This is the best way to make enemies.
- *Have good sources of referral at hand.* A few psychiatrists, some

clergy, and many family agencies are available to carry on family and marital work. Get to know people you can trust to do good work with your patients. After successful intervention with you, many patients will want to go further in therapy. From the start, some problems may be beyond the time and/or expertise you possess. If you have good referral sources to turn to, it will support your own attempts to make positive changes in the families you treat.

BIBLIOGRAPHY

Guerin P: Family Therapy; Theory and Practice: New York, Gardner Press, 1976, 553 pp.

This is a multiple-author book that includes and reviews Murray Bowen's contributions to family therapy and summarizes other theoretical positions and practical approaches.

Minuchin S: Families and Family Therapy. Cambridge, Mass, Harvard University Press, 1974, 268 pp.

This book is the "primer" for the structural approach to the family and is a most useful and readable introduction.

Minuchin S, Rosman B, Baker L: Psychosomatic Families: Anorexia Nervosa in Context. Cambridge, Mass, Harvard University Press, 1978, 350 pp.

The treatment of the family of anorexia nervosa patients is specialized beyond the training of most family practitioners. However, this book outlines an approach to the psychotherapy of children with somatic problems and is of general interest and importance for the family practitioner.

Alexander Levay, M.D.
Lawrence Sharpe, M.D.

9

The Management of Sexual Disorders

Patients expect their physicians to be knowledgeable about sexual functioning. This is consistent with their view of the physician as the only individual to whom they can entrust complete access to their bodies and their most intimate concerns, relying on the doctor–patient relationship as one of strict confidentiality.

Physicians, however, have always been aware of their limitations in this area. The individual physician has often been handicapped by a lack of teaching about sex in medical school, and by a prevalent professional attitude that our concern is with sex solely as a procreative act. Physicians, therefore, have readily assisted patients with fertility problems but have considered the pleasurable and interpersonal aspects of sexual activity at best, too private or recreational and, at worst, lewd or immoral, and thus outside the physician's domain. The importance of healthy sexual functioning to the total well-being of the individual and the emotional pain and suffering of patients with sexual problems have usually been ignored.

The past decade has brought revolutionary changes in attitudes, knowledge, and treatment approaches to sexual problems. Patients now have even greater expectations of their physicians' knowledgeability about human sexuality and competence to handle problems in all areas of sexual functioning. They also expect that their doctors will approach these problems with the same nonjudgmental, informed attitude they would display toward the psychological and physical aspects of any other medical condition. Studies of the effectiveness of postgraduate courses show that once inhibiting and conflictual attitudes are recognized and resolved, physicians are able to use their clinical skills to deal effectively with the sexual problems of the patients in their practice.

THE NATURE OF SEXUALITY

The vast majority of sexual problems seen by physicians can be viewed along six parameters, which are not mutually exclusive: physical, psychological, interpersonal, informational, circumstantial, and psychiatric. A degreee of overlap between these categories is almost always present, but it is helpful for the physician to elicit and organize the clinical data along these lines to facilitate the understanding of the problems and to organize a treatment plan.

The Physical Aspects of Sexuality

In the anatomically and physiologically intact, mature adult, the sexual response cycle consists of four sequential stages. Assuming a healthy sexual drive and the presence of sexual desire, adequate stimulation leads to an initial arousal stage involving penile engorgement and erection in the male, and genital engorgement and vaginal lubrication in the female. This continues into the plateau stage, in which high levels of sexual arousal and continued pleasurable tension are maintained and magnified, followed by the orgasmic phase, in which the high levels of tension are released by orgasm in the female and the orgasmic–ejaculatory response in the male. The final phase is one of resolution, in which the genitalia return to their previously nonstimulated state. During the arousal, plateau, and orgasmic stages, there are concomitant physiological changes in other parts of the body, producing muscular hypertonia, substantial rises in blood pressure and pulse rates, and an increase in respiratory rate.

Developmentally and functionally the male and female genitalia are strikingly similar, though their anatomical forms bear little similarity. The major areas of pleasurable stimulation are the glans and the frenulum of the penis in the male, and the clitoris, the periclitoral area, and the mons in the female. These are the areas of maximal nerve ending concentration. The vagina is supplied with a few nerve endings which transmit pain, temperature, and proprioception, but do not transmit pleasurable stimuli similar to those perceived by the clitoris. The pleasurable sensation of penile containment is probably mediated by proprioceptive receptors of the vaginal walls and in the surrounding musculature.

Thus, direct and/or indirect clitoral stimulation is essential for a woman, so that she may experience maximal pleasurable sensations and reach orgasm. However, the small size of the clitoris, the fact that it is largely covered by the clitoral hood, its anatomical position proximal to the vaginal introitus, and its disappearance behind the symphysis pubis at the height of arousal, means that it is not so readily stimulated and is not automatically stimulated during intercourse.

Such stimulation in intercourse can be obtained by mutual thrusting producing indirect stimulation of the area; by the female pressing and rubbing her pelvis against her partner's body, and by direct manual stimulation of the clitoris.

In both sexes, the arousal stage of the sexual response cycle is mediated by the parasympathetic nervous system and orgasm (and ejaculation) is mediated via the sympathetic system. The functional importance of this physiological fact is that the sexual response cycle is not subject to voluntary control. In addition, affects such as rage, fear, and anxiety are also mediated through the autonomic nervous system. Therefore, if these affects occur prior to or during the sexual response cycle, the naturally occuring sexual responses can be interfered with, blocked, or aborted.

External factors can similarly cause interference with the autonomic nervous system pathways, resulting in impaired sexual functioning. Direct injury during surgical procedure can occur in any operation involving the abdominal or perineal autonomic plexi. For example, radical prostatic surgery and abdomino-perineal resection invariably result in extensive autonomic plexus damage that is irreversible and invariably leads to impaired sexual functioning.

Ganglionic blocking agents and certain psychotropic medications that have a direct effect on the autonomic nervous system can produce impairment in sexual functioning (See Table 9-1). Certain metabolic and vascular diseases, such as diabetes mellitus, can also affect the autonomic nervous system directly, causing impairment in sexual functioning.

The role of hormones in sexual functioning is not yet fully known. However, an adequate level of testosterone secretion appears essential for adequate sexual desire to occur in both sexes. Testosterone is secreted by the adrenals in females. There is some evidence that the peaking of the estrogen level associated with ovulation has an effect on the initiation of sexual behavior by the female, but this interaction is still to be elucidated.

In the healthy male, testosterone has no pharmacological role in the treatment of functional sexual disorders. The amount of testosterone produced saturates all available central and peripheral receptor sites, and the introduction of further amounts of testosterone does not produce a therapeutic effect. In fact, exogenous testosterone leads, via a feedback mechanism, to a reduction in the naturally produced hormone. However,

Table 9–1
Drugs that May Affect Sexual Functioning

Drug	Effects on		
	Libido	Arousal	Orgasm
Antihypertensives			
Alpha-methyldopa	++	+++	+
Spironolactone (Aldactone)	+	+	0
Thiazides, alpha-blockers	0	+	0
Sympathoplegic drugs	0	+++	++
Beta-blockers	+	+	0
Quaternary NH_3 compounds	0	+++	+
Anticholinergics	0	+	0
Hormones			
Androgens, estrogens[a]			
Progesterone	0	0	0
Adrenal steroids	+	0	0
Psychotropics			
Sedative–hypnotics[b]	+	+	+
Antianxiety drugs	0	0	0
Narcotics[b]	+++	+++	+++
Phenothiazines[b]	+	+	+++[c]
Butyrophenones	+	+	0
Tricyclics	0	+	0
MAO inhibitors	0	+	++[d]
Lithium carbonate	+	+	0
Amphetamines[b]	+++	++	+++[e]
L-Dopa	Increased desire	0	0
Others			
Clofibrate (Atromid)	++	++	0
Disulfiram (Antabuse)	0	+	+
Tryptophane	++	++	0

Notes: 0 = absent, + = occasionally reported, ++ = occur with some frequency, +++ = frequent. These effects occur only in males except where effects on the female are explicitly stated. Orgasmic problems in the male invariably mean retarded ejaculation.

This list is not meant to be all inclusive. Physicians should always refer to reference books and should not hesitate to inquire directly of the drug company for supportive evidence that a medication may have otherwise unreported sideeffects on the sexual system.

[a] See text for detailed information.
[b] Affects functioning only when taken in high doses.
[c] See text for discussion of orgasmic difficulties reported with thioridazine (Mellaril).
[d] Affects both males and females.
[e] Has greater effect on females.

there is evidence to show that some male patients with complaints of erectile dysfunction have lowered blood testosterone levels due to abnormalities in the hypothalamic–pituitary–gonadal hormonal axis.[1] Consequently, it is essential that, as a part of a complete examination, blood testosterone levels be measured.

In the hypogonadal male, the introduction of exogenous testosterone leads to an increase in sexual drive and a restoration of sexual functioning. In females this occurs in both the healthy female and those suffering from disorders such as Addison's disease, in which there is a diminution of secreted testosterone. The use of testosterone as a therapeutic agent in the otherwise healthy female is contraindicated due to its rapid masculinizing effect.

In cases of occult hyperthyroidism with elevated serum testosterone, a high percentage of patients complain of loss of libido and a decrease in potency; these symptoms respond to appropriate treatment of the hyperthyroid condition.

Psychological Aspects of Sexuality

The greatest inhibitions on healthy sexual functioning are feelings of guilt and anxiety and a negative attitude toward sexuality. For example, females often fear that it is not proper for a woman to be sexual or to respond overtly to her partner's efforts to stimulate her.

> Mrs. T had been married for over two years. On a routine gynecological examination she revealed that she was concerned about her reactions when lovemaking. For the first 18 months of marriage, she occasionally had an orgasm, which she described as a "so-so experience." In the last six months, she had found that she became so excited that she lost all control of herself, screamed, moaned and shouted and was overwhelmed when she had her orgasm. Her husband encouraged her in this type of response, but she felt that her behavior was unfeminine and unlike herself and was concerned that her loss of control might indicate that she was a potential nymphomaniac. Mrs. T needed to know that her responses were not "unfeminine" but actually healthy expressions of female sexuality and that what she called "loss of control," was, in fact, full sexual responsiveness. When her behavior was thus relabeled and she was reassured of its normality, she was able to see herself as healthy.

The healthy and sexually comfortable woman is able to accept full responsibility for her own sexuality, is knowledgeable about sex and about her own body's responsiveness to sexual stimulation, and is able to satisfy her needs in a sexual relationship. Such a woman understands that her arousal and satisfaction will also be arousing and satisfying to her partner and will add to their joint sense of pleasure and closeness.

By necessity, both members of a couple have to focus on their own personal pleasure in the sexual experience, communicate this pleasure to the partner, and be cognizant of and responsive to the needs and pleasures of the chosen partner. The sexual experience is a moment-to-moment pleasure activity involving many forms of activity, including oral and other touching stimulation as well as intercourse. The pleasure of the experience is greatly enhanced if the couple are highly intimate and loving and thus are able to communicate freely to each other about their innermost sexual desires, fantasies, and preferences, and able to please each other without compromising their own pleasure.

If sexual activity is used to satisfy aims other than mutual support and pleasure, the sexual relationship is invariably placed at risk and negative feelings can be created in one or both partners. This occurs when, for example, the sexual act is undertaken to prove the individual's masculinity or dominance or to impose a degree of control over the partner for any one of a variety of reasons, or where the sexual act merly fulfills the sense of duty of one partner toward the other.

> Mr. and Mrs. S, who had been married for 18 months, presented themselves for a joint consultation. Throughout their marriage, sexual activity had been limited to once every 10 or more days. Mr. S always took two or three drinks beforehand, although he never drank otherwise. Mr. S's sexual activity was aggressive and domineering, and initially Mrs. S played into this scenario with mutual satisfaction. More recently, Mrs. S had been asking for more sensitive and romantic love-making, which did not occur, and she found that the aggressive type preferred by Mr. S was no longer satisfying. Both she and her husband were concerned that he can only be sexual when drinking, and wondered if this could mean that he is an alcoholic.
>
> When the physician pointed out to Mr. S that it would not take away from his masculinity to be less aggressive sexually and more tender and loving, he seemed to become less anxious. He and his wife then started a series of sexual exercises in which this role was relearned to their mutual satisfaction, with the concomitant diminution in his need for alcohol.

An unfortunate persistent negative attitude in our society is the prohibition against masturbation. Most men masturbate as a normal aspect of sexual maturation and a partnerless existence. Women do so less frequently, although this seems to be changing as acceptance of female sexuality has increased. The negative attitude in females is often associated with negative feelings about one's body image and sexuality. A woman may not only find it impossible to contemplate masturbation but find it difficult either to allow her partner to fondle her genitals manually or for her to handle his genitals.

Associated with these attitudes are others in which the woman perceives the penis as a threatening or disgusting object and her own vagina as "nonexistent" or revolting. Men frequently believe that their penises are inadequate in size and perceive the vulva and vagina as a threatening "terra incognita." Similar misconceptions are often held about other aspects of one's body, such as breasts and facial appearance, which can interfere with one's understanding of one's own desirability.

Once anxiety, guilt, or other affects interfere with sexual functioning, both partners begin to think of sex in terms of performance. Three phenomena become apparent at this stage in the development of dysfunction: (1) *performance anxiety,* in which the individual is highly anxious about moment-to-moment performance and activity; (2) *goal orientation,* in which the individual or both members of the partnership direct their concerns to the achievement of a specific goal, usually that of orgasm; and (3) *spectatoring,* in which either or both partners of the couple start checking their own and their partner's current state of excitement and response. The treatment of these problems is discussed later.

Interpersonal Relationships and Sexuality

Free communication without anxiety is the basis of the best interpersonal relationships, yet it is often particularly difficult for a couple to communicate about sexual matters. Frequently, partners know little about one another's sexual fantasies, preferences, dislikes, fears, and vulnerabilities. In many relationships, certain aspects of an individual's preferences are never revealed to the spouse and are either totally repressed or allowed expression only outside the relationship. Obviously, the presence of such surreptitious behavior is potentially damaging to the relationship. The difficulties that may be present vary. A common factor to all however, is that a particular behavior or behavioral mode is desirable to one member of the couple but considered either unacceptable or "perverted" by the other and/or is perceived by one as desirable but as likely to produce negative reactions on the part of the partner; examples include different frequencies of sexual activity, sexual contact in positions other than the male-superior one, oral–genital contact, mutual masturbatory activity, or the use of sexual fantasies or pornographic material to enhance sexual activity.

On the other hand, sexual dysfunction may be the presenting symptom of an interpersonal problem that has yet to be identified in the marriage. The presence of a serious characterological difficulty may appear first in the sexual area; for example, the need of one partner to totally dominate the other in a situation in which the partner refuses to accede.

Mr. U kept an appointment made for him by his wife, who complained that he had become "impotent" in the last year. They had been married for ten years, without problems in the sexual area. A complete physical examination did not reveal any disorder to account for the erectile difficulties. Mr. U described his wife as a most attractive woman, who was very desirable to most men. She was from a prominent political family with wealth and social position, and he felt fortunate to have married her. With her family's help, he became a successful minor politician, but was not reelected and recently had lost two elections to less prominent positions. He had exhausted their funds, and his wife's family was pressuring him to abandon his political career and take a minor position in the family law firm. He saw this as a loss of independence.

His wife was always sexually assertive, which he appreciated, but now he perceived her continuing insistence on daily sexual activity and being brought to orgasm as a chore. He recalled that the first incident of loss of erection occurred when his wife remarked during lovemaking that in spite of everything else in his life, he was still a good lover. More recently, with repetitive loss of erection, sexual intercourse had become less frequent and she had tended to make such remarks as "if you can't be a proper man, you had better see a doctor."

Mr and Mrs. U both needed help in separating his career problems from his sexual problems. With counseling, Mr. U was able to shift his energies into a more fruitful business enterprise of *his* own choosing, which restored his wife's respect. This so improved their situation that, with only minimal specific sex therapy, their sexual and marital problems were successfully resolved.

Sexual dysfunction almost invariably leads to interpersonal problems, which then further aggravate the sexual difficulties. This can create uncertainty as to whether the sexual difficulties are primary or secondary to the marital distress. When the sexual problems are primary, resolution of the problems rapidly brings the couple into harmony. However, when the sexual problems are secondary to an underlying interpersonal disharmony, signs of a successful and incipient resolution of the sexual problem often, ironically, aggravate the interpersonal problem. Because the sexual dysfunction has served as an unconsciously determined symptom that stabilized a dysfunctional relationship, the sexual aspect is difficult or impossible to treat by itself. Referral of these patients for marital therapy is indicated.

Effects of Information on Sexuality

People still do not know much about sex. They still maintain myths and negative attitudes as well as major misconceptions that often lead to constricted, if not dysfunctional, sexual lives. Even when accurate information is available, many people will not and cannot put the information to use in their own personal sex lives, possibly because of uncertainty or outright guilt. The physician can handle many of these problems. He acts not only as an educator but as an authoritative permission-giver and supporter of these patients. In many cases, reversal of the sexual problem can be accomplished by this type of encouragement, with specific correction of false information and the provision of knowledge.

The dissemination of information regarding contraception is an example of how knowledge can enhance sexual satisfaction. Contraception is a shared responsibility in a sexual relationship, but all too often it has been viewed as the sole responsibility of the male or, currently, of the female. Although the individual's responsibility cannot be minimized, the assumption of responsibility by both members of a couple enhances their total relationship.

The physician is in an excellent position to see both members of the couple and to explore their attitudes about birth control. Both members should be given factual information about each method, its efficiency and its potential side effects and dangers. Although in the young female (under 30), the "pill" is less dangerous than pregnancy, the couple should be told of the potential dangers for the female above the age of 30. The unpleasant side effects of menorrhagia with the use of an intrauterine device (such as the "coil"); the diminished penile sensation that results from the use of a condom by a male; and the lesser degree of reliability with the use of foam should all be noted and discussed.

The high level of reliability of the diaphragm, combined with the use of a spermicidal gel, should be explained to the couple. It should be pointed out to those who choose the diaphragm as the method of contraception that in some situations, both members of the couple can participate in the use of the diaphragm as a regular part of their lovemaking. If the couple are interested, the male partner can be instructed on the use of the diaphragm and encouraged to be both an active participant as well as an observer in its insertion. This allows him to share the responsibility in the prevention of pregnancy, and it avoids the resentment the woman might otherwise feel if she were to insert the diaphragm on her own initiative and then no sexual activity or penetration were to take place.

For those individuals requesting a more permanent type of contraception, such as tubal ligation or vasectomy, the physician should be able to discuss with both partners the physical and possible psychological consequences of the procedures and to explore the potential negative and positive effects of such a procedure on the interpersonal relationship. Although evidence of blood clotting problems as a side effect of hormonal adjustment therapy in the female has been widely reported, less well-known and less well-documented evidence is accumulating that vasectomy may lead to an autoimmune reaction involving the sperm and its breakdown products. The combination of antibody plus sperm fragments appears to attach to the walls of the major arteries, leading to an acceleration of atherosclerotic processes. Although these effects have only been documented in rhesus monkeys, this evidence must be considered significant enough to suggest that vasectomy is not the simple, and totally safe procedure that it has been considered.[2]

The Circumstantial Aspects of Sexuality

Many sexual problems seem to be associated with extraneous and circumstantial problems of daily living; other aspects of daily life—for example, work, children, hobbies, and sleep patterns—intrude into the time available for sexual activity. In some cases, when such conflicts exist they may be symptomatic of severe interpersonal relationship problems, but where the problems are truly circumstantial, simple advice is eagerly accepted and adopted by the couple. A most common phenomenon is the inability of couples to schedule their time together so that sexual activity may occur. The pressure of work and work-related activities often takes priority over interpersonal activities. The physician is in an excellent position to aid the couple in getting their priorities in order so that work pressures do not interfere with their interpersonal lives.

Many couples fall into the habit of having sex at night, before they fall asleep, which is the time when they are most tired and least open to lovemaking. It is a time when there is a potential for making sex a duty instead of a pleasure. Another area of potential conflict occurs when one member of a couple is an early-to-bed, early-to-rise individual and the other a late-to-bed, late-to-rise person. Methods of dealing with these problems will be presented in the section on "Management".

Variations in sexual activity during the life cycle clearly occur in both sexes. The sudden explosion of sexual awareness in adolescence is severely modified by societal factors, availability of partners, and attitudes toward sexuality. Changes in sexual responsiveness during the menstrual cycle and at the menopause are thought to occur but are still open to investigation. The idea that sexual ability and activity must necessarily disappear after middle age has proven to be a myth, and although sexual activity alters with advanced age, there seems to be no reason why it should not continue throughout one's life. The female does tend to lubricate less after menopause and with aging; the male tends to take longer to achieve an erection. In those couples who are able to adapt to these phenomena and make use of ancillary methods, such as oils and lubricants, sexual functioning continues to be enjoyable and satisfying.

At times of severe emotional stress, such as following the loss of parents, children, or spouse by death or the breaking up of a relationship and divorce, alterations in one's sexual desires and abilities are likely to occur. In one group of individuals such circumstances lead to an increase in their need for sexual expression; some apparently need the warmth, reassurance, and emotional feeling that comes with close contact. Others need to reaffirm the continuity of life by symbolically and nonemotionally performing the sexual act. In other groups, the loss of libido is a common part of the bereavement process. The physician who is aware of these possibilities is able to reassure these patients that their behavior is not uncommon and is part of the process of mourning.

The Psychiatric Aspects of Sexuality

Changes in sexual desire, functioning, and activity are often indicative of a more serious psychiatric disorder. Patients with a depressive disorder often present with decreased libido or erectile difficulties as a principal symptom. This phenomenon can be misdiagnosed, by patients and doctors alike, as exclusively a sexual problem. The sudden appearance of excessive sexual desire, increased sexual activity, and promiscuity may be indicative of a manic disorder. Bizarrely diverse sexual behavior may be part of a schizophrenic disorder. Exhibitionistic sexual behavior in the elderly may indicate the presence of a dementia. Other inappropriate sexual behaviors, such as the compulsive seeking of new sexual partners, may be precipitated by a variety of severe life stress stituations.

Homosexual behavior is a complex phenomenon. In some patients it may be related to as yet undefined intrauterine hormonal influences. In these individuals there appears to be a lifelong pattern of homosexual interests. For others, homosexual behavior appears to be related to psychological influences in the patient's early development. Here the patient's problem appears to be based on a fear of heterosexual relationships which then produces a secondary homosexual orientation. When the homosexual relationship is an expression of a nonsexual conflict it is called *pseudohomosexuality*.[3]

The physician must realize that homosexuality is not necessarily associated with "femininity" in the male or "masculinity" in the female. A sexual history is the only way to obtain reliable data as to homosexual behavior. Homosexual relationship patterns can also vary from extreme promiscuity to stable, long-term marriage-like relationships. Homosexuals of both sexes may thus present with all the sexual concerns and problems in interpersonal relationships presented by people who engage in heterosexual activity, and they should be treated accordingly.

There are also patients who seek help for the distress they experience specifically from their homosexual concerns. These include adolescents who have not acted on these homosexual impulses; adolescents and adults who have been functioning homosexually but wish to function heterosexually; patients functioning heterosexually who are disturbed by homosexual impulses; and heterosexually functioning adults who mistakenly develop fears of homosexuality because of the presence of problems in their sexual functioning such as loss of sexual desire and the inability to become aroused in a heterosexual setting.

Many of these patients can be treated with simple reassurance. Others, however, should be referred for treatment. It is important that the referring physician understand that some well-motivated patients may be helped to shift to a heterosexual orientation but that psychotherapy for others, who are fixed in their homosexual pattern, may mean helping them deal with the problems their homosexuality entails. The prognosis for a shift in orientation is good for a male homosexual if the patient is well motivated, still has heterosexual dreams or fantasies, has had one or more successful heterosexual encounters, and had his first homosexual experience after age 16. About one in three patients with these good prognostic indicators can be helped to become heterosexual.[4]

While manual and/or oral sexual behavior appears to be the preferred mode of homosexual expression, anal intercourse is practiced and can produce a variety of related medical problems, which makes it essential that the physician be comfortable in exploring his or her patient's sexual history.

Many physicians still maintain a negative attitude toward homosexual patients. Such negative attitudes may interfere with their ability to maintain their usual objectivity, take an adequate history, or provide the usual concern and support given their other patients. This can lead to misdiagnoses and other medical errors. A physician who is unable to approach such patients with a nonjudgmental, therapeutic attitude is best advised to refer these patients to a physician whose behavior is not so encumbered.[5]

Paraphiliac sexual behavior includes activity involving nonconsenting partners, for example, children or animals; the use of pain or severe humiliation in the sexual relationship; exhibitionism; or the use of fetish objects to achieve sexual satisfaction. When either partner reports these sexual activities, the physician should attempt to determine whether sexual dysfunction would occur in the absence of the paraphiliac behavior. In the milder form, these conditions can often coexist with healthy sexual functioning. In these instances, the paraphilia seems to serve the dual function of reducing anxiety associated with the sexual act, as well as enhancing sexual arousal. Patients and their partners often attach shame and humiliation to this aspect of sexual behavior, and therefore, usually do not voluntarily report their behavior to the doctor.

In the mildest forms of fetishism—for example, a husbands' need for his wife to wear a garter belt—where the fetish object is integrated into the sexual and love play of the couple, it is often the partner's anxiety about the meaning and consequences of this fetishistic behavior that requires reassurance. Minimal couple therapy is often quite successful in these cases. If the physician assesses that such paraphiliac behavior is seriously interfering with healthy sexual functioning or with other aspects of daily life for either partner, referral for more specialized care is recommended.

THE SEXUAL DYSFUNCTIONS

Male Sexual Dysfunctions

Male sexual dysfunction is often associated with anxiety derived from the misconception and expectation that all sexual activity must lead to vaginal penetration by the penis, ejaculation, and the achievement of an orgasm by the partner. If this expectation is not met, the sexual act is considered a failure. Since the sexual response cycle is not under voluntary control, people with this self-imposed expectation are particularly vulnerable to anxieties, which can preclude full male arousal and thus set up a self-fulfilling prophecy of failure.

Premature ejaculation is probably the most common sexual dysfunction and the most easily treated. It occurs in men who, once aroused, cannot regulate their level of sexual stimulation or time their ejacualtion.

> Mr. V was 39 and had been married for 15 years. Although he thought he had a happy and successful sexual life, he had been recently told by his wife that he had never aroused her enough in his lovemaking and that her orgasms were "faked." Since then he had tried to prevent himself from ejaculating soon after penetration, which was his habit, and to monitor his level of arousal and his wife's responses. However, he found that he was unable to control the ejaculation and that on some occasions he ejaculated before entry. Recently, he had found that he did not desire sex as often as he used to.
>
> Mrs. V's "revelation" had brought on what is called "performance anxiety" and "spectatoring" in Mr. V. When patients are not able to cope with these manifestations of their anxiety, sexual functioning deteriorates further and their anxiety can even lead to cessation of desire.

Performance anxiety arises as a result of the inability to control the length of time spent in the arousal and plateau stages and an inability to choose the point of ejaculation. Characteristically, men who experience this type of anxiety ejaculate immediately prior to or immediately after penetration. This is often associated with frustration on the part of the partner, who is denied sufficent arousal time, especially if all sexual activity terminates with the male's ejaculation. This situation escalates and creates secondary problems centered around the maladaptive attempts to control the ejaculation and the partner's lack of satisfaction in intercourse. The persistence of the premature ejaculation frequently leads to sexual interaction becoming a dreaded and frustrating experience, to be avoided by both members. Erectile difficulties start to occur, and either or both members experience a lack of sexual desire. Either partner's frustrations and dissatisfactions may lead to seeking help as an individual or as a couple. Frequently, the female is presented by the male as being unresponsive, or the female may present herself as being frustrated and/or unable to experience sexual desire. The couple may present for marital counseling for nonsexual problems even though the major need is a therapeutic approach to the premature ejaculation.

Retarded ejaculation is also an inability to time the ejaculation. Here the erection is maintained for an excessive length of time. When ejaculation occurs, although satisfaction is experienced, the timing of the orgasm is experienced as unsatisfactory for the male, and occurs at a point when the female is often exhausted and no longer in an aroused condition. In some cases, in spite of continued erectile ability, ejaculation does not occur at all. The maintenance of an erection for too long a period of time is mythologically desirable but clinically disturbing. In actual experience, this condition can be distressful to the individual and to the partner. The inability to time the point of ejaculation, the striving for the ejaculation, and the female's perception that she is inadequate to help the spouse, can lead to distress not only in the sexual act, but also in the relationship. Such individuals may present with the problem of being unable to ejaculate intravaginally, but also may present with the complaint that the female is unable to conceive.

At a deeper psychological level, these individuals often have problems about committing themselves to the relationship and about sharing and intimate involvement with their partners. Fears of impregnation or dominance of the partner may also play a part, as well as the fear that the final orgasmic–ejaculatory response is a form of aggression, over which the individual must maintain control.

Retarded ejaculation is not as significant for the individual when it occurs during solitary masturbation; however, in rare cases, total inability to ejaculate occurs under all circumstances. These primary and totally inhibited nonejaculators are a separate pathological entity with more serious interpersonal psychopathology.

Erectile dysfunction refers to the inability to achieve and maintain penile erection. Anxiety interferes with the arousal process and can be encountered at any time during the arousal and plateau stages of lovemaking. Some individuals are unable to respond in a normally sexually stimulating environment; other individuals experience anxiety later on in the arousal stage. The inability to maintain the erection may become apparent at any stage: at the point of disrobing, of touching the partner, or of expected penetration, or, after penetration, of approaching ejaculation. In some individuals these symptoms occur in all situations with any partner, but in others they occur only in more specific situations, for example, on attempting an extramarital affair. In some cases, the condition is primary, and the individual has never had an erection in an interpersonal relationship but is able to have one in masturbation.

Men with erectile problems usually display spectatoring and are constantly monitoring the size of their erection. They are particularly sensitive to their partner's comments and their partner's activity and attitude toward the penis. This symptom may lead them to avoid sexual encounters and they can develop a loss of sexual desire. The reluctance to admit to this problem may lead a man to present to his physician with vague somatic complaints or seek the help of a physician who does not know him. In other instances, the spouse may present with complaints about her own lack of sexual attractiveness, her inadequacy as a sexual partner, her concern over her husbands's lack of sexual interest, or her inability to conceive.

Female Sexual Dysfunction

The most significant difference between male and female sexual dysfunction is that women can perform sexually and simulate the overt phenomena of orgasm, whereas the male finds it impossible to simulate erection. However, with increased awareness in women of their "sexual rights," the level of performance anxiety is now raised in both sexes. The female has a greater capacity for physiological responsiveness in sexual activity than the male, enabling her to become orgasmic early in the arousal stage and, due to the absence of the male postorgasmic refractory period, to have more than one orgasm during the same sexual activity. This natural physiological response combined with the female's anatomy should give the healthy female greater protection against developing sexual dysfunction than the male. However, certain societal attitudes regarding sexual activity in the female have contributed to a variety of sexual dysfunctions.

Anorgasmia is the most common female sexual dysfunction. Anorgasmic females are unable to experience the orgasm phase of the sexual response cycle physiologically or psychologically. This problem is analogous to the male ejacualtory disorders in that it is the inability of the female to time the point of the orgasm. With the changes in cultural attitudes toward female sexuality and the dissemination of corrective information regarding sex, most women now expect to be fully responsive and orgasmic. They are therefore concerned if they are not, and are likely to seek professional help.

Mrs. W was a 24-year-old woman, married for three years, who claimed never to have experienced orgasm. She was a mild, soft spoken woman, whose only knowledge about sex came from her husband and her mother. Recently she had read in some women's magazines about female orgasm and felt she had missed something important. She could not discuss this with her friends or her mother and did not want to burden her husband with what she saw as her own problem. The physician encouraged her to confide in her husband, who the doctor knew to be a very helpful and sensitive man. This was indeed the case and, with appropriate couple-oriented sexual therapy, Mrs. W rapidly became orgasmic.

There are three different types of anorgasmia. In the *primary* type, the woman has never been orgasmic in any sexual situation, including masturbation; paradoxically, this type is the most responsive to treatment. In the *secondary* type, a woman who has been orgasmic in the past becomes anorgasmic. This is more difficult to treat with sexual therapy alone since intrapsychic and interpersonal factors not directly connected to the sexual experience usually play a role. In the third type, actually a subtype of the secondary condition, the anorgasmia is situational and occurs only under specific conditions (e.g., when the children are still awake) or with specific individuals. Frequently, these anxiety-provoking concomitants are easily identified and are subject to therapeutic approaches.

In some instances, the male partner develops a high level of anxiety because he perceives his partner's inability to climax as a sign of his own sexual inadequacy. The striving, anxious female and the striving, anxious male can create a stituation in which a specific goal orientation becomes the principle reason for sexual activity. This invariably leads to frustration in achieving the desired result.

Arousal stage problems are reflected in the degreee of lubrication experienced. Physiological changes in the degree of lubrication can occur with physical illness, medication, aging, and the like, and can be treated successfully by the use of creams, oils, and artificial lubricants. However, complaints about inadequate lubrication in the healthy, premenopausal woman reflect either psychological problems associated with sexual response or the use by the partner of inadequate arousal techniques. Such individuals can also present with complaints of pain on intercourse (dyspareunia) and a lessening of sexual desire.

Dyspareunia is the presence of persistent and/or recurrent pain in the genital region during intercourse. It is a rare condition in the male, when it is usually associated with penile pathology. When it occurs in the female, an organic basis for the symptom must be fully investigated. Among the more common organic causes of this condition are recurrent vaginitis, recurrent urethrocystitis, localized vaginal scarring (as occurs after episiotomy), broad ligament injuries, prolapse of the uterus, endometriosis, and ovarian tumors. Functional dyspareunia is usually associated with other forms of sexual dysfunction, especially vaginismus (see next paragraph) or inadequate lubrication. Often there is a generalized aversion toward all sexual activity but particularly sexual intercourse.

Vaginismus is the sudden contraction of the musculature of the outer third of the vagina, which can occur at any point in the sexual response cycle. In some females it can occur prior to the sexual response cycle and is precipitated by the knowledge that her partner is about to begin sexual activity. Usually vaginal penetration cannot occur. Dyspareunia becomes a frequently associated sympton when penetration is forced, and further contraction occurs.

Mr. and Mrs. X were a recently married couple in their 20s who were in good physical health. Mrs. X stated that prior to marriage she was interested in sex and had masturbated to orgasm but had never allowed penetration by her fiance to occur. Since the marriage she had been avoiding any type of sexual activity. Although her husband was initially sympathetic, he had now reached the point at threatening divorce unless medical advice was sought.

History revealed that intercourse was not achieved on the honeymoon because of pain on attempted penetration. Penetration occurred with much pain about three weeks after the wedding. Since that time, Mrs. X had submitted to her husband's sexual advances out of a sense of duty but with no desire on her part and no pleasure. Penetration had rarely occurred as she became tense and was certain that she would again experience severe pain. In the last four months of the marriage no sexual activity had occurred and she had even rebuffed his attempts to touch her in an affectionate, nonsexual manner. Mrs. X had tried to masturbate but found that when she approached her introitus she became too tense and fearful.

Mr. X was initially concerned that it was his fault that his wife was responding negatively to his lovemaking, and he acted in a gentle, nondemanding manner. Recently he had become less tolerant of her behavior. Experiences prior to marriage and several extramarital encounters had convinced him that he was not at fault.

When physical examination determined the absence of pelvic pathology and confirmed the presence of vaginismus, the physician was able to reassure the couple that the problems stemmed from the initial painful intercourse experience. With the introduction of a series of graduated dilators and the concomitant use of graded sex therapy exercises, there was a rapid establishment of pleasurable intercourse and the disappearance of the marital strife.

The underlying mechanism of vaginismus, as in the other dysfunctions, is anxiety, though this may be present at an unconscious level. The causes of the anxiety are varied and include fears associated with previously experienced pain caused by localized conditions; painful intercourse in rape or rape-like situations; and fears of penetration associated with injury, violation, or impregnation. In spite of the difficulty in elucidating the psychological causes, the condition of vaginismus responds very well to treatment.

MANAGEMENT

Diagnosis

In some cases, patients may present with overt complaints of sexual problems. However, many patients with sexual dysfunction present with vague, somatic complaints, that may become the focus of unsuccessful treatment unless the underlying sexual dysfunction is identified and given correct prominence. Most of these patients are willing and even relieved to answer questions about their sexual lives if the physician is professional in his concern and sensitive regarding the patient's feelings.

One must realize that in the presentation of a sexual problem, lack of knowledge, guilt, or anxiety may cause the patient to misplace the responsibility for the problem. For example, the female patient complaining of anorgasmia may have a male partner with premature ejaculation; the male patient complaining of premature ejaculation may have a partner with anorgasmia. Thus a detailed history will be essential to an accurate diagnosis.

In those patients in whom the physician suspects sexual dysfunction as a symptom of a medical disorder, direct questioning about the sexual problem should be part of the investigation of the presenting illness. The introduction could be: "Some patients with your symptoms also have symptoms affecting their sexual functioning; do you have any problems in that area?" In other patients, where the physician feels the response would be negative and that the questions may elicit an iatrogenic development of sexual dysfunction, the connection between the presenting complaint and the inquiry about sexual symptoms should be postponed to the routine review of systems.

In the absence of special concern regarding potential sexual dysfunction, questions relating to sexuality should be part of the general systems review. All the information need not be gathered at one interview, though eventually the physician should know the patient's sexuality in the same detail as the other areas of the patient's life.

With male patients, questions about sex follow naturally after the review of the urinary system. The concluding questions in that area usually deal with such things as the presence of pain or burning sensations on micturition. The next question should be, "Do you have any problems with your sexual life?" The patient is then given the opportunity he may have been hoping for to discuss his problem.

With female patients, questions about sexuality should follow the review of the female reproductive system and questions about menstruation. The first question can be, "Do you have any problems in your sexual life?" A positive response then leads to a detailed sexual history.

The physician should not assume that the single, partnerless patient is celibate and should phrase the questions in such a manner as to obtain the necessary information without causing embarrassment to the patient. For example, "Are you sexually active?" is open enough to require a response without being unduly threatening. Additional questions regarding birth control methods can be asked where indicated. By this time the patient should realize that when sexual problems do arise he or she can consult you without embarrassment.

Physicians should always be aware that patients may not understand the precise meaning of technical terms used for sexual activities and the sexual parts of the body, and should know what terms may be more appropriate for any individual patient. It is not recommended that these terms be used routinely, as that tends to alter the professional relationship in a negative fashion. However, the physician should be able to use these terms if the patient does not comprehend the use of the more professional ones.

In those cases where the physician is aware that sexual functioning is likely to become problematic for the patient and the partner in the near or distant future, routine questioning in this area requires amplification, so that a detailed baseline of current healthy activity and preferred sexuality is obtained. In such instances, the sexual advice that the physician will be able to give the patient with a progressively debilitating disease or after an acute condition, will be based on an accurate perception of the previous level of healthy functioning. In these instances, information should be obtained regarding the current and preferred frequency of sexual activity; preferred positions used in intercourse; preference in sexual interplay; attitudes concerning self-pleasuring; the degree of satisfaction in both partners; and sexual experience prior to and outside the partnership. Attention should also be paid to prior instances of sexual dysfunction and the circumstances in which it may have occurred, and any early sexual experiences involving physical, sexual, or emotional trauma, as the anxieties associated with such occurrences may reemerge.

The information gathered from the patient and the partner should be organized according to the categories mentioned at the beginning of this chapter: To what extent do these symptoms represent physical disorder? a psychological condition? problems in the interpersonal functioning of the patient and the partner? false information or belief in sexual myths on the part of the patient or the partner? problems in the current circumstances of the patient? or an underlying psychiatric disorder? Obviously, the symptoms may be organized to fit more than one category and frequent overlap is the rule, requiring treatment and management to be directed in more than one direction.

In many cases, information from a patient should be corroborated by the partner. This is particularly important in the differential diagnosis of erectile dysfunction, where the presence on any occasion of an erection adequate for penetration usually rules out an organic basis for the problem. To confirm this, the patient must be asked about erectile dysfunction on masturbation; the partner must be asked to confirm the absence of erectile function during lovemaking, and the partner should also be asked to monitor whether the patient has penile tumescence during REM sleep. If the patient sleeps without night attire, REM sleep penile tumescence should be observable during the first two hours of sleep or just prior to waking. In the absence of this confirmation, the use of a portable penile tumescence apparatus is indicated or the use of a sleep laboratory setting. In a sleep laboratory, penile tumescence and REM sleep can be easily monitored. Because the anxieties associated with the unusual setting and the knowledge that erectile functioning is to be measured, it is recommended that three nights of testing occur, and that psychogenic erectile dysfunction be diagnosed only when one or more full erections are directly observed, each one of which would be adequate for vaginal penetration, and maintained with this degree of rigidity for five or more consecutive minutes.[6,7]

In the absence of any recording of adequate penile tumescence, the probability of an associated organic condition should be fully investigated, including endocrine evaluation and glucose tolerance tests. The diagnosis of an organic basis for the symptom does not mean that the condition is irreversible.

General Principles of Treatment

Where sexual dysfunction is based on a general physical disorder or psychiatric condition, or reflects side effects of some medication, treatment should obviously be directed toward the precipitating cause. Where the condition is considered to be mainly psychological, and in those patients with a psychological element superimposed on an underlying organic physical disorder, treatment should be considered along the lines of the PLISSIT model, introduced by Annon.[8] This model, which outlines a progression of interventions that are to be followed according to the patient's needs, is briefly summarized in Table 9–2.

The preferred mode of treatment for all sexual problems utilizes a couple situation, in which both members take a degree of responsibility for the sexual activity. After the problem has been delineated by the patient, it is helpful to see the partner, in order to evaluate his or her

Table 9–2
The PLISSIT Model of Treatment for Sexual Problems

Intervention	Procedures
Permission	The physician assures the patient that it is medically safe and psychologically sound to engage in a particular sexual activity.
Limited information	The physician expands the patient's information by giving him or her all the necessary facts of basic sexual functioning, dispels false beliefs and myths, puts the patient's sexual difficulties and concerns into language the patient can understand, and lays the groundwork for psychotherapeutic intervention should it become necessary.
Specific suggestions	The physician recommends specific sexual exercises to aid the patient in achieving a resumption of normal sexual functioning.
Intensive therapy	If the first three steps—which can be taken by any physician, whether the problem is organic or functional—are insufficient, the physician refers the patient for expert psychotherapeutic and sexual counseling.

Adapted from Annon J: The Behavioral Treatment of Sexual Problems, Vol. 1, Brief Therapy. Honolulu, Enabling Systems, Inc., 1974.

contribution to the problem and bring the partner into the treatment process. Both members of the couple should then be seen together, and the physician's summary of the problem should be shared with them. Some of the more obvious myths can be dispelled at this stage. The role of anxiety in sexual problems can be explained in the context of performance anxiety and goal orientation.

Permission

In an atmosphere of interest and acceptance, the physician is in a unique position to reassure patients about their sexual concerns. As an authority and permission giver, he can promote a patient's right to express his or her sexuality in a way that is pleasurable, mutually agreeable, and not harmful to either patient or partner. Specifically, this includes reassuring the patient that sexual activity such as masturbation and/or oral–genital contact is not harmful. Other kinds of permission are suggested in Table 9–3.

The physician's own value system and moral standards, whether more liberal or conservative than a patient's, should not interfere with these permission giving reassurances. In fact, an understanding respect and acceptance of the patient's value systems will allow the physician to

Table 9–3
Common Forms of Permission

- Assuring parents of young children that exploration of the genital area and playing with their genitals is normal and healthy for children.
- Assuring adolescents that interest in sex is natural and occurs in all adolescents; and that using self-pleasuring (masturbation) to relieve sexual desire is common and not unhealthy.
- Informing the adolescent that close friendships and loving feelings towards members of the same sex are common and do not indicate homosexual inclinations.
- Supporting an individual's right to sexual experience and activity in a relationship before marriage or a commitment as well as their right to avoid sexual activity, despite peer pressure.
- Assuring both members of a couple that experimentation with various modes of sexual stimulation and behavior is healthy and beneficial to the couple's sexuality, as long as neither member experiences pain or distress.
- Encouraging each member of the couple to satisfy the other, if and when the other member requests it, without feeling obliged to have a personal arousal or engage in coitus.
- Encouraging each member of a couple that if the partner is incapacitated, unavailable, or unprepared to join in sexual activity, self-pleasuring (masturbation) is not unhealthy and may be used without disrupting the relationship.
- Reassuring elderly individuals and couples that continuing interest in sexual activity is not unhealthy, occurs frequently and with pleasure, and that there is every reason to continue sexual activity with increasing age.
- Reassuring both members of a couple that the use of fantasy during lovemaking is not unhealthy, can be an added pleasurable stimulus for either partner, and does not necessarily mean that the other partner is less than adequate.

support one patient's regular premarital sexual activity and another patient's unwillingness to contemplate such actions.

When both members of a couple are seen together, the physician can reassure the more conservative member that the partner's sexual interests or variations are commonly accepted, as well as help the more experimental member to be respectful of the partner's anxiety that usually underlies his or her reluctance. In this way, permission is given to move slowly and gently into new sexual activities if they so choose. Both members of the couple can also be reassured that their sexual fantasies can be shared and used to enhance their relationship either by including the fantasized activities in the couple's sexual repertoire or by simply discussing them. When these special desires are listened to with acceptance, there is usually a reduction in anxiety that promotes an increase in warmth, closeness, and love in the relationship.

Limited Information

The physician must also assume the role of the giver of accurate and pertinent information, limited to the needs of each patient. In fact, this aspect of the physician's role may become the most important part of his or her relationship with some patients. Some information, such as the universality and safety of masturbation in men and its growing universality in women, is given as part of the permission to masturbate. Similar information, relevant to each partner's specific symptoms and concerns, is given as part of the specific suggestions in treatment. The role of anxiety or other disruptive affects in the generation and maintenance of sexual problems is information that should be given to most patients. Imparting any information that a specific physical disorder is *not* associated with sexual dysfunction (e.g., a benign prostatic nodule or prostatic hypertrophy) is essential and in many instances may remove the symptom. Similarly, in the physically disabled, the information that positions other than the traditional male-superior one are indicated may allow sexual intercourse to occur in a stress free situation. Types of information commonly needed by patients are described in Table 9–4.

Table 9–4
Common Areas of Information-Giving

- Explaining to cardiovascular patients the concept of workload and how this applies to sexual activity.
- Explaining to adolescents and other patients who may have regular sexual activity with different partners, the common signs and symptoms of sexually transmitted diseases, and the prevention and treatment of such diseases.
- Explaining to couples in which one member has a genital infection the possibility of repeated passage of the disorder between each member, the chances of reinfection, and how to minimize these chances.
- Explaining the relationship between the use of drugs and alcohol and erectile failure and dissatisfaction with the sexual experience.
- Clarifying for patients undergoing pelvic surgery the changes that the surgery will interfere with postoperative sexual activity.
- Detailing for older patients the natural physiological changes that occur with aging and their effects on sexuality.
- Emphasizing the absence of sexual dysfunction after those surgical procedures in which the patient may imagine sexual sequelae, such as simple hysterectomy and prostatectomy for benign hypertrophy.
- Indicating the occurrence of side effects of medications that might affect sexual functioning before a dysfunction appears.
- Informing the patient who has had a major surgical procedure, a serious medical disorder, trauma, or is experiencing a chronic debilitating disease about effects the disease or trauma may have on future sexual functioning and about the help available to minimize the effects when they occur.

Many couples may not have a sexual dysfunction per se. Their symptoms may reflect a lack of knowledge about anatomical details and the physiology of the sexual act. In this case, the doctor's role is to inform them as to such matters as the anatomical position of the clitoris, the types of clitoral and penile stimulation required, and the various stages of the sexual response cycle for each partner. In the older patient, information regarding the longer period of stimulation required often reduces the concerns of the elderly about achieving and maintaining an erection, adequate lubrication, and/or satisfying orgasm.

The couple should also be given some basic information on techniques of communication. Beginning sentences with "*I* need" or "*I* feel" or "*I* fear" is self-descriptive and thus minimizes blaming the partner and misunderstanding each other. Anger, disappointment, or disapproval directed at the dysfunctional partner is likely to increase the partner's low self-esteem and frustration and may reinforce both the sexual and marital dysfunction. The explanation of such destructive cycles of interaction is part of the essential therapeutic process and can often lead to their modification and elimination. The angry, demanding partner can be helped to learn to ask for expressions of love and sexual affection in ways that do not require intercourse, while remaining sexually inviting and pleasing to the temporarily dysfunctional partner. Such changes in communication require time and patience before they become consistent. Both partners should be made aware of how goal orientation, performance anxiety and spectatoring produces high levels of anxiety and tension that can sabotage their desired aim. The physician should not be discouraged if he or she has to repeat these principles many times in the course of a couple's treatment.

Specific Suggestions

When sexual dysfunction does not respond to permission or limited information, the physician must become more specific and directive in treatment. The most important and helpful instruction the physician can give the couple is *not* to have intercourse. This dictum usually diminishes anxiety quickly, especially for the dysfunctional partner, and prepares the couple to begin to experience the pleasurable aspects of other sexual activity. Both partners may require reassurance that the suspension of intercourse is only temporary and will not significantly deprive the functional partner of his or her sexual expression.

The second instruction is to tell the couple to find a time for themselves free from outside interference or diversion when they are both relaxed and alert, and to use this time to be together sexually. Point out that sex should not be a duty but a form of pleasure, an expression of love, and a method of relaxation. When people come home from work or their daily housework is over, they need to unwind and relax and be with their partner. Lovemaking in these circumstances is not unusual, and having sex before having dinner can be a normal extension of their wish to be together. Sexual activity in the morning before going to work, when the body is refreshed by sleep and there is a greater facility in sexual arousal, or sexual activity on weekends are also potential alternatives. Concerns about interruptions in the middle of activity by children or visitors can easily be handled by locking the bedroom door and insisting that everyone in the family has a right to some degree and place of privacy. The use of a pseudo-vacation where the couple stay at home, but inform their friends and relations that they will be out of town, is another simple and practical method of breaking through the apparently unsurmountable problems of daily circumstances.

The third instruction is to introduce the sensate focus exercises[9] (outlined in the next section) in which each partner has a period of time in which to give and to receive sexual stimulation; each is encouraged to be himself or herself sexually and to do what each wishes to do for himself or herself with the partner. In this manner, anxiety levels are reduced and pleasurable activity is increased. And by discussing sexual questions with the physician, the partners enhance their communication with each other. Other common specific suggestions are given in Table 9–5.

The Specific Sensate Focus Exercises

Sensate Focus I. Each partner is required, for 15–20 minutes, to be totally receptive while the other partner explores, stimulates, and caresses *all* of his or her body, using all types of manual and oral stimulation BUT omitting stimulation of the genital areas and the breasts. The touching should include all types from light touch to stroking and rubbing and can include other parts of the body besides the hands such as the lips and hair. Partners should be instructed to take turns in initiating sensate focus exercises.

Sensate Focus II. The exercises are continued but now include the genital areas, and some feedback from the partner is encouraged so that those aspects of stimulation found most pleasurable are integrated into the stimulating exercises. Orgasm and penetration are still prohibited. Oral–genital contact is allowed and in some cases is encouraged.

Sensate Focus III. The exercises are continued, and penetration and continued activity to orgasm is encouraged, depending on the specific sexual dysfunction.

The sensate focus exercises in the recommended sequences are valuable procedures on resuming sexual activity for any couple who have had periods of sexual inactivity. They are also of value in enhancing

Table 9–5
Common Specific Suggestions

- Suggesting specific coital positions for those patients with dysfunction and limited knowledge.
- Suggesting that medication be taken prophylactically before sexual activity by those cardiac patients who also use prophylactic vasodilators prior to other strenuous physical activities.
- Suggesting that the routine use of medication with hypnotic or other side-effects, which would interfere with sexual enjoyment, be postponed till after the sexual activity has occurred.
- Suggesting that a partner with physical limitations due to pain on movement can still enjoy sexual activity if the coital position is chosen carefully and additions, such as cushions, are used to minimize the pain and obtain the greatest flexibility of movements.
- Suggesting to patients for whom sexual intercourse is suspended for medical reasons that manual and oral sex play can be a valid and satisfying alternative sexual experience.
- Suggesting the use of other sexual positions for those patients who cannot engage in their usual mode, such as the female-astride position for the couple, the male member of which is incapacitated and on his back.
- Suggesting to the partner of a fully incapacitated or absent patient, and to the patient, that self-pleasuring is a valid alternative to inactivity.
- Suggesting to couples, when surgical disfigurement has occurred in one member, that the environment can be altered to minimize the initial impact of the disfigurement on both members of the couple, by such simple means as lowering the lights or wearing appropriate clothing, such as a kimono.

sexual activity when it has become routine and nonimaginative. At each appointment the doctor reviews with the couple their experience with the sensate focus exercises they are using. Where difficulties have occurred, the problem is fully investigated and the couple are encouraged to repeat the procedures until they have mastered the exercises. Couples are not recommended to proceed to a succeeding stage until mastery of the current stage has been achieved.

Specific Disorders

Dysfunction in the Male

Premature ejaculation. Treatment of premature ejaculation depends on the presence or absence of secondary factors such as loss of desire and erectile dysfunction. As sexual activity in these circumstances almost invariably becomes goal directed and is no longer pleasurable for either member, the couple should be told to stop aiming for intercourse in their lovemaking. All other forms of lovemaking are encouraged in whatever way the couple finds comfortable. Instructions are given to the couple to experience their sexual activity in terms of moment-to-moment sensory pleasure rather than genital performance, and also to eliminate spectatoring. Permission should be given for the male patient to stop worrying about pleasing the partner and to concentrate on his own sense of sexual pleasure. It can be explained to the couple that ejaculatory control is just a matter of learning, something that can easily be mastered when secondary anxiety is removed. The male is further informed (where appropriate) that, if there is control in masturbation, the mechanisms are already in place and simply require generalization to sex with a partner. The aim of treatment is consistently to reduce anxiety so that the new techniques can be practiced.

Remember, during Sensate Focus I, the couple is told that NO intercourse must occur or be attempted. Each partner is stimulated by the other, but genital stimulation is not allowed. In most instances the male is surprised that, under these circumstances, he has been able to maintain the erection for up to 15 minutes of stimulation without ejaculation.

When the genital area is included, in Sensate Focus II exercises, the male is instructed to become aware of the immediate preejaculatory phenomena. This is the period when he feels that ejaculation requires only a "few more thrusts" and/or limited added stimulation. This leads, within seconds, to the emission phase of ejaculation, in which there is an accompanying feeling of inevitability that ejaculation will occur even if all stimulation ceases. It coincides physiologically with the bolus of semen entering into the membranous urethra. Once these phenomena are identified, the male can assume some control, since stopping thrusting activity and/or stimulation during the first part of the preejaculatory phase will lower the level of excitation and prevent ejaculation from occurring.

There are two techniques which can then be utilized: the *stop and go* technique and the *squeeze* technique.

In the *stop and go* technique, the male requests cessation of manual stimulation when he experiences the first sensations of the preejaculatory phenomena. This prevents ejaculation from taking place, and after 15–30 seconds, stimulation can be resumed until the preejaculatory sensations again occur.

Once the male is secure in his identification of the preejaculatory phenomena, the cessation of stimulation should be practiced randomly three or four times before the preejaculatory phase occurs by either the patient or his partner. This prevents undue concentration on the preejaculatory phenomena and allows full involvement in the pleasurable aspects of lovemaking. If the preejaculatory phenomena occur between random stops, the male is instructed to request cessation of stimulation as well.

As the male obtains a sense of control over the point of ejaculation, he is encouraged to decide when he wishes to ejaculate. Generally one recommends that there should be four occasions when the male asks the female to stop genital stimulation before allowing the fifth stimulation to carry through to manually caused ejaculation.

When mastery has been obtained in this fashion, oral–genital contact is recommended for those couples who consider this activity acceptable. The purpose of oral–genital contact is to stimulate a more vaginal-type environment than can be provided by the hand.

Sensate Focus III exercises are based on essentially similar principles. The exercises are the same, but the female assumes the female-astride position and controls the penile stimulation by her movements, under the direction of the male. Again four approaches to ejaculation and away from it are recommended, until the fifth occasion, when the male is encouraged to ejaculate intravaginally. By the time this third sensate focus exercise has become part of the couple's regular sexual activity, the premature ejaculation has disappeared, and sexual activity in which the male takes the male-superior or other positions can occur without ejaculation being immediate. In uncomplicated cases, this process usually takes about six to eight weeks of twice weekly exercises. There is a high percentage of success for this type of therapy.

In severe cases of premature ejaculation, when the male ejaculates immediately or before he achieves an erection, it is useful to begin treatment with the *squeeze* technique and then gradually switch to the stop and go technique as progress occurs. The squeeze technique is applied by placing the thumb diagonally across the frenulum with the index and middle fingers straddling the ridge of the glans on the opposite side. A firm squeeze is applied for two to four seconds during the preejaculatory period. The degree of pressure should depend on the degree of erection present, since the penis in the unerect state may be sensitive while the erect penis is essentially insensitive to pain. If properly applied, the squeeze will reflexly prevent ejaculation, giving the couple a sense of mastery that they did not possess before.

Sometimes in response to the cessation of stimulation or the squeeze, the erection may diminish or disappear. The couple should be prewarned and reassured that this frequently occurs and all that is required is a resumption of manual stimulation.

Occasional instances of ejaculation occur during the early stages of the exercises, in spite of the couple following the instructions. This is not to be considered a failure of the couple's efforts, the technique, or the doctor's instructions. With reassurance and some more practice this problem usually disappears.

Retarded ejaculation. The principles of treatment for retarded ejaculation involve reduction in anxiety and goal orientation; the teaching of techniques of control over the timing of ejaculation; and in most cases, a therapeutic involvement in the psychodynamics of the interpersonal relationship.

Initially, permission is given for the patient to be "selfish" and to concentrate on his own feelings and pleasure and for the partner to do the same. The man is told that anxiety has replaced the pleasurable aspects of lovemaking. The patient and the partner are encouraged to experience in full the stimuli they are receiving and assured that in an anxiety-free situation this should reach the required physiological level for ejaculation to occur spontaneously.

The same senate focus exercises are suggested for this disorder as in all other sexual disorders, including the initial prohibition of intercourse.

When the couple has achieved a pleasurable state of lovemaking with low anxiety, emphasis is placed on encouraging the man to demonstrate, in front of his partner, whatever methods he uses to experience ejaculation by masturbation. In Senate Focus II exercises, the woman is encouraged to become more active in the lovemaking and in particular to stimulate the penis and to utilize the techniques the patient uses himself. When mastery of these techniques has been achieved, so that ejaculation occurs with manual and/or manual plus oral play by the partner, the patient and his partner can move on to Sensate Focus III. In Sensate Focus III exercises the woman is put in charge of inserting the penis into the vagina at the point of ejaculatory inevitability. Furthermore, to facilitate this, the woman should adopt the female-astride position. Once this exercise has been completed, male-superior intercourse is introduced so that the male may continue the exercises in a position where he can thrust the best and start to take control over the moment of ejaculation himself. During male-superior intercourse, it is helpful if the woman learns to use her pubococcygeal muscles as well as pelvic movements and varying forms of thrusting, which may be new for her and are particularly helpful in reinforcing penile stimulation. Some women require considerable permission-giving and encouragement in order to overcome their reluctance to adopt such an active role in intercourse.

At the same time the exercises are being prescribed, the therapist must investigate psychodynamic issues between the couple, such as pregnancy fears and desires, communication problems, and other issues leading to discord in the relationship. However, involvement in this area may require intensive therapy with an experienced psychotherapist.

Erectile dysfunction. Treatment must be initially directed to the alleviation of the secondary anxiety that has begun to operate. So severe is this anxiety that the initial establishment of a nonthreatening, pleasurable milieu generally takes longer than in patients with other male dysfunctions. Constant attention must be paid to the mechanisms of performance anxiety, goal orientation and spectatoring.

Permission here, as in the other dysfunctions, means the patient may experience disappointment and anxiety but not feelings of being "inadequate as a man." Similarly, the partner may be disappointed but must not consider herself to blame or inadequate. Continued intimate contact and maintenance of emotional warmth is encouraged, without the "need" for intercourse. In fact, permission is given *not* to have intercourse, so that other forms of intimate contact can be encouraged.

Where the dynamics of the dysfunction are obvious and do not involve deep psychological factors, these should be discussed with the patient. For example, erectile dysfunction following one or two episodes of heavy alcohol consumption is invariably due to the combination of alcohol and anxiety. Explaining this to the patient can often lead to a rapid diminution of anxiety and resumption of sexual activity. With physical illness and aging, an explanation of the relationship can reduce the secondary anxiety and permit more effective treatment to be prescribed. All such information should be shared directly with the partner, as the partner's anxiety plays an important part in the maintenance of the symptom.

The same sensate focus exercises are prescribed as in the other male sexual disorders, with an emphasis on prohibition of intercourse. In some patients the reduction of anxiety and the prohibition of intercourse is enough to enable erectile functioning to recur. Once erectile functioning occurs the patient is told to allow the erection to disappear by cessation of stimulation and to return by renewed stimulation in order to demonstrate that erections can come and go and that the pleasurable aspect of lovemaking is paramount. This method also demonstrates that the erection is not under conscious control but is the most obvious outcome of adequate stimulation in a relaxed, nonanxious male. The partner's role is to help provide the nonanxious environment and to maintain such an atmosphere. She should also learn to accept the other pleasurable aspects of lovemaking and not to demand intercourse and an erect penis from her partner.

Where pleasurable, moment-to-moment sensations are difficult for the patient to attend to because they invariably lead to spectatoring, other methods of avoiding spectatoring should be suggested, such as concentrating on the partner's attractiveness, her enjoyment, or even the freckles on her forehead. When even this does not work, the pleasuring of the individual with erectile dysfunction should be terminated and he should concentrate on pleasuring his partner to her orgasm by nonpenile means. In this way the functional partner is not left disappointed, and the dysfunctional partner and the couple are not traumatized by the "failure" of the experience. These exercises are continued until the anxiety is reduced and the normal sexual response cycle can again be established.

For those patients who have true organic erectile dysfunction, Small-Carrion penile prostheses are available. There are two types, one of which is a semi-rigid silastic rod that allows a semi-rigid penis to function and penetrate. The other is a hydraulic implant that allows the male patient to bring about tumescence and detumescence of the penis as he wishes.

Long term follow-up of these patients is not as yet sufficient to warrant definitive statements about their use. Implants do not interfere with residual intact functioning and can be removed at any time.[10]

Dysfunction in the Female

Arousal disorders. The inability of the female to respond to adequate sexual stimulation with lubrication and the vasocongestive response, causes problems in vaginal intercourse. The apprehension this entails often leads to the female discouraging further sexual activity.

Information should be given about fluctuations that occur in lubrication with age, illness, and psychological attitudes, and specific information and suggestions about the use of lubricants should be offered. Further information should be given about adequate clitoral stimulation and the advantages of varying sexual positions for providing such stimulation. For example, the female-astride position provides for more clitoral stimulation than the traditional male-superior position. Some females also have fears about conception and the adequacy of their birth control methods. Such anxiety inhibits their sexual responsiveness. This area should, therefore, be explored and the necessary information provided.

The sensate focus exercises mentioned earlier form the basis of treatment. The increased period of stimulation that the exercises provide, the greater attention paid to the female's sexual needs, and the reduction in anxiety can allow a normal arousal response to be established.

After the establishment of the sensate focus exercises it is also valuable for the subject of self-stimulation to be discussed. If a woman has not previously masturbated, and assuming she is not personally opposed to it, she should be encouraged to have periods of time during which she can stimulate herself and experience those sensations that are most pleasurable. Assurance must be given that being sexual is consistent with being feminine. The technique of self-pleasuring is used to emphasize the female's control of her body and her sexual responsiveness and to educate her in an understanding of her own body. Females with strong negative attitudes about masturbation require encouragement to help them achieve a state of mind where they can use masturbation as a therapeutic and self-pleasuring tool. After the establishment of such self-pleasuring exercises, the patient should bring them into the partnership exercises, demonstrating them to her partner and encouraging his participation in specific activities such as clitoral stimulation. These exercises encourage the woman to play a more active role in achieving sexual satisfaction and emphasize the woman's responsibility for gratifying her own sexual needs.

Orgasmic disorders. The inability of the female to reach orgasm is often associated with goal orientation and spectatoring. The primary form of this disorder, in which the woman has never experienced an orgasm, tends to be more successfully treated than the secondary forms, in which the more complex psychological factors and interpersonal difficulties are often present.

The woman with a primary preorgasmic condition is generally less informed about her own sexuality and is often apprehensive about expressing her own sexual needs. Such women respond rapidly to the permission and limited information aspects of the treatment. In fact, good responses have occurred in women's groups, in which the main thrust is toward education about female sexuality, assertiveness in expressing one's own sexual needs, and the use of masturbatory exercises. The latter help women become comfortable with their sexuality.

In individual therapy the physician's initial aims must be the same; that is, for the patient to become assertive and knowledgeable about her sexual needs and responses and to use self-pleasuring as a therapeutic exercise to these ends. The initial sessions should emphasize the educational aspects of sexuality; it is often useful to recommend reading material to the patient such as Lonnie Barbach's *For Yourself* (see the Bibliography to this chapter). The woman is given permission to be sexual and to explore her own anatomy and physiological responses. The use of models of the genitalia and educational anatomical drawings are useful adjuncts, but most important is to persuade the patient to examine her own genitalia by hand and with the use of a mirror, and to identify the position of her clitoris and her other anatomical features. It is also useful for the patient to identify and learn to use the pubococcygeal muscles and to become fully conversant with their physiological capacities.

A suitable method of identifying these muscles is to ask the female to insert two fingers in the vagina and tighten the gluteus maximus muscles for thirty seconds. On conscious relaxation, she should feel the pubococcygeal muscles relax because they are automatically contracted with the glutei. Exploration of the physiological responses to sexual stimulation is encouraged by self-pleasuring at periods of time when the woman is free from interruption and other concerns. The increased knowledge of her own sexual responsivity, plus the repetitive solo exercises, assists the majority of women to become orgasmic by self-pleasuring.

During these procedures, sexual activity with the partner should be continued and sensate focus exercises by the couple instituted. This allows the female to introduce into the couple's activity the knowledge she is gaining through self-exploration and self-stimulation; it also avoids resentment on the part of the spouse, who may be feeling blame for the partner's lack of responsiveness. The partner should be made knowledgeable about female anatomy and about his partner's needs and responses and should learn to integrate this knowledge into his techniques. Most important is to ensure that clitoral stimulation continues during vaginal penetration. This can be established by using manual stimulation by either the woman or the partner, while penetration is occurring. Other methods of increasing clitoral stimulation include the use of alternate positions for penetration. The female-astride position not only allows this to occur but is a position in which direct manual stimulation of the clitoris is easier. For many couples a return to pleasurable intercourse is facilitated by first establishing orgasm by manual and/or oral stimulation.

Variations in the sensate exercises should be allowed, based on the preferences of the patient and the partner and, particularly, on the orgasmic stage the patient displays. Women who are easily orgasmic on self-stimulation but not in intercourse should be encouraged to bring the self-pleasuring exercises rapidly into activity with the partner, showing the partner her preferences and encouraging the partner to take over a role in the manual (and oral) stimulation, prior to integrating this into intercourse. Women who find self-pleasuring unacceptable and who resist the plan of treatment suggested above, insisting on direct partner involvement from the start, can best be helped by encouragement to become more active during sexual activity; they can be taught to use the pubococcygeal muscles and encouraged to seek additional clitoral stimulation during intercourse.

As goal orientation and spectatoring are quite common in orgasmic disorders, in both patient and partner, emphasis on the process of lovemaking and the pleasurable experiences of moment-to-moment stimulation must be employed and the inevitability of the orgasmic response emphasized.

Many partners view the lack of orgasm in the female as a personal shortcoming and as a result are anxious about their own performance. This situation requires attention, preferably in the setting of the couple's treatment. Reassurance is essential that it is not the male's responsibility and that no male can give his partner an orgasm. The role of the male is to provide adequate stimulation for the partner while participating in the sexual activity for his own pleasure.

In those patients where these techniques are unsuccessful, deeper psychological and intrapersonal factors are usually at play and more intensive psychotherapy is required. This usually requires referral to a specialist.

Vaginismus. Spontaneous contractions of the vaginal musculature, when not due to organic factors, are usually treatable by the use of dilators, or in milder cases, the patient's and the partner's own fingers. The pelvic exam will usually demonstrate this response. The husband should be told that this vaginal contraction is an automatic response outside his wife's control. With some couples, this can be demonstrated in the examination room. It should be emphasized that it is neither the spouse's nor the patient's fault, nor exclusively a sexual problem. The physician should demonstrate that the conscious use of the pelvic musculature by "bearing down" movements can help the patient relax the introitus and minimize the vaginismus.

The husband should be directly involved in the treatment, which should occur at home, although the final responsibility must rest with the female patient. Each day she inserts one of a set of graduated dilators and maintains it in position for at least 15 minutes without discomfort. She is encouraged to be active with the dilator in place. After she uses the dilators she is also encouraged to insert her own fingers and to allow her husband to insert his fingers into the vagina, to desensitize the painful stimuli and resensitize the vagina to pleasurable stimuli. In the meantime, the couple are also instructed to continue the sensate focus exercises mentioned above. The insertion of dilators and fingers and the use of sensate focus exercises are coordinated so that by the time the patient is able to tolerate a size #5 dilator without discomfort, the couple is ready to experience penile penetration. The most efficacious manner is for the female to insert the penis while she is in the astride position, and the husband is instructed not to thrust but to allow the female to control her own movements. As she becomes familiar with this experience and the sensation of penile containment, the husband is encouraged to take a more active role. The establishment of full sexual activity and enjoyment is usually rapid, once the initial aversion to penetration has been overcome.

Dyspareunia. Once the presence of an organic etiology is ruled out, the treatment of dyspareunia is geared initially toward providing adequate stimulation and lubrication prior to vaginal penetration. Then, since the continued perception of pain is usually associated with apprehension and increased muscular tension, this condition should respond to the desensitization and resensitization methods described for vaginismus.

Desire Disorders in Either Sex

A significant number of patients experience a lack of sexual desire, while their actual physiological sexual functioning remains intact. Although lack of sexual desire is a commonplace outcome of other sexual dysfunctions, in this disorder the individual can continue to function well but lacks any appetite for sexual activity. The factors leading to the onset of this condition are wide ranging and multiple, leading to severe obstacles to successful treatment.

Abnormalities associated with hormonal problems are considered rare. A full physical examination and adequate history should identify those patients where a more detailed hormonal assessment is required.

Secondary lack of sexual desire following physical illness, as in post-myocardial infarct patients or post-hysterectomy patients, is often associated with fear and apprehension. These elements must be directly identified and discussed.

Although a small percentage respond to sensate focus exercises and treatment based on the PLISSIT model, the majority of patients with lack of sexual desire—more than patients with any other sexual disorder—experience interpersonal and/or intrapersonal problems and should be referred for pyschotherapy.

Summary

In all the treatment programs described, the exercises must be continued on a regular basis twice to three times a week. Regular discussions should be held with the physician. This repetitive and consistent practice should occur over several months, until the new sex behaviors have become established as a regular part of the couple's activities. The couple must realize that the goal of treatment is the removal of the anxiety and the anxiety-producing behavior that are inhibiting natural sexual activity from occurring. Treatment is *not* directed primarily to the symptoms of which they complain.

There are patients who do not respond to the above approach and who require referral for more specialized care. Among the indications for such referrals are (1) the presence of severe interpersonal difficulties that directly interfere with treatment, so that instructions are not followed or are actively sabotaged by one or both partners; (2) indications that treatment has made the problems more severe or the appearance of new symptoms; (3) improvement in sexual behavior but deterioration in nonsexual interaction and cooperation; (4) the appearance of overt and persistent psychiatric symptoms in either partner, or the recognition that the sexual symptoms are associated with a psychiatric illness such as depression or schizophrenia; and (5) the physician's decision that the problem is beyond his level of interest, information, expertise, or comfort.

SEXUAL DYSFUNCTION AND PHYSICAL ILLNESS

Sexual functioning can become disrupted by direct infection or injury to the genital area. Of course, during the active phase of venereal infection, intercourse should not occur. A more recent development is the increase in the prevalence of herpes simplex of the genitalia. No entirely satisfactory treatment is available for this viral condition. The patient must be told that the infection can be transferred so that sexual activity should be minimized during the acute stage of the infection and intercourse should not occur. The use of a condom is recommended in the healing stages, and intercourse should not occur if penile or introitovaginal pain is experienced.

The presence of urethrocystitis in the female is often exacerbated by intercourse, and this in turn may lead to sexual dysfunction. Acute prostatitis in the male, because of the associated pain, is often the source of sexual problems.

Any operation in the genital and perineal areas involves posttraumatic vasocongestion of the area that leads to painful spontaneous erections in the male and the more generalized feeling of sexual urgency in the female. Explanation of these distressing physiological responses prior to surgery will minimize the associated distress and suggest means of minimizing the phenomena.

Certain disorders that do not directly involve the genitals may present with sexual dysfunction. Foremost of these is diabetes mellitus. In its early stages, the uncontrolled disease has a direct effect on the autonomic innervation of the sexual system that leads to a disruption of the neural impulses. Arteriolar sclerosis can affect the small arterioles supplying the autonomic nervous system as well as the larger arterioles supplying the corpora cavernosa and the corpus spongiosum. These vascular effects do not appear to be reversible when the diabetic condition is stabilized.

In 30 patients between the ages of 30 and 56, with a history of one year or longer of erectile dysfunction, arteriography of the penile arterial bed demonstrated occlusive lesions of various degrees to be present in the internal pudendal artery, and the penile artery and its branches, a condition similar to claudication. Among this group of patients, 12 had diabetes mellitus; 2 had hypertension; 2 had previous pelvic trauma, and 14 had no demonstrable disorders. The angiographic findings, which were not demonstrated in 4 patients with obvious psychogenic impotence, correlated with the absence of pulsation in the dorsal penile arteries but, except for two patients with mild ischemic heart disease, no other vascular disease was demonstrable. Interestingly, although 46 percent of these patients had nocturnal emissions, 53 percent reported complete absence of erections; 33 percent had weak morning erections no more often than weekly; and 14 percent reported frequent morning erections of reasonable turgidity but short duration.[11]

Adequate control of the diabetic condition can lead to a reemergence of full sexual functioning in males with erectile difficulty, if irreversible effects on the autonomic nervous system and the corpora have not occurred. In those instances where dysfunction persists even though the diabetes is under control, the symptoms may be due to the organic pathological process or to the superimposed anxiety about the illness and sexual functioning.

In a recent study of nocturnal penile tumescence in 57 male diabetics with sexual dysfunction, 30 percent were found to have an organic etiology, 20 percent a psychogenic etiology, and 44 percent a mixed organic, psychogenic etiology.[12]

While it is plausible to suspect that diabetes may also affect sexual functioning in the female, no good evidence has yet been presented confirming this. In many chronic female diabetics, a vulvovaginitis develops that is resistant to treatment and can lead to a cessation of sexual activity. To avoid the problem, advice regarding stricter diabetic control and hygiene to avoid infection can be helpful.

Endocrine disorders such as Addison's disease in women, primary and secondary hypogonadism, hyperprolactinemia, hyperthyroidism, pituitary tumors, and disorders that disrupt the nervous impulses in the spinal cord frequently have an effect on sexual activity. Sexual symptoms are also encountered in the arteriosclerotic cardiovascular disorders; uremia; disorders of the musculoskeletal system, such as disc lesions and myasthenia gravis; and such systemic conditions as chronic alcoholic neuropathy and lupus erythematosis. In some cases, adequate treatment of the primary condition leads to a reversal of the sexual dysfunction.

In all acute disorders, such as myocardial infarction, sexual functioning and concerns are suspended by the severity and life-threatening aspects of the condition itself. Questions regarding sexual activity become important in the convalescent stage, when the issue of resumption of sexual activity should be raised. At this time patients and their partners are usually concerned about the possible deleterious effects of sexual activity on the damaged organ. The physician should be able to advise the patient and the partner when and how to resume sexual activity.

Dr. S was concerned when he was informed by the nursing staff that, two weeks after his patient's coronary occlusion, a nurse interrupted the patient and his wife in the act of fellatio. Dr. S's initial response was one of anger toward the patient for taking such risks in his convalescent period and also anger on behalf of the nurse who was horrified at being a forced witness to a sexual act. On secondary consideration, the physican realized that he had never discussed sexual activity with the patient, or its effect on the cardiac condition. Rather than confront the patient with his mixed feelings about the behavior, he asked for a psychiatric consult.

The psychiatrist confirmed the physician's own realization that the patient had not been informed of the dangers of sexual activity in his convalescent period. Furthermore, the patient had become extremely anxious about his continued sexual functioning in the face of his myocardial infarction and had indulged in "testing behavior" to reassure himself, without realizing the potential dangers. Open discussion about sexual activity after a myocardial infarction and reassurance that sexual functioning would not be affected, allowed the patient's anxiety to diminish and the need for testing behavior to cease. The wife was also seen and the situation was explained to her, reducing her anxiety and securing her cooperation. Full and satisfactory functioning was reestablished under the physician's guidance within three months of the myocardial infarction.

It has been generally thought that post-myocardial infarct patients could resume sexual activity with safety if they could master the workload involved in climbing two flights of stairs. That viewpoint, however, must now be modified. Some cardiologists believe that all post-myocardial infarct patients should first have a limited treadmill evaluation in hospital prior to discharge. Those able to achieve 3 mets* without symptoms, arrythmias, or ECG changes suggesting ischemia should be able to resume some sexual activity after they have returned home, after allowing several days to pass to become comfortable again in the home environment. Patients must realize that their bodies have been weakened by the inactivity of the hospital, and a plan of conditioning should be instituted.

Before the patient leaves the hospital, the spouse should be brought into the plans for resuming sexual activity. Initially, sensate focus exercises can be prescribed if you believe the couple will be comfortable with them. This allows the physician to monitor the return to full sexuality and limits the pressure on the patient to "perform" and the associated cardiac stress. With no complications, the patient and the spouse should be able to complete the full sexual cycle to sexual intercourse within three weeks after discharge, having gone through five or six sensate focus exercise sessions.

Those patients with persistent and recurrent angina should avoid sexual activity immediately after discharge and should not resume any

* One met is a measure of the energy expenditure per kilogram of body weight per minute of an average individual sitting quietly in a chair at rest.

activity until the angina is under control with the use of nitroglycerine. Sexual activity is then resumed gradually, perhaps through the sensate focus route, with nitroglycerine being given prophylactically.

A similar regimen is recommended for patients on antiarrhythmic agents. The patient should be warned that sexual activity under unusual circumstances or emotional stress is to be completely avoided. This precludes sexual activity with a nonregular partner, in stressful surroundings, or in positions that are unusual or emotionally disturbing for the patient. Ambulatory (Holter) monitoring during the patient's first few sexual experiences may be advised if the physician is concerned that arrythmia may occur during sexual activity.[13] The physician should bear in mind that the use of the Holter might itself be stressful for many patients. Many cardiologists find it useful to teach patients how to monitor their pulse and check it before and after any physical stress, including sexual relations. Some cardiologists suggest that the production of a heart rate greater than 70 percent of the "maximal predicted heart rate"* should be an indication that return to full sexual activity should be delayed. Once sexual activity is re-established to the couple's satisfaction without the recurrence of cardiac symptomatology, more active and stimulating activity can be introduced.

The most essential element in the management of the post-myocardial infarction patient is to be sure to discuss sexuality. You can be sure it is on the minds of most patients and their spouses, but they may not ask their questions unless you encourage them. With your help these patients should be able to return to satisfactory relations.†,[14–16]

In the convalescent stage of all operations and trauma, the resumption of sexual activity is usually of great concern to the patient and partner. Preoperatively the physician should inquire about sexual functioning and should advise when sexual activity should be resumed and what limitations should be imposed. This preoperative discussion should maximize the patient's return to full sexual functioning. It is important that the physican offer the appropriate information and not wait to be asked.

In all medical and surgical conditions in which the resumption of sexual activity is likely to be limited by anxiety and/or physical impediment, the physican should spell out very specific steps as to how the sexual activity should be resumed gradually. Physicians should base their recommendations on their knowledge of the natural course of the con-

---

* The maximal predictable heart rate is calculated by subtracting the patient's age from 220. Thus a 40-year-old patient has a "maximal predictable heart rate" of 180/min. Seventy percent of this is 126/min.

† A pamphlet, written for patients and in a very light-hearted manner, discusses sex after myocardial infarction. You might write for a copy and decide if it would be useful in your practice *The Sensuous Heart,* Pritchett and Hull Associates, Inc., 2122 Faulkner Road, N.E., Atlanta, GA 30324).

valescence of the specific illness or surgical procedure, the patients' overall health, their special anxieties, and their premorbid sexual history.

In postoperative cases, specific attention should be addressed to the degree of sensitivity of scar tissue, to residual pain, or to other adverse sensations.

Radical surgical procedures, such as transperineal prostatectomy or abdomino-perineal resection invariably lead to sexual dysfunction due to interruption of neural pathways. Patients must be informed preoperatively that they are to expect permanent cessation of the genito-sexual responses, so that the necessary adaptation to this condition can be begun prior to the operation. They can be reassured that alternative nongenital forms of sexual activity and pleasure can be developed.

In cases where patients have undergone surgical procedures, such as a mastectomy or ileostomy, that result in disfigurment, they often need advice on how to minimize the unpleasant aspects of such changes to the spouse as well as to the self. In such situations it is recommended that the couple be seen prior to the operation and the postoperative disfigurement discussed openly with both partners. This procedure facilitates the patient's need to ventilate the underlying anxiety and concerns and provides the spouse with an equal opportunity to ventilate similar concerns. The surgeon is also given an opportunity to explain to both the patient and spouse the reality of the potential disfigurement and ways in which it can be minimized in future sexual activity. Moreover, such a discussion gives the physician an opportunity to assess the likelihood of postoperative sexual problems and to suggest ways of coping with them. An appropriate referral is indicated if the patient's and the spouse's concerns are strong enough that the physician feels psychotherapeutic help is required.

It is useful to advise the ileostomy patient about the use of deodorants and perfumes before and during sexual activity, and the use of a relatively loose but enclosing garment covering the operative area. The postmastectomy patient can be advised that, until both she and her partner are comfortable with the sight and sensation of the absence of a breast, a padded bra and mini-negligee may be worn during lovemaking.

The sexual needs of hospitalized patients have not been acknowledged by the medical, nursing, and administrative staff of hospitals. In the recuperative stages of trauma, operations, and many illnesses the patient does not remain asexual. In hospitals, the lack of privacy and the apparent assumption that all patients are asexual or "should control themselves," means that any activity beyond inconspicuous kissing and touching is usually considered inappropriate and objectionable by the hospital staff and by other patients. The patient's sexuality should be accepted as basic and legitimate.

When specific physical disorders such as emphysema, arthritis, and cardiac failure, reach the chronic disabling stage, sexual activity is often the first function the patient relinquishes. Your understanding of the problems that these patients encounter in sexual intercourse and encouragement that they seek alternative forms of lovemaking should allow the patient and the partner to continue to experience some form of satisfying and meaningful sexual activity. Even patients with complete paraplegia are able to learn to obtain some degree of pleasure without a genital response, and to perceive and experience the mental and emotional aspects of the sensations of orgasm without a genital orgasmic response.[17]

The treatment of sexual dysfunction associated with a physical disability must involve the partner. Both partners should be encouraged to continue warm, emotional behavior, such as kissing and petting, even though this may not lead to sexual arousal on the part of the afflicted individual. These activities in themselves are intrinsically satisfying and pleasurable, and the fact that arousal cannot occur and intercourse and climax are unobtainable does not mean that the pleasure associated with closeness and intimacy should be lost. The pessimistic abjuration of all forms of sexual activity is pathological and should not be encouraged.

The physician's role is to suggest and help implement alternate forms of sexual activity. Your goal is for the healthy partner to obtain pleasure and gratification, while the ill spouse accepts modifications which insure some pleasure within the limitations created by the physical disorder. For example, different positions for intercourse, such as the female-astride position apply less physical stress on the male and may allow intercourse to continue when the male-superior position is not longer feasible. Alternate forms of reaching orgasm for both partners should also be explored with the patient and the spouse and the possible use of oral and manual stimulation explained. The astute physician, however, must be aware of the psychological stresses that may be engendered by the adoption of such new techniques. Males may find the female-astride position emasculating, while females may find it too assertive. Oral sexual activity may be an anathema to many individuals. In such cases, psychotherapy is indicated to assist the patient and the partner in adapting to such new techniques. In selected cases of penile dysfunction, referral for a penile prosthesis implant should be considered.

Many of the drugs used in general medical practice can affect sexual function. Table 9–1 summarizes these effects. The physician has an obligation to inform the patient that these sideefects (along with others) may occur; that they are not necessarily present in all people who take the medication; and that if these symptoms do appear, adjusting the dosage, the timing of the doses, or changing the medication may minimize or eliminate the distressful symptoms. Obviously, during the course of treatment, the physician should regularly inquire whether these side-effects do appear.

REFERENCES

1. Sparks RF, White RA, Connolly PB: Impotence is not always psychogenic. JAMA 243:750–755, 1980
2. Clarkson TB, Alexander NJ: Long-term vasectomy effects in the occurrence and extent of atherosclerosis in rhesus monkeys. J Clin Invest 65:15–25, 1980
3. Ovesey L: Homosexuality and Pseudohomosexuality. New York, Science House, 1969
4. Lief H: Medical Aspects of Sexuality in Beeson PB, McDermott W, and Wyngaarden JB (eds): Textbook of Medicine. Philadelphia, Pa, WB Saunders, 1979
5. Owen WF: The clinical approach to the homosexual patient. *Ann Intern Med* 93: 90–92, 1980
6. Magee M: Psychogenic impotence: A critical review. Urology 5:435–1980
7. Wasserman MD, Pollack CP, Spielman AJ, Weitzman ED: Theoretical and technical problems in the measurement of nocturnal penile tumescence for the differential diagnosis of impotence. Psychosom Med 42: 575–585, 1980
8. Annon, J: The Behavioral Treatment of Sexual Problems, vol.1. Honolulu: Enabling Systems Inc., 1974
9. Masters WH, Johnson V: Human Sexual Inadequacy. Boston, Little, Brown, 1970
10. Scott B. Byrd GJ, Karacan, I. Olsson P; Beutler LE, Attia SJ: Erectile impotence treated with implantable, inflatable prosthesis. JAMA 241:2609–2612, 1979
11. Michal V, Pospichal J: Phalloarteriography in the diagnosis of erectile impotence. World J Surg 2:239–247, 1978
12. Abel G, et al.: Paper presented at Sixth Annual Conference of the International Academy of Sex Research, Tucson, Ariz, 1980
13. Sex and the heart patient: Portable ECG finds arrythmias. Sexual Medicine Today, March 1979
14. Sex and the Heart Patient. A brochure published by Burroughs Wellcome Co, Research Triangle, NC, 1977
15. Cole CM, Levin CM, Whitley JO, Young SH: Brief sexual counseling during cardiac rehabilitation. Heart & Lung 8:224–229, 1979
16. Green AW: Sexual activity and the postmyocardial infarction patient. Am Heart J 89:246–252, 1975
17. Comfort A: Sexual consequences of disability. Philadelphia, Stickley, 1978

BIBLIOGRAPHY

Barbach L: For Yourself: The Fulfillment of Female Sexuality. Garden City, NY, 1975

Comfort A: The Joy of Sex. New York, Crown Publishers, 1972

Kaplan HS: The New Sex Therapy. New York, Brunner/Mazel, 1974

Kaplan HS: The Illustrated Manual of Sex Therapy. New York, Quadrangle, 1975

Kaplan HS: Disorders of Sexual Desire. New York, Brunner/Mazel, 1979

Levay A, Kagle A: Overcoming premature ejaculation: "Stop and go" versus "squeeze technique." Med Asp Hum Sex 11:104–112, 1977

Lief HI (ed): Sexual Problems in Medical Practice. Chicago, AMA, 1981

Masters W, Johnson V: Human Sexual Response. Boston, Little, Brown, 1966

Masters W, Johnson V: Human Sexual Inadequacy. Boston, Little, Brown, 1970

Spark R, White R, Connolly P: Impotence is not always psychogenic: Newer insights into hypothalamic–pituitary gonadal dysfunction. JAMA 243:750–755, 1980

Zilbergeld B: Male Sexuality: A Guide to Sexual Fulfillment. Boston, Little, Brown, 1970

Richard A. Gardner, M.D.

10

The Management of Psychiatric Problems of Childhood

The primary care physician is in an excellent position to treat many forms of psychiatric disturbance of childhood in their earliest phases and thereby to prevent them from developing into more severe forms of pathology. Not only does the primary care physician have an excellent opportunity for early intervention, but he or she generally has developed an ongoing relationship with the patient that is not enjoyed by the psychiatrist to whom the physician might refer. Most therapists agree that a good doctor–patient relationship is crucial to successful psychotherapy and that without it, it is not likely that treatment will be successful.

This chapter describes some of the more common types of psychiatric disturbance of childhood that may initially come to the attention of the primary care physician. For each disorder, some of the psychotherapeutic approaches that the primary care physician might be able to utilize successfully are examined. Finally, the chapter provides guidelines for determining when referral to a child psychiatrist (or other mental health professional trained to treat children) is warranted.

MINIMAL BRAIN DYSFUNCTION

In this chapter, the term *minimal brain dysfunction* (MBD) is used to refer to mild neurological disease of the brain. Although this may appear to be a very loose definition, unbecoming of a physician, in the author's opinion it describes more accurately than any other definition what we are talking about when we use the term. The vague definition is also a reflection of our ignorance about this disorder, or more accurately, group of disorders in that we are not talking about a single entity when we use the term. I would prefer that we use *the group of minimal brain dysfunction syndromes,* a term that more accurately describes what many of us in the field conceive MBD to be.

Hyperactivity has traditionally been considered one of the cardinal signs of MBD. In fact, there are some who prefer that term to MBD. The author, however, views hyperactivity as one possible sign of MBD; it may or may not be present. It seems unreasonable to label a disorder by one common sign; One might as well call appendicitis *fever* or brain tumor *headache.* Assessing the significance of hyperactivity is further complicated by the fact that children with purely psychogenic problems can be hyperactive—their hyperactivity being a concomitant of their tension and anxiety. One of the major problems in MBD diagnosis has been that subjective criteria have often been utilized to decide that a child is hyperactive. A teacher, for example, will decide that a boy is hyperactive because he appears to move around in his seat more than other children his age. The parents are contacted and soon the child is in the physician's office. Although the physician has not observed the hyperactivity himself or herself (these children are typically more subdued in the one-to-one situation), the child is placed on psychostimulant medication (the dose is guessed) and told to return in 6 months or a year. An analogous situation would be one in which a man walks into his internist's office and says that his wife thinks that he has high blood sugar. Without any further examination or testing, the physician decides the man has diabetes mellitus, prescribes 50 units of insulin to be injected every morning, and fails to recommend any monitoring of either the insulin dose or the diet. Although there are probably few (if any) adults who have been administered insulin this way, it is common practice to place children on psychostimulant medication in this manner and to maintain them on such medication for years.

The evaluation for MBD cannot be made in ten minutes. Such an evaluation should include testing for a wide variety of auditory and visual processing deficits (that often contribute to the learning disabilities seen in many of these children), fine and gross motor coordination problems, mild dysphasias and dyspraxias, soft neurological signs, and intellectual deficits. In addition to evaluating for hyperactivity, the examiner is deficient if assessment for other manifestations of MBD are not included.

The twelve subtests of the Wechsler Intelligence Scale for Children–Revised (WISC-R) can provide the physician with a wealth of information about a wide variety of deficits seen in MBD.[1] Each subtest, viewed as an instrument in its own right, accesses at least a few of the possible functions that may be impaired in MBD. The Reversals Frequency Test is a useful screening device for neurologically based reading disability (dyslexia) in that there is a high correlation between a high reversals frequency and organic reading disabilities.[2-4] The Bender Visual Motor Gestalt Test is much more likely to detect dyspraxia than visual perceptual problems (its initial intent) and is especially useful if one quantifies the scores with Kippitz normative data.[5-7]

Fine motor coordination can be evaluated with the Purdue Pegboard,[8] utilizing normative data collected by this examiner.[2,9] The Balls and Basket Test assesses gross motor coordination.[2,10] The Steadiness Tester measures hyperactivity and/or the ability to sustain attention.[2,11,12]

The ability to hold the stylus steadily depends upon an activity-level factor as well as the capacity to sustain attention. Recent work has demonstrated that these factors may be operating interdependently in MBD children. The hyperactivity may be viewed as secondary to an impairment in sustaining attention. Because they cannot maintain attention long on a particular stimulus, they flit from stimulus to stimulus—thus the hyperactivity. Psychostimulant medication helps them sustain concentration and thereby reduces the hyperactivity. The traditional view that such medication acts "paradoxically" in these children is not upheld by research. Rappoport has demonstrated well that the action of dextroamphetamine sulfate is the same in normal and MBD children.[13] Both groups react with reduced activity level, improved concentration, shorter reaction time, and improved performance on other neuropsychological tests.

The basic screening battery just described can be administered in 2 to 3 hours. If a child shows no evidence of deficiency on any of these instruments, MBD is extremely unlikely (if not entirely ruled out).

If deficits are revealed on any of these tests, further evaluation is warranted. For example, if the child does poorly on the Purdue Pegboard, other tests of fine motor coordination should be administered in order to determine whether or not a deficit in this area is present. Or, if the child does poorly on the Reversals Frequency Test, other tests of longterm memory (especially for linguistic material) should be administered. Elsewhere, this examiner describes the full MBD battery he utilizes and discusses the various tests that one can administer to access MBD in greater depth.[2]

If the physician is willing to take the time to train himself to administer the aforementioned tests and to set aside two or three 1-hour examining sessions (it is unwise to administer the battery in one prolonged testing session), he will be performing a valuable service for patients being screened for MBD. If he does not wish to involve himself this deeply in MBD diagnosis, he should have such an evaluation performed by someone interested in and trained to perform MBD assessments. If the practitioner's practice includes a large number of such children (and this is likely in group practices), having such a person in the office one or more days a week can be useful.

Whether or not the physician involves himself in primary diagnosis, he may become involved in treatment. In counseling parents, the author generally provides them with a copy of *MBD: The Family Book About Minimal Brain Dysfunction*.[14] The first section of this book is for parents; it provides them with basic information about the disorder and advises them on how to deal with the more common problems. The second part is designed to be read by the MBD child himself or herself and is accompanied by informative and attractive illustrations. Other books this author has found useful are two by Doreen Kronick: one advises parents on how to deal with MBD children,[15] the other advises them on how to deal with MBD adolescents.[16] Physicians themselves may learn much from reading these books.

The physician may also be called upon to provide medication. Other diagnosticians may have made the diagnosis, but nonmedical people have to rely on the physician to administer medication. Hyperactivity, concentration impairment, and impulsivity are the target symptoms which have been traditionally considered to warrant psychostimulant medication. The author's present studies (as yet unpublished) suggest that Ritalin may improve short-term auditory memory, short-term visual memory, visual-motor coordination, and compliance capacity. The instruments devised for these studies are designed not only to assess the effects of Ritalin on the aforementioned functions but also to quantify changes that may occur. As an initial dose, I commonly try either 5 mg of dextroamphetamine sulfate (Dexedrine) or 10 mg of methylphenidate hydrochloride (Ritalin). During the period of evaluation (two to three sessions), I obtain Steadiness Tester scores. This gives me a baseline curve. (It is rare for there to be more than a 10–15-percent variation among baseline scores.) I then have the mother bring the child early in the morning, get another Steadiness Tester score, and immediately afterward give a dose of one of the aforementioned medications. Repeat scores are obtained after 1, 2, 3, 4, and (if necessary) 5 hours. For the child who responds, there will be a decline in the total touch time as the medication helps him concentrate and maintain steadiness. A sample response curve is shown in Figure 10-1. If the dose has not been great enough, the Steadiness Tester will record no change. If the dose has been too high the child's score will be higher. Thus the physician can use objective criteria for monitoring medication. About 25 percent of children, in the author's experience, become more agitated no matter how small the dose of psy-

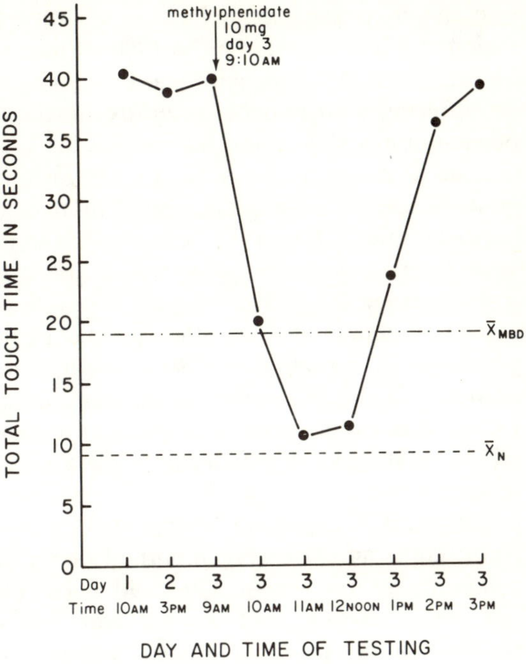

Figure 10–1. Response to psychostimulant medication as measured by the Steadiness Tester. This 10-year-old patient's total touch time averages 40.3 sec. The normal boy his age scores 8.80 ± 7.33 sec. The patient's score is 4.3 S.D. above the mean for normals and is far below the 10th percentile level for normal boys (10th percentile = 20.17 sec.). The average 10-year-old MBD boy scores 18.30 ± 17.45 sec. The patient's score is 1.26 S.D. above the MBD mean and is approximately at the 15th percentile level for MBD boys.

chostimulant medication. Such children's hyperactivity is probably not related to a concentration impairment. Rather, these children seem to have "revved up motors"; they appear to be "driven from within," and the medication only agitates them more. Educational tutoring by someone specifically trained to teach MBD children (either in the school system or privately) can also be useful, if a learning disability is present.

PSYCHOGENIC LEARNING DISABILITIES

Prior to the twentieth century, children who had difficulty learning in school were generally categorized as being either morons, imbeciles, or idiots. These forms of mental retardation were viewed as organic in etiology and were considered to represent either low levels on the bell-shaped curve of intellectual capacity or intellectual deficits due to brain disease. In the early part of the twentieth century, especially as a result of the psychoanalytic movement, many children's learning difficulties were considered to have a psychological etiology. This was especially the case for children whose learning problems were mild and who did not seem to show the massive degree of intellectual impairment seen in those traditionally considered to be mentally retarded. The psychogenic explanation reached its peak in the 1950s. Since that time, an ever-increasing percentage of children with learning problems have been considered to be suffering with minimal brain dysfunction. In the author's view, the pendulum has shifted too far back in the organic direction—so much so that we hear little today of the psychogenic learning disabilities. Yet this group of disorders is probably much more common than the organic learning disabilities. One of the reasons for the popularity of the MBD diagnosis is that psychostimulant medication can often be helpful, whereas, if the learning disorder is viewed as psychogenic, a time-consuming and expensive course of psychotherapy may be indicated. Unfortunately, the psychogenic learning disabilities appear to be becoming "extinct." This section will discuss some of the more common (but certainly not all) factors that can contribute to these psychological learning disorders and will suggest ways in which the primary care physician might be of help to such children.

First, it is important to appreciate that the family's attitude toward education is an extremely important factor in determining the children's committment to learning. The child whose parents hardly ever read, find little joy in learning, and rarely if ever show curiosity about the world is not likely to be strongly motivated to learn in school. If the parents view the school as a place where the law requires all children to be until their mid-teens and think that the best thing one can do is tolerate it until one is free to remove oneself, then the child is not likely to learn very much. In such family settings there may be little, if anything, that physicians can do, and they do well to recognize their impotence here. Sometimes a child therapist, who has the opportunity to work with such a child over a long period of time, can be helpful. Probably more successful would be a series of teachers, each of whom enjoys learning and thereby serves as a model for the child's identification and emulation. Unfortunately such teachers are not too common—there are only a small percentage in most school systems—so this chance of help is lost to most children.

Poor school performance can be a manifestation of a hostility problem. Children who are very angry at their parents may find that school failure is an excellent way to hurt them. Most healthy parents get pride in their children's doing well in school and are disappointed when they do poorly. Children who are inhibited in overtly expressing anger toward their parents may release their anger through school failure. In this way, they hide from themselves the fact that they are being hostile to their parents and thereby protect themselves from the guilt they would suffer and reprisals they anticipate they would receive were they to express their resentment overtly. The physician does well to try to ascertain, by means of interviews with both the child and the parents (alone and in family sessions), what the sources of the anger are. Physicians do well also to help such children feel less guilty about their anger and express it in more direct and appropriate ways. Family interviews, especially when older siblings are involved, can be very helpful here. Such children have to be helped, as well, to appreciate that in order to gain the gratifications of this type of vengence, they must blind themselves to how self-destructive they are being in the process.

Some parents are overcommitted to the educational process. Often such parents have not had the opportunity to reach their own educational goals and hope to satisfy their aspirations vicariously through their children. Other parents, who actually have reached their educational objectives, wish their children to be involved in an academic program to an inordinate degree. Such parents may place undue pressures on their children to excel in school. And the children may rebel by doing poorly. These parents are even better targets for hostility than are parents with the average degree of committment to education. As is true of all children with educational problems, it is useful to get an IQ score. The Wechsler Intelligence Scale for Children–Revised is probably the best and most widely used IQ test. If the child's intelligence is in the below average or average range, parental pressures are even more inappropriate. In any case, the physician should try to help such parents relax and pull back. The children of pressuring parents may become very perfectionistic, and may not tolerate even occasional mistakes. Such perfectionism may stem from the parents' intolerance for error and their inability to admit deficiencies within either themselves or their children. In such cases, family interviews may be useful in helping all become more comfortable with human imperfection.

Parental overprotection can contribute to children's poor school performance. There are parents who check their children's homework in order to detect errors in advance so that they will be protected from getting lower grades on their homework assignments than they might otherwise get. Others go further and almost *do* the homework for the child. This is a terrible disservice to the child. Children are much more likely to be motivated to do well if they have some mild (but not paralyzing) fear of poor performance. In addition, children are much more likely to master material when they have to do it on their own. Ideally, parents do well to be available to help their children learn how to do the work on their own. This is truly what education is all about. An old proverb says it well: "Give a man a fish and you've given him a meal. Teach a man how to fish and you've given him a meal for life."

Overprotective parents can contribute to their children's learning problems in other ways. The parents may deny that their child is anything but perfect and explain all criticisms away with rationalizations such as

"The teacher has it in for him," "She just won't see how bright he is," and "She's prejudiced." With parental denial, the child is not confronted with deficits and is not likely to correct many of them. Some overprotective parents may profess interest in their childrens' progressing academically, but unconsciously they may really want the opposite because they may dread the day when the child finally leaves the home. As a result, their committment to the child's academic progress is ambivalent. Their ambivalence may be reflected in a relatively mild concern over failures; basically, they do not want the child to reach the point of self-sufficiency, their statements to the contrary notwithstanding. Other overprotective parents indulge every illness, keep the child home from school over the slightest physical complaint, and thereby contribute to academic deficiency. The physician should try to help overprotective parents gain insight into the ways they are contributing to their children's academic difficulties. Here, direct work with the child alone is not likely to be successful. The child is often so comfortable with the pampering that he or she is not likely to be motivated to change. Accordingly, the treatment is likely to be successful only if the parents change.

Another factor that can contribute to psychogenic learning disabilities is a family atmosphere of suppression (conscious) and repression (unconscious) of feelings. All physically and psychologically healthy children have unbounded curiosity and freely express their feelings. There are parents who suppress these displays either overtly or covertly. They may communicate to the child that such expression is unacceptable in "fine and proper" households, and that only cruder people are so open and free with their feelings: "Big boys and girls don't cry" (even at funerals); "Nice people don't talk so loud"; "Children should be seen and not heard"; and "Don't ask so many questions. Don't you know it's not polite?" Such parents may serve as models for emotional inhibition as well. They may rarely, if ever, fight. All frustrations are handled with a facade of equanimity. It is no surprise, then, that the children of such parents will not exhibit the curiosity and spontaneity so crucial to a rich and successful educational experience. They may do better in such subjects as science and mathematics, where the expression of feelings is not only frowned upon but may be considered to interfere with learning. But in such subjects as literature, drama, poety, music, and art—where emotional expression is crucial—their inhibitions may interfere significantly. The physician should try to help the parents of such children appreciate how stultifying their attitudes are. However, he or she does well not to expect significant changes since these personality traits are deep-seated and have been many years in the making.

Space has permitted the discussion of only a few of the more common types of psychogenic learning disabilities, and even these have been discussed somewhat superficially. A more detailed discussion of this topic is presented elsewhere.[17]

SEPARATION ANXIETY DISORDER (SCHOOL PHOBIA)

Some children exhibit morbid dread and severe panic states when required to attend school. Usually there is a past history of some hesitation about going to school. The child may have complained of stomachaches, headaches, and the like in order to avoid going to school. Nevertheless, in spite of such procrastination, the child has managed to attend successfully. Then a specific traumatic event occurs—an event that threatens the security of the child's bond with a parent, usually the mother. The most common such traumas, in this author's experience, are maternal illness (especially when hospitalization is required); birth of a sibling; death of a significant relative; and parental divorce. Typically, the child provides endless rationalizations for fearing to attend school: For example, "The teacher is mean and yells a lot," "The kids there hit me," "The kids tease me," "The work is boring," "The bathroom smells," and "The food in the lunchroom is terrible." Although there may be varying degrees of truth to such complaints, other children are still attending. Attempts to convince the child that he or she is exaggerating these discomforts, or that they are nonexistent, prove futile. As fast as the parents and school personnel are able to refute these excuses, the child comes up with new ones. In addition (and this will be discussed further), children may express the fear that something terrible will happen to their mothers while they are in school.

The typical pattern is one in which the child provides a variety of excuses for refusing to get out of bed in the morning. Once out of the house, the closer the child gets to the school the greater the panic. Once in the school building, cries and blood-curdling shrieks may fill the halls. Teachers may come running out of their classrooms in fear that someone is being murdered. The panic element is often combined with a refusal factor. When the panic is predominant, the term *school phobia* is often used to describe the problem. When the refusal element predominates, then the term *school refusal* is warranted. An important diagnostic criterion for determining if a school phobia exists is whether the child still panics when the mother is allowed to remain with the child in the classroom. Generally, the school phobic child is not fearful of staying in school if the parent (usually the mother) is allowed to remain with him or her in the classroom. In fact, with the mother present all panic may be gone and the child may be able to function normally. This phenomenon has led most psychiatrists to the realization that the term *school phobia* is a misnomer. The child only appears to be afraid of the school (or the people in it). The real fear is separation from a parent (usually the mother). It is for this reason that the term *separation anxiety disorder* has recently been substituted and is the term used in the American Psychiatric Association's new edition of *Diagnostic and Statistical Manual of Mental Disorders* (DSM-III).[18] It is to be hoped that the new term will prevail.

Another common phenomenon observed in the families of children with this disorder is the parental overprotection, especially the mother's. These mothers may not let their children ride bicycles on streets where other children of the same age are permitted to ride. They may not let their children swim in water as deep as the water in which the child's peers are swimming. When their children are playing in the street they are ever observing, ever warning their children to be careful. Commonly, mothers of school phobic children view mothers of these other children as negligent and unloving. The basic message that such mothers are giving their children is, "The world is a dangerous place. I am the only one who can protect you from such dangers. If you stay ever at my side, no harm will befall you. If you are out of my sight, terrible things (even death) are likely to occur." This message may not be communicated directly, but it is certainly gotten across through the aforementioned behaviors. No surprise, then, that school becomes a threatening place. There the child is not only removed from the mother but such separation is enforced. There the child may feel that he or she is in a prison. The mother's overprotection usually feeds into the perpetuation of the symptoms, in that she may be very ambivalent herself about sending the child to school. She may be indulgent to the point of allowing the child to stay home with every minor physical complaint and may look upon parents who send their children to school under such circumstances as negligent of their own children's health and as exposing healthy classmates to dreaded diseases. She may consider the physician incompetent who recommends that these minor illnesses be ignored.

Interestingly, the fathers of these children are often passive individuals who view their wives as being very good mothers and thereby support, in a passive way, their wives' overprotectiveness. Another consequence of the overprotectiveness that contributes to the school problem is the narcissism that it engenders. These children are often viewed as "God's gift to the world" by their mothers, and they may develop the same opinion of themselves. Teachers and classmates, however, do not share this delusion and therefore treat the child as a mere human being. The pampered child may find this lack of respect and indulgence intolerable and may avoid school and remain home where he or she is more appreciated.

An important psychodynamic factor that contributes to these children's symptom is the repressed anger that they feel toward their mothers. These children have good reasons to be angry at their mothers. The overprotectiveness may serve as a reaction formation to the mother's basic desire to reject and abandon the child. Such hostility cannot be overtly exhibited by the mother. The overprotectivenss, however, provides her with an acceptable vehicle for the expression of such anger. Each time she envisions calamity befalling her child she is satisfying, in fantasy, her hostile wishes. Although presented as a fear, the basic imagery is still hostile. Each time she deprives the child of age-appropriate growth opportunities (under the guise of protecting him or her from danger), she satisfies her desire to restrict the child from pleasure. Although the child may not consciously appreciate that the mother's concerns are motivated more by hositility than love, the child does know that he or she leads a restricted life and suffers embarrassment and harassment in relationships with peers. This causes anger. But the anger cannot be easily expressed because of the risk of alienating the person whom the child has been taught to believe is necessary for his or her very existence. The child's hostility is then repressed and it exhibits itself in the excessive fear that something will happen to the mother. Having her ever by his or her side reassures the child that she is still alive, that hostile impulses toward her have not been realized in reality.[19,20] Although other psychodynamic factors are certainly operative, the aforementioned are the more important in producing the separation anxiety disorder.

The primary care physician may be able to treat mild cases of this type of separation anxiety disorder, but the more severe cases may require the help of a child psychiatrist. Of paramount importance in the treatment of such children is the physician's taking the strong positon that unless there is bona fide evidence for significant physical illness, the child must go to school each day. If the child is not able to tolerate remaining in school throughout the whole morning, he or she still must return for the afternoon session, and when at home the child must not be allowed to watch television or engage in other pleasurable activities. A minor tranquilizer like diazepam (Valium), in doses of 2–5 mg q2h may be useful. Such medication is given less for pharmacologic than for psychological value. I usually tell the child, "This medicine will help you become less scared of going to school. When you come here, after school hours, I will try to help you with this trouble." *After* school the therapist can discuss with the child and family the various psychological factors that are contributing to the child's illness. The mothers of these children are notoriously unreliable in following this advice. They will profess willingness to comply with the above recommendations, but they usually rationalize keeping the child home anyway. Accordingly, any insight they can be helped to gain regarding their own participation in the child's illness can be useful. The fathers may not be particularly useful here in that they tend to view their wives' protectiveness as desirable. The assistance of school personnel must also be enlisted. Without their cooperation it is not likely that the child will be quickly returned to school. The physician does well to appreciate that such cooperation may not be so quickly forthcoming, in that it is easier for the school to place the child on home instruction (an extremely antitherapeutic measure) than to suffer the hassles associated with trying to keep the child in school.

There are some who hold that the above approach is cruel, exposing the child as it does to enforced confrontation with the phobic situation. This program is indeed difficult for the child. However, in the long run it is undoubledly the more humane. Allowing the child to remain away from school until the problems are worked out may initially appear to be the more benevolent course. However, in practice if often results in a deepening of the pathology. Protected from the anxiety-provoking situation, the child becomes even less motivated to return to school and the problem becomes even more deeply entrenched. The enforced return (up to the point of panic) allows for desensitization to and increasing toleration for separation. In time the child comes to appreciate that separation from the mother does not result in her death, and more important, he or she comes to grow more independent of her. Allowing the child to remain at home (often with home tutors provided by the school in misguided benevolence) only deepens the pathological dependent tie with the mother. The therapy must not only help the child grow up but help the mother lessen her needs to be overprotective.

Gittleman-Klein reports imipramine (Tofranil) to be especially effective treatment for this pathlogical form of separation anxiety, especially where other methods have failed.[21,22] The doses needed are variable, although most children require at least 65 mg/day. A daily dose of 200 mg should not be exceeded. The drug can be given twice a day or at bedtime. Children usually respond in 6 to 8 weeks. The drug should be continued for 4 weeks after remission, then gradually withdrawn. Most children maintain their improvement. I agree that imipramine can be useful in ameliorating the panic symptomatology but consider working through the aforementioned psychogenic difficulties (especially the overprotection problem) crucial if one is to provide long-term alleviation of this kind of separation anxiety syndrome. The use of imipramine in the treatment of panic disorders in adults is discussed in Chapter 5.

In adolescence the picture may appear to be more one of a school refusal than a school phobia problem.[23] However, the refusal may be only a facade for the fears that the adolescent is less prone to reveal overtly. In such cases, the onset is usually more chronic and insidious and the prognosis much poorer. Without extensive psychiatric intervention the adolescent may ultimately drop out of school.

DIVORCE

In an age of an ever-increasing divorce rate, the primary physician is being increasingly consulted by separating parents regarding how to deal with the various problems with which they are confronted in their new situation. This section will focus on the counsel the physician can provide to help such parents alleviate and prevent psychopathological reactions in their children.

A common question that divorcing parents will ask is whether the divorce will be psychologically detrimental to their children. In response to this question, the author first advises parents that divorce per se is not necessarily so detrimental. The child of divorce, however, is at greater risk for the development of untoward psychological reactions than the child living in an intact and relatively stable home. With regard to whether the child of divorce is at greater risk for developing psychopathology than the child living in an intact but unstable home, no one can answer with certainty. Some children do better when the parents stay together, even though this involves ongoing exposure to and possible involvement with the parents' conflicts. We are dealing here with a choice between two undesirable alternatives, and it is inappropriate and even grandiose of anyone to say that he or she knows in advance which of the alternatives is worse.

The author's next advice to parents is that the way they relate to their children—at the time of and following the separation—is the main determinant of whether the children will suffer. If the separation is a relatively civilized one and the children are not brought significantly into the parental conflict, they may be spared psychological difficulty. If, however, they are exposed unduly to the parental strife, the children are probably going to suffer. In addition, the absent parent's involvement with the children *after* the separation is another important determinant of whether the children will develop pathology. If that parent is reliable and affectionate and if he or she maintains an ongoing, predictable, and loving relationship with the children, they are not likely to suffer. If, on the other hand, the absent parent does not maintain such a relationship with the children, they will suffer psychologically from the separation.

It is important for the physician to take a strictly neutral position regarding the question of whether or not the parents should separate. It is misguided benevolence to encourage people to stay together, whether for their own sakes or for the sake of the children. For some people the separation may be one of the healthiest decisions they have made, and urging them to stay together may result in the entrenchment of pathological ties. On the other hand, encouraging people to part because the physician views the relationship as extremely pathological may not be in the parties' best interests either. The pathological tie, as horrendous as it may appear, can sometimes provide a stablizing influence. Once separated, people who have developed such a tie are likely to find others who will provide the same neurotic—even psychotic—gratifications, A new liaison is then formed, and the main change that has occurred is that the children now have to live with a nonparent. Or the separation may result in psychological decompensation as the partners find themselves unable to function without the pathological tie. The counselor's job should be to help the individuals clarify the issues that are contributing to their wish to separate and to reduce and alleviate pathological behavior. With clarification and symptom reduction the individuals should be in a better position to make a judicious decision regarding whether to separate.

In advising separated parents, the physician does well to avoid providing two bits of common but, in the author's opinion, misguided advice: (1) one parent should never criticize the other to the children, and (2) the parent with whom the children live should always reassure them that the absent parent still loves them, even though he or she has left the home. With regard to the first statement, children generally do best in a home in which both parents are stable enough to admit their deficiencies to their children. We all do best when we view our parents realistically, as people with both assets and liabilities. To view one's parents as perfect makes it difficult to relate to other mere human beings who inevitably reveal their deficits. Such unfavorable comparisons are likely to result in difficulties with peers, spouses, employers, and employees, as well as others whom the individual may encounter. It can also contribute to dissatisfaction with oneself as one invariably exhibits imperfections that one believes one's parents do not possess. This principle holds whether the child grows up in an intact or a divorced home. Accordingly, both parents do well to try to help the child gain a balanced and accurate view of each other, and divorced parents do well to try to overcome their animosities in order to help their children gain such a realistic picture of each parent. And the physician can help with such clarification as well as encourage the parents to provide it.

Reassuring children that the absent parent still loves them is certainly warranted in most cases. But what about the situation, for example, in which a father has abandoned the household and has not been heard from in years? The mother who has been left behind may still reassure the children that their father still loves them from the belief that to tell them that he does not might be psychologically devastating. Such a mother is bound to disillusion her children as they ultimately come to realize that she has not been truthful with them. She is also likely to confuse them about love, because they have been told that love can exist without involvement. Such a mother does better to tell the children that their father does not love them. However, she should not stop there. She does well to tell the children that the defect lies within their father—the man who cannot or will not love. It does not lie within them, because they are lovable. She should then enumerate the people who do love the children. The children should also be encouraged to develop relations with others who can provide gratifications to compensate for the loss of their father.

But what about the more common situation, where there is no total abandonment but where the father, for example, is unreliable, does not show up when he promises, and only sporadically sends presents yet still wants, on occasion, to see the children? The children of such fathers have to be helped to appreciate that love is not a yes–no proposition. It is not like the on–off switch of the electric light. Rather it is like the dimmer and can range from very little to very much. They have to be helped to appreciate that such a father is limited in the degree to which he can provide affection. They have to assert themselves and try to gain as much love and affection as their father can provide, and they must be discouraged from trying to extract more than he is capable of giving. They then have to involve themselves in other relations that are more promising. Again, they have to be helped to appreciate that the defect lies within the parent, not within themselves.

Space does not permit a detailed description here of the many problems for which divorcing parents may need counseling. The interested reader can find such a description elsewhere.[24] Because telling children about a separation raises issues that it is helpful to explore when counseling parents with regard to other problems of divorce, this section will focus on four questions in this area that parents commonly ask.

How Old Should the Children Be Before Being Told?

All the children, regardless of age, should be told together. To exclude younger children because "they won't understand" is to risk engendering distrust of the parents at a time when the children can least afford to become distrustful. Being excluded from a conversation, or finding out that one has been excluded, is bound to produce feelings of resentment and distrust. Of course, with children of different ages present, the explanation may have to be repeated to suit their varying levels of comprehension. Less important than the child's full understanding of what is being told is the experience that the parents are open and honest, that the atmosphere is one in which revelations are made openly and questions are answered directly. If a parent chooses not to answer a question, he or she should, directly and honestly, give a reasonable explanation for not providing a response. As the younger children grow older, as they become more capable of understanding what they are being told, they will have the ongoing experience that their questions will be answered.

When Should the Children Be Told?

The younger the child, the less capable he or she is of appreciating the passage of time. To tell younger children very far in advance (a few months, for example) about an impending separation is not very meaningful. The child is not likely to appreciate such a time span. Because the event is then viewed as occurring at some time in the remote future, it is more likely that denial mechanisms will begin to operate. But to provide too short notice (as one parent is ready to leave the house with packed bags, for example), does not provide the children with sufficient time for adjustment and working through their reactions. The optimum time, in the author's opinion, is a few weeks before the actual separation. This is not long enough to encourage denial and not short enough to deprive the children of time to work through their initial reactions and begin the adjustment process. Older children can be given longer advance notice, but denial mechanisms may still operate—sometimes even after the departure.

Who Should Tell the Children?

Ideally both parents *together* should tell the children. In this way they both establish for themselves the reputation of being the providers of information. It is not simply the immediate task of giving information that is important to accomplish here. The parents also want to get across the message that they will both be available for subsequent discussion (so vital to the working-through process), even though one parent will no longer be living in the household. Such ongoing discussions are invaluable in preventing a host of untoward psychological reactions that children of divorce may exhibit.

What Should the Children Be Told?

The children should be told the major reasons for the separation. All too often parents hide this information, frequently rationalizing such withholding with reasons like, "They're too young to understand," "It's better that they don't know," and "It will upset them too much." Sometimes specious explanations are given, explanations that really provide no real new information. To tell the children, for example, that "Mommy and Daddy are going to get a divorce because we don't love each other any more," provides no new information. Obviously, at least one of the parties doesn't love the other (and possibly both have little or no affection for one another), or else there would be no separation. It's like saying, "They buried Mr. Jones today because he was dead." Parents often cover up in this way because they are ashamed of revealing certain details or actually believe that such withholding will protect their children from psychological trauma. Such parents do not seem to appreciate that they are doing their children more harm than good by their failure to disclose the major reasons for the separation.

First, the children usually sense that they are not being given all the vital information and this can increase feelings of distrust of the parents. A parent is soon to abandon them (as the children view it); adding further sources of distrust is unwarranted and unnecessary. It is common for children to develop delusions that the divorce was their fault. One contributing factor to this notion is the failure of the parents to provide the real reasons. There is a kind of mourning that many (if not most) children of divorce must experience if they are to adjust optimally to the separation. (Although this mourning is not identical to mourning when a parent has died, there are similarities.[24]) Just as it is impossible to truly mourn if one does not know whether or not the loved one has died, the post-separation mourning process is impeded if significant information is not provided. This is not to suggest that every single detail of the parents' personal lives be given. The parents still have a right to certain privacies. But the major reasons for the separation must be given.

Many children have been helped by reading *The Boys and Girls Book About Divorce,* which is written at the child's level of comprehension and provides explanations and advice for many of the more common problems that children of divorce face.[25] Its companion, *The Parents Book About Divorce,* has been useful to many parents, and the primary care practitioner may find much in the latter book that may be useful to him or her in counseling divorcing parents.[26]

DEATH OF A PARENT

The death of a parent is one of the greatest traumas that can befall a child. And the younger the child, the greater the likelihood that the child will suffer untoward psychological reactions. A child whose parent has died will not automatically suffer psychopathological reactions, but such a child is at increased risk for the development of such difficulties. The main determinants of whether such children will exhibit psychological problems are the way the death itself is handled by the child and the way the surviving parent deals with the child afterwards. In both of these areas the physican's advice can be useful.

Helping children deal with the imminent death of a parent cannot be separated from the question of how the dying parent is dealing with his or her forthcoming demise. The way one deals with the child depends on whether denial mechanisms are being utilized to a significant degree or the parent is openly discussing his or her death. When the dying parent uses denial, it behooves the nearest of kin to help support such an adjustment. To do otherwise is, in the author's opinion, cruel. I am not in agreement with those who claim that all dying people are better off openly discussing their illness. Some are better off and others are not. True respect for the patient involves respecting his or her wishes regarding the handling of the death, rather than imposing a theory of what the physician believes would be best. If the dying parent is denying, the adults generally can be relied upon not to reveal the true prognosis; the child, however, cannot be so relied on. In such situations the child usually should be told exactly what the dying parent has been told: "It's chronic inflammation," "They got it all out," "The radiation treatments are going to work," and so on. Although this method of dealing with the parent's death does little for the child, it does protect the parent from the danger that his or her denial mechanisms will be jeopardized by a child's disclosure of the illness's true prognosis.

In the situation in which the parent is openly discussing death, it is most often useful to draw the child into the discussion. In this way the child is provided with the opportunity to experience what is sometimes referred to as "anticipatory mourning." In this process the child is protected from the acute shock of the death; he or she is eased into adjustment to the loss. Piecemeal desensitization is a far better way to cope with a trauma than to do it "all at once." Also, the emotional expression attendent to such anticipation is likely to be salutory. Parents who believe that they are doing their children a service by protecting them from such disclosure are really doing their children a disservice. Such "coverups" can be psychologically detrimental to the children. The conspiracy of silence not only deprives children of the aforementioned benefits to be derived from anticipatory mourning and predeath working through but, worse, creates an atmosphere of distrust. The older the children, the more likely they will come to appreciate that important information is being withheld from them. This creates an atmosphere of distrust at a time when the child can least afford to have such an experience. The forthcoming death will be traumatic enough. It is adding an unnecessary burden to the child to bring about distrust of the surviving parent. The physician does well, therefore, to encourage the family to give the child this important information and to provide, as well, the opportunity for discussion, desensitization, and working through.

The question of whether the child should attend the funeral is often asked. There are times (such as when the death is by accident) that rational discussion of the matter is almost impossible. Some family members are insistent that the children not attend because they believe that the experience will just add another psychological trauma. Others firmly hold that the child attend. In general, the child should be *invited* to attend both the services and the burial. If the child refuses (rarely, in the author's experience) this refusal should be respected. For young children, it is best to bring along someone who is not that close to the family—someone who can watch over the children and remove any who might be disruptive.

There are a number of important reasons for the child's attending the funeral. Children are concrete; they learn far better from direct experience than explanations. To actually see the coffin (and possibly the exposed dead body) and to see it lowered into the ground provides the child with a very concrete experience of what has happened to the parent. The exposure helps the child accept death's finality, a crucial appreciation if healthy mourning is to occur. At the funeral the child will have the best opportunity to observe the mourners expressing their sadness and grief. Such observations make it more likely that the child will freely express his or her own feelings, the suppression and/or repression of which not only interferes with successful mourning but may contribute to the development of psychopathological reactions to the death as well. Parents who believe that the child's attending the funeral will cause psychological trauma are only seemingly benevolent. By protecting the child from the discomforts of attending they are contributing to the development of untoward reactions.

Another common form of misguided benevolence is the surviving parent's not being truthful with the child in regard to the hereafter. A common way of dealing with the situation is to tell the child that the deceased parent is in heaven and leading a pleasant and even happy life there. I have no strong objection to this if the parent has the genuine conviction that this is the case. The parent, however, who does not really believe this but tells the child this story in order to protect him or her from a more painful explanation, is doing the child a disservice. The parent's lack of conviction may be detected by the child, and this will engender distrust and confusion. The death of a parent, in itself, produces distrust in that the child feels abandoned and is not likely to fully appreciate that the deceased parent wished the child no pain and loneliness. Such contrived explanations may produce additional, unnecessary distrust. The physician does best to encourage the surviving family to tell the child exactly what they believe regarding the hereafter. They should describe exactly what they envision it to be. If they have no belief in afterlife, they should say so. If they are unsure, they should say that. Since the child may be hearing different opinions on this subject, it is usually helpful to tell children that it is understandable that they will be confused by these different explanations and that as they grow older they will be in a better position to decide for themselves what theory seems most reasonable to them.

Parents do well to appreciate that it is extremely important that children be given every opportunity for open expression of their feelings about the death. The parent who says, "Big boys and girls don't cry," and "See how brave you can be" is likely to contribute to suppression of feelings. The surviving relatives who praise a bereaved mother, for example, with such comments as "Mary's holding up well," are presenting for the child an unhealthy model for emulation. It is also important for the family members to appreciate that healthy children are by nature playful and optimistic and may not exhibit the degree of grief and depression that the adults deem appropriate. To chastise children with a comment like, "How can you laugh and joke at a time like this? Why your father's body isn't even cold in the grave," is likely to produce unwarranted guilt and add to the child's burden at this unfortunate time in his or her life. Adults must also appreciate that some children may work through their reactions to death through the vehicle of play. By playing such games as "hospital," "accident," and "funeral," the child is attempting to adjust to the loss.

In the early phases following the death, the child may exhibit denial. Denial is one of the more primitive mental mechanisms, and children almost universally utilize it. Sigmund Freud describes a boy who said, "I know father's died, but what I can't understand is why he doesn't come home for supper."[27] One can simply hope that, with the passage of time and the continuing experience of the absence of the parent, such mechanisms will no longer be utilized. Anger reactions are also common. All of us have some angry feelings toward a loved one who died "on us." The more loving the relationship, the greater the loss and sense of frustration, and the greater the likelihood that angry feelings toward the deceased will be present—even though we appreciate that the deceased did not wish to abandon us. And the child is no different. Accordingly, angry reactions should be tolerated, and the child should not be made to feel guilty over them.

It is the ultimate aim of the working-through process that the child not only accept the reality of the death, but recognize that life goes on and that his or her life can still be a gratifying one in spite of the loss. This is more likely to happen if the child both gains gratifications from the surviving family members and substitutes both present and future relationships for that with the dead parent. In the service of helping children reach this goal, the reader may find it useful to provide children in this situation with reading material such as *The Boys and Girls Book About One-Parent Families*.[28] A more complete theoretical discussion of children's dealing with parental death is presented elsewhere.[29]

ADOLESCENT ANTISOCIAL ACTING OUT

Before physicians can counsel acting-out adolescents and their parents, it is important that they understand some of the basic psychological conflicts with which the adolescent is dealing.

Identity

The adoescent is part child and part adult—not completely either. The adolescent would like to believe that he or she is an adult, but reality factors force lingering doubts about his or her exact status. The physician should avoid falling into the trap of viewing the adolescent as an adult just because of physical maturity. He or she does best to view the adolescent as having the body of an adult and the mind of a child.

In order to help solve this problem of what he or she is, the adolescent tries to establish a separate identity from parents. Accordingly, we see special styles of dress and language that quickly identify the adolescent as different. Special tastes in music may also be used to establish this separate identity. In our society, the healthy adolescent establishes an identity as a "good student," a "good athlete," a "good musician," or as someone who gets along well with others and has many friends. If, because of personality problems in the formative years, the youngster is not successful in attaining a healthy identity in at least one of these important areas, he or she may resort to obtaining an identity somewhat quickly, an identity that is likely to produce a sense of notoriety: for example, he or she may become "The kid who's always in trouble with police," "The biggest flirt (or slut) in school," "The one who set all those fires," or "The guy who's on drugs." The heavy price paid for the label is well worth it because of the compensatory gratification it provides.

Dependence versus Independence

Because the adolescent is half way between being a child and an adult, he or she is confused regarding dependence on parents. The adolescent is big enough to fend for himself or herself physically but unprepared to take on the responsibilities of adulthood because he or she has not had the opportunity to attain the skills necessary to function in our highly complex social structure. The youngster would like to be and feel independent but lacks the wherewithal to be so. Rebellion is one way to achieve a sense of independence. One way is to eschew parental values, religion, life styles, and so on. In a sense this is healthy. If not for such adolescent rebellion, we might all still be living in caves. The physician must help the adolescent differentiate healthy from unhealthy rebellion. He or she must support the former and discourage the latter and must help the youngster's parents to make similar distinctions.

Potency versus Impotence

The adolescent feels weak in comparison to adults. A boy may be as strong if not stronger than his father, but is still weaker with regard to his ability to cope with the complex world into which he would like to venture. Rebellion provides a sense of power to compensate for this impotence. Anger and rage can also provide a feeling of power, as can antisocial behavior.

Adolescents are very much group persons. They are slavishly dependent on the opinions of their peers, their professions of independent thinking notwithstanding. The group provides them with clues as to what methods of rebellion and independent style are in vogue. The group provides them with the strength that they alone do not possess. Antisocial groups may provide "loner" types with the first "friends" they have had. It is in early adolescence that the fringe youngster first forms strong group affiliations. There the friendless find others who have been similarly unsuccessful in gaining a sense of self-worth. The price of admission to such groups of people on this fringe of the mainstream is generally a willingness to overcome one's fears and hesitations about involving oneself in some form of antisocial behavior. Such involvement is often regarded as a small price to pay for a cessation of loneliness and social alienation.

Helping Parents Deal with Adolescent Antisocial Acting Act

The physician does well to inquire into possible sources of a youngster's anger. Perhaps the parents are being too punitive. Or they may be pressuring a youngster inappropriately. For example, divorced parents may be treating each other in the most primitive fashion and serving thereby as models for their child's acting out. It is unrealistic to expect youngsters to discontinue their acting-out behavior when their parents are still involved in their own. Or, one parent may be using the child as a weapon against the other (again, often the case in divorce situations). Unless one deals with the parental contribution, one is not likely to help the child. Often family interviews can be useful in bringing to the surface such parental involvement in the adolescent's acting out.

In working with the parents of these youngsters it is useful for them to become firmly committed to the advice of Reinhold Niebuhr:

> O God, give us serenity to accept what cannot be changed,
> courage to change what should be changed,
> and wisdom to distinguish the one from the other.[30]

Parents have very little control over their adolescent's companions outside the home, but they do have the power to decide who shall come into their home. They cannot stop a youngster from using drugs outside the home, but they can certainly confiscate (by flushing down the toilet in front of the youngster) what they find in the home. Although the adolescent's right to privacy is generally important to respect, when it comes to harboring illegal substances, drawers should be freely searched. However, parents should be discouraged from making fools of themselves by calling up the homes of their adolescent's friends, at all hours of the night, trying to find the youngster. This not only irritates the neighbors, but causes the parents unnecessary humiliation as well. But, most important, it perpetuates the antisocial behavior because it provides the youngster with the hostile gratification he seeks.

Parents should be helped to differentiate between innocuous and destructive forms of antisocial behavior. They should provide youngsters who exhibit harmless forms of acting out with the negative verbal and gestural feedback they crave, but nothing else. If they react too punitively to the innocuous behavior, the adolescent may resort to the more destructive. In the 1960s, long hair came into vogue as a method of rebellion for adolescent boys. The person (or persons) who introduced this style should have been awarded the Nobel peace prize. It was one of the most innocent forms of rebellion ever invented. Wise parents at that time recognized it for what it was, provided their youngsters with the disgust reactions they craved and thereby lessened the likelihood that the youngsters would utilize destructive and/or dangerous forms of rebellion.

Many communities (especially the larger ones) have facilities for the placement (either short-term or long-term) of incorrigible youngsters. The most common of these are hospitals, residential treatment centers, and foster homes. These facilities are generally used for adolescents who have not committed bona fide civil crimes; rather they exhibit little or no respect for parental and/or school authorities. They are in constant trouble and give their parents or teachers little or no peace. Although communities vary with regard to the steps to be taken for the placement of such youngsters, the parents usually have to initiate the process. The physician should not pressure parents to do this. Rather he or she should learn about the nature of the local facilities and the steps that need to be taken for placement. This information should be given to the parents and youngster. Merely providing such information can sometimes serve as a deterrent to antisocial behavior. When, and only when, the parents have reached the point at which they can no longer tolerate the adolescent's behavior they should take steps to have the child placed. Most parents are going to feel significant guilt over such a step. It is only when the pain of the youngster's remaining in the home becomes great that they will be willing to tolerate such guilt. And only they can know when this point is reached.

Generally, there is a two-step process to such placement. The first involves psychiatric and psychological evaluation as well as interviews with a social worker. The second involves an appearance before a judge who must then render a decision. Sometimes a warning is given, sometimes therapy is ordered (which is not often useful if it must be ordered), and sometimes placement for observation is ordered. (It is rare for long-term placement to be ordered early in the youngster's career). Because of the usual slowness of most bureaucracies, this process usually drags on for months, even years. In many cases, such delays prolong the parents' burden. However, in the less severe cases the delays are useful. They serve as a deterrent to the youngster's antisocial behavior in that he or she generally fears the judge and the courtroom scene. Only a small percentage of such children actually end up in placement. The whole system, however, is most therapeutic in that it serves to provide strength for the parents. It is a clear message to the youngster that his or her parents are not impotent, and that when they have exhausted their own resources to limit the antisocial behavior they can resort to agencies outside the home, agencies that have the power to restrain the youngster in a meaningful way. Although no actual therapy (in the formal sense) is provided by the application process and the court appearance, it is definitely therapeutic. This may be the only therapy that such youngsters may have in that many refuse treatment and those who are ordered to receive it are not likely to gain much (if anything) from it under such circumstances.

When an antisocial adolescent is to be brought before a court for illegal (as opposed to incorrigible) behavior, the parents often engage the services of an attorney. If the latter is like the overwhelming majority of lawyers, he or she will do everything possible to get the clients "off." Lawyers may try to discredit the veracity of witnesses, if they possibly can. They may try to prove that their client was not involved. The "better" the attorney, the more ingenious will be his or her ways of protecting the client from punishment. Such attorneys are doing antisocial youngsters a terrible disservice. They are only encouraging perpetuation of the antisocial behavior. The more times they are successful in this regard, the more deeply the problems are likely to become entrenched. Parents do better to get an attorney who will protect their youngster's rights but encourage the judge to impose the fine or penalty that is usual and proper for the particular crime—no more and no less. This is the best way to discourage repetition of such behavior.

Helping the Antisocial Adolescent

Crucial to counseling such youngsters is the development of a good relationship. If the adolescent does not basically respect and admire the physician, it is not likely that he or she will be able to be of much help to such a youngster. The primary physician has an advantage here over the psychiatrist to whom the physician may be inclined to refer the patient. The psychiatrist is, at first, at a great disadvantage in helping such youngsters because he does not have the prerequisite relationship. The family physician often has just the kind of relationship that may serve as the basis for effective counseling.

In family interviews (often useful in such counseling), physicians do well to establish for themselves the reputation of being equally receptive to taking the side of the youngster and the side of the parents. Otherwise they will be viewed as the parent's ally against the youngster and little will be gained. They should not, however, be artificial. They should strictly support the healthy position, regardless of who exhibits it; and criticize unhealthy behavior—again, regardless of who manifests it.

The physician should try to help antisocial youngsters appreciate that in their desire to hurt their parents they must be blind to the harm they are doing themselves. A typical comment in this regard might be: "Let's say that you're 100 percent successful in hurting your parents. You have them writhing on the floor, tearing their hair out, and crying in pain over what you've done to them. Yes, you've gotten vengeance. But what you don't appreciate is the price you're paying for such gratification. You're ruining your own life in order to enjoy your vengeance. Someday they'll be dead and gone. And where will you be with your vengeance? You'll have given up your education for it. You've already been in trouble with the police, and no one but you can determine how much more trouble you'll have with them. What a price to pay for vengeance!"

The treatment of such youngsters may be quite difficult; psychiatrists themselves cannot claim a great rate of success in therapy with antisocial youngsters. If referral is warranted, the physician does well to refer to someone who has an adolescent group. As mentioned, adolescents are very much group persons and exquisitely sensitive to the opinions of their peers. Accordingly, they will take advice from peers that they might not so readily take from the therapist, whom they view as an adult like their parents and thus not to be trusted. Peers, in a therapy group, may take on a maturity that they do not actually possess and may preach what they do not actually practice. In the traditional individual session, adolescents may be very uncomfortable. They may not wish to spend 45–50 minutes talking about themselves. In the group they can talk when they wish and be silent when they are so inclined. Silences then do not cause them discomfrot because there is likely to be someone else who will speak up and fill the silence.

The reader interested in more detailed descriptions of psychotherapeutic treatment of antisocial children would do well to refer the works of Redl and Wineman, [31] Bettelheim, [32] and Holmes.[33]

EATING DISORDERS

Obesity

Obesity problems are extremely common in twentieth-century America, and it is no surprise that children as well should suffer with this disorder (although less commonly than adults). Although there have always been (and may always be) those who hold that obesity is primarily a physical problem, as long as the theory of conversation of mass (matter can neither be created nor destroyed, but it can be changed from one form into another) holds up, the author will consider obesity to be primarily a psychogenic problem. In short, since matter cannot be created from nothing, people cannot get fat unless they eat excessively. Even in rare metabolic disorders associated with obesity, the individual must still eat in order to provide the molecules to make the fatty tissue. If one views obesity as a psychiatric problem, treatment with diet alone is not likely to help. One must look into the psychological problems that are at the root of the problem. It is through alleviating these that one has the greatest chance of helping such patients.

In looking for the pyschological sources of obesity problems in children, one does well to investigate the family. In many families, heavy eating is a part of the living pattern. Mother routinely cooks large meals as a matter of course and may never have given thought to the possiblity of providing less. All family members are overweight. Putting such a child on a diet is ludicrous. Yet changing such a family pattern may also be impossible. In such cases there may be little that can be done for the obese child.

A common source of obesity in children is maternal overprotection. Although there are many factors involved in maternal overprotection, an important one is compensation for maternal inadequacy, either real or feared. The mother who feels basically inadequate (either consciously or unconsciously) may try to compensate for her deficiency by overfeeding her child. The fat, well-fed baby is a symbol to her and to the world (as she views it) that she is a good, loving, concerned mother. The worst possible thing for such mothers is a skinny baby, one who clearly has not been well fed. Again, working directly with such children, or simply placing them on a diet is not likely to be successful. One must try to help the mothers gain confidence in themselves as mothers and overcome their feelings of inadequacy. They must be helped to see that stuffing children with food is not a bona fide way of demonstrating one's maternal capacity and that, to the contrary, the sensitive observer considers it a sign of maternal inadequacy. If such a mother can be helped, then it is more likely that the child will be helped.

Food lends itself well to symbolizing mother's love. Mother is the first and primary source of food, and it is reasonable for the child to associate food with mother's affection. Even the child without an overprotective mother may utilize this compensatory method of gaining mother's affection in a symbolic way. But the child with a mother who overfeeds is even more likely to use food as a substitute for affection.

Some mothers contribute to the problem by using false criteria for determining whether the child should eat. They may decide that the child must eat a certain number of meals and snacks per day if it is to be healthy. When a mother says, "It's time to eat," she is using the clock on the wall as the criterion for eating rather than hunger pangs within the child's stomach. Similarly, when she says, "You haven't eaten enough food," she is also using external criteria for making a decision about an event which lies primarily within the child. This is not to suggest that we dispense with the concept of mealtime altogether, but rather that the too frequent use of such external criteria for when a child should eat can cause the child to ignore internal cues for eating and come to rely on external ones. As Bruch has pointed out, many obese people rely on such external cues, do not necessarily eat when they are hungry and, sometimes, even say that they are hungry when they are not.[34]

In some families the concepts of big, strong, and powerful are associated with being fat; whereas smallness, weakness, and impotence are associated with being thin. In such families terms like "big and fat" are heard as well as comments like, "He's a skinny weakling." This notion goes beyond family idiosyncrasy. Business moguls and tycoons are generally envisioned as being corpulent. With such programming the child may view his or her obesity as a source of protection and power. Such children may feel strong when obese and taking off weight may symbolize susceptibility to attack and inability to defend themselves. Obviously trying to convince such a child to lose weight is likely to prove futile unless some of the aforementioned distortions about weight, protection, and power are corrected.

Eating can provide pleasure. One need only look at the euphoric expression on the face of the just-fed baby. Children who are unhappy may resort to food as a method of compensation. Most of us do this to some extent, but the obese child is addicted to food because other pleasures are not forthcoming. In such cases, one has to help the child deal with the underlying problems that are causing unhappiness. As a euphoria-producing substance, food shares much in common with the narcotics. Both can be psychologically addicting. And like the narcotics, food can desensitize one to pain. Again, it is only by reducing the pain that one is likely to lessen the child's need to use food as an analgesic. Narcotics are also tranquilizers. Children may use food to lessen unpleasant feelings of anxiety and tension. One must try to help the child reduce tensions and anxieties if one is to lessen the need to use foods as a tranquilizer. The latter use of food is one of the more common and can be particularly difficult to deal with because life (even for the relatively stable) is so filled with tensions and anxieties.

As can be seen, many factors can contribute to a child's becoming obese. We have focused here on some of the more common ones. The primary treatment approach must utilize information about the underlying psychodynamic factors that are causing the obesity. Diet is indicated but is not likely to be effective if the basic problems are not dealt with. The sight and smell of foods makes eating particularly tempting, and so every reasonable effort should be made to reduce such exposure. Rather than specifying a particular diet, however, the author generally suggests that a mother restrict the eating of sweets and other high-caloric foods. Strict diets promote power struggles, which should be avoided lest they add to the child's misery and thereby increase the likelihood that he or she will eat excessively. Most important to avoid are crash diets. These are not only medically unhealthy but promulgate the notion that once a certain lower weight has been reached the child will then be able to return to the previous eating habits. The child and the family have to be helped to appreciate that keeping one's weight low is a life-time battle and requires a basic reorientation toward eating.

Anorexia Nervosa

Anorexia means a lack of appetite that may result from any cause, physical or psychological. *Nervosa* suggests a psychogenic (or "nervous") type of anorexia, but the term *anorexia nervosa* usually refers to a specific type of psychogenic eating disturbance that can be so severe that the patient may literally starve to death. The term *anorexia* is misleading because the failure to eat less often reflects loss of appetite than it does factors that have little to do with hunger. The disorder is much more common in girls; in fact, it is extremely rare in boys. (Accordingly, for ease of presentation I will refer to these patients in the feminine gender.)

Typically, the symptoms begin in the pubertal period. In full-blown cases the girl becomes obsessed with losing weight, and no matter how thin she is, she is still not satisfied. Reassurances by others that she is not too fat are usually of no avail. The youngster is ever on a diet, is preoccupied with the caloric content of every food ingested, and hardly speaks of anything else. The food-weight issue becomes an all-consuming obession. But the girl is not alone in her deliberations over what she should and should not eat. Her parents (especially the mother) also get drawn into the problem. Typically, the mother is also constantly involved in trying to get the girl to eat. Every possible method is utilized—bribery, threats, and trickery. Power struggles become the family pattern, as the child manages to thwart every attempt to get her to eat. A common maneuver of such a youngster is to say that she is in the mood to eat a certain food and if the mother would only prepare that food, she would eat every bit. After the mother has prepared the particular food (often in great haste and at no small expenditure of time and energy), the child calmly states that she has changed her mind and no longer feels like eating that particular food or any other food either. Worse, the parents may be sent out at all hours of the night searching for a place where a particular food can be purchased. Again, when the food is finally obtained the child blithely decides that she no longer feels like eating.

It is important for the physician to understand some of the basic psychodynamic factors that contribute to this disorder if he or she is to deal properly with it. One factor involves fear of sexual development. The reduction in food intake generally impedes breast growth and the development of subcutaneous fat that produces sexually attractive curvaciousness. This lessens the likelihood that boys will be attracted to the girl. Cessation of menses, or failure to initiate menstrual cycles is also accomplished by the anorexia. But it is not simply sexual fears that are dealt with by the anorexia. A general fear of growing up is also contributing to the problem. The anorexia can interfere with the height and weight gain that is part of the process of maturing into adulthood. The symptom serves other purposes as well. An important one is the expression of hostility. Refusing to eat is a good way to upset parents, especially if they are excessively involved in the child's eating patterns (a common parental manifestation in these families). And the various maneuvers that tantalize the parents also serve as vehicles for hostile expression. Power over the parent is gained. Rather then being dependent children, totally in the power of the parents, these girls literally enslave their parents. By what they do (or promise to do) with food they can manipulate their parents into granting any wish or performing any service. Their ambivalence over what they will eat and their parents' involvement in their deliberations gain them a degree of attention and parental involvement that they would probably not otherwise enjoy.

Lastly, they gain a sense of control over what most consider to be a relatively uncontrollable aspect of their lives. Most girls resign themselves to the way their bodies will develop. Within reason they accept the fact that they will be of a certain height and weight, will have a certain breast size, will or will not have those body configurations that are generally considered sexually attractive, and will menstrate. Most accept the fact that there is only minimal to moderate control over these factors. Anorexic girls cannot tolerate leaving these matters to nature. They must control these functions themselves. All these factors (and there are others, but we have focused upon the most important and common) can produce such a severe psychiatric disorder that the child may starve herself to death. Interestingly, in the terminal stages, these young girls often exhibit a grandiose delusion that no matter how low their weight goes, they will not die.

Like most diseases, anorexia displays a whole range of severity, from the mildest to the most severe. And as in many diseases, mild cases are much more common than severe ones. The primary physician may be of help in treating the more common, mild cases, but he or she should refer to a child psychiatrist (especially one with particular experience treating these children) those who do not respond early to more superficial therapy. In these early cases it is important to try to dissuade the parents from getting involved in the obsession and the power struggles. They must restrain themselves from counting calories and watching the child's weight. The mother should cook reasonable amounts of food, three meals a day, and avoid offering restaurant services in the hope that she will have something available for the child. The parents must neither submit to unreasonable demands nor get involved in bribing, threatening, and coercing. The youngster herself must be helped to gain a healthier attitude toward sex, growth, and adult life. If referral to a child psychiatrist is warranted (and the primary physician should not hesitate to make this referral because anorexia is a dangerous disease), he or she is likely to continue with a similar program but in greater intensity and depth. In the more severe cases, hospitalization is often indicated. Preferably this should be done at a center with experience in the treatment of this disorder. Otherwise, the hospital personnel are likely to get involved in the same power struggles and games that the parents did.

The reader who is interested in a detailed description of eating disorders may want to refer to Bruch's comprehensive work on the subject.[34]

ELIMINATION DISORDERS

Enuresis

Enuresis is traditionally defined as the involuntary passage of urine, without the presence of physical disorder, in children who are old enough to control their urination voluntarily. One problem with this definition is its lack of specificity with regard to the age at which children are supposed to be able to control their micturition. Most people would not label as enuretic a 1-year-old who has not yet been trained. But the 8-year-old who wets the bed at night is usually considered to be enuretic. Generally, children stop wetting at 2½ to 3 years (girls are usually trained earlier than boys). Most physicians, however, do not get concerned when 4 year olds and even 5 year olds are still wetting. In fact, the prevalence of enuresis among children over 6 is still so great that it is not generally considered a significant form of pathology. Most agree that by puberty a high percentage of enuretic children stop wetting the bed, but there are adults (the number is unknown) who still wet at night. Another problem with the aforementioned definition is that the term is supposed to be reserved for children who do not have a physical disorder. This definition is fine if we are referring to demonstrable pathology of the traditional kind, for example, spina bifida and chronic cystitis. But what about neurophysiological abnormalities that might result in a neurodevelopmental lag in bladder control or hyperirritability? Isn't this a form of physical disease as well? Some would say yes; others would consider the latter forms of disorder to be physical manifestations of a psychogenic disorder.

With regard to the organic versus psychogenic issue, it is premature for anyone to say that he or she knows with certainty whether most children's enuresis is physical or psychological in etiology. Primarily as the result of the great sway that psychoanalytic teachings had over American psychiatry from the 1930s through the 1960s, the view generally held during that period was that enuresis is psychogenic. Since that time, with the general shift of the pendulum back to organic explanations for many psychiatric phenomena, the neurophysiological explanation is coming back into vogue. Although I do not totally reject psychoanalysis, as many people do today, I have for many years considered enuresis to be primarily a neurophysiological disorder.

The author's main reason for holding this view is that these children suffer a terrible amount of embarrassment and discomfort because of their illness. They cannot enjoy overnight visits with friends nor go to sleep-away camp. And when they are brave enough to chance such experiences they may fear (and justifiably so) the terrible scorn and mockery of their peers. The psychological gratification that is allegedly derived from the symptom does not seem worth the trouble it causes these children. In addition, many of these children have little or no evidence of other psychological disturbance. It is rare to see true psychogenic symptoms in isolation from other forms of psychopathology. Furthermore, the traditional psychoanalytic explanations in which the enuresis is explained as a manifestation of hostile and/or sexual problems (especially with regard to the child's relationship with parents) have not seemed to hold up with the vast majority of the patients the author has seen. If one stretches the data and uses one's imagination, it is possible to apply just about any psychoanalytic explanation to anyone. With a cautious and conservative approach to the acceptance of psychoanalytic explanations, the author has not found the theory applicable to most of his patients with enuresis. These observations and considerations have led to serious questioning of the theory that enuresis is psychogenic. In the absence of gross psychopathology (the usual situation) the author has considered the vast majority of his enuretic child patients to be suffering with a neurophysiological development lag and/or bladder hyperirritability.

Psychogenic factors, however, can play a role in intensifying the enuretic problem. The bladders of such children are more prone than other organs to react to stress. All of us have such "weak" or "target" organs that react inordinately to stress. Some react to stress with elevation of blood pressure, others with rapid heart rate, shortness of breath, sweating, or spasm of the gastrointestinal tract (producting vomiting or diarrhea). The bladder is another organ that can react strongly to stress. Accordingly, it is not surprising that the enuretic child is likely to wet more when tense, such as when sleeping in a strange place or the night before the first day of school. Although the presence of enuresis as an isolated symptom supports the conclusion that it is neurophysiological, the presence of other psychogenic symptoms does not rule out the possiblity that the enuresis may still be organic. Children with psychological disturbance of any type can still have, in addition, an enuretic problem on a neurophysiological basis, just as they can inherit or acquire any other physical problem.

With regard to the treatment of enuresis, a first suggestion is that the parents try a *combination* of strict fluid restriction after supper *plus* the ingestion of a highly salty snack before bedtime. Potato chips or pretzels are generally chosen. Because these foods may leave an unpleasant aftertaste and residuum in the mouth if not taken with fluids, the child can rinse his or her mouth with water, without swallowing (obviously), following ingestion. In the author's experience, about a third of children will reduce their enuresis on such a program. One cannot know whether it is really being successful unless the reduction in the frequency of enuresis extends over a number of weeks. Even then one cannot be completely certain that it was the program and not psychological suggestibility that caused the improvement. The reader should note this treatment may *reduce* the enuresis (and it may reduce it significantly), but it will not often *cure* it completely (although this has happened on a few occasions).

If the program fails, one can suggest that the parents consider purchasing an electronic device that wakes the child up on the passage of the first drops of urine. The principle is a simple one. A unit that contains two perforated thin metal plates separated by a porous pad is placed beneath the child's sheet. The first drops of urine (a good conductor of electricity) seep through the perforation of the top plate, expand through the porous pad, and complete electrical contact between the two electrical plates. This completes a low voltage electrical circuit that sounds off an alarm. The alarm rings until manually turned off. Once awakened, the child goes (or is taken) to the bathroom. The main drawback of the system lies in the fact that it may have a greater effect on the rest of the family than on the child. Although the alarm is generally quite loud (obviously, if it is soft it will not serve its purpose of awakening the child and thereby interrupting micturition), it may still not awaken the child (some consider heavy sleeping to be a contributing factor in enuresis). In fact, the whole family may be awakened by the shrill of the alarm while the child remains deeply asleep—lying all the while in a pool of warm urine. For a small percentage of children the method works. They do wake up on the passage of the first drops of urine, turn off the machine (sometimes before it has caused more than minimal family disturbance), and go to the bathroom. Many of these successful children need to use the machine for only a few weeks and then find that they remain dry without it. In such cases of "cure" there are, in my opinion, three main possibilities:

- The trial with the device occurred coincidentally at the time at which the child would have stopped wetting anyway.
- The instrument worked by negative conditioning; that is, the noxious alarm served as a negative reinforcement, thereby inhibiting the symptom.
- The instrument worked by suggestion: the physician, a powerful authority, has told the child that this instrument will cure the enuresis. This somehow has brought about the cure (rather as hypnosis works).

If both programs described fail (or if the parents do not wish to try the alarm device), one can suggest a trial on imipramine (Tofranil). If a starting dose of 25 mg 1 hour before bedtime is not successful after 4 to 5 days, it can be increased to 50 mg. If still not successful after another 4 to 5 days, it can be increased to a maximum of 75 mg. The mechanism of action of imipramine in enuresis has been thought to be the production of spasm of the internal urethreal sphincter. Recent work suggests, however, that the reduced bladder responsivesness to filling may be related to a central midbrain effect.[35] In the author's experience, about a third of children with enuresis will improve on imipramine. Of course, this rate can be increased by combining it with the aforementioned water restriction/salt ingestion program.

If none of the treatments described work (and this is still the case in a significant percentage of children) *and* if there is no evidence for significant psychopathology in other areas of functioning, one can recommend that the parents do nothing and hope that the child will gradually outgrow the symptom. One can reassure the child and family that the likelihood of this happening is very great and that the older the child grows, the greater the chance the symptom will disappear. If the child does have psychological problems that warrant treatment, one can try to reduce sources of tension that might be contributing.

Encopresis

Encopresis is defined as the failure to retain feces, in the absence of demonstrable physical disease, after the child has attained the age when most children are doing so. Like the definition of enuresis, this definition raises certain operational problems. Although the age by which children are supposed to be bowel trained is generally considered to be 2 years (girls again usually being trained earlier than boys), few would label a child as encopretic who was still not bowel trained at 2½ or 3 years of age. However, unlike enuresis, there is a much earlier cut-off point at which one would apply the label. One could stretch normality for bladder control to puberty, but most would not go beyond 4 or 5 years of age as the upper limit or normality for bowel control. In the definition of enuresis, the word involuntary is used. The word is not so frequently used when defining encopresis because it if often difficult to determine whether or not the failure to train is voluntary, involuntary, or a combination of both. Enuretics wet at night, when it is easy to assume that the passage of urine was involuntary; encopretics "do their thing" in the daytime when it is often difficult, if not impossible, to ascertain the degree to which the act was voluntary.

With regard to the organic vs. psychogenic question in encopresis, it is the author's opinion that encorpresis over the age of four or four and a half is psychogenic. (Of course, organic disease must be ruled out.) Although developmental lags and bladder irritability may play a significant role in most children's enuresis, these factors do not play a significant role in most children's encopresis. For some of these children it is a hostile act. In fact it is one of the most hostile acts in the child's repertoire. What better way to upset, enrage, and disgust parents and other significant figures than to fill the room with the odor of a fresh bowel movement. For some of these children the anger element seems to be combined with an attitude of "who cares" or "why be bothered." Many of these children are neglected or otherwise maltreated. Their motivation to inhibit or restrict themselves is very low because there has been little affection forthcoming when they have inhibited themselves and tried to "be good." Many do not anticipate enjoyable relationships with friends and so the scorn and jeering by peers does not serve as a deterrent. This is especially the case for borderline or schizophrenic children. Some children with minimal brain dysfunction seem to be encopretic as part of their attentional deficit, to neither external nor internal stimuli. Or they may have trouble understanding the meaning of stimuli, internal and/or external, and so do not associate the sensation of a full lower bowel with the importance of going to the bathroom as soon as possible.

In summary, in the author's view, the child who is significantly encopretic beyond the age of five is suffering with moderately severe to severe psychopathology. By significantly encopretic is meant four to five or more such episodes a week (that is, almost daily). One should then consider the possible diagnoses of mental retardation, minimal brain dysfunction (with encopresis, not so minimal), schizophrenia, autism, borderline psychosis, and severe behavior disorder. Most often, the primary care physician should refer children with significant encopresis to a child psychiatrist for detailed evaluation and appropriate treatment.

WHEN SHOULD CHILDREN BE REFERRED TO A CHILD PSYCHIATRIST?

Throughout this chapter the author has recommended referral to a child psychiatrist (or other mental health professional qualified to treat children's psychological disorders) when the primary physician considers the problem to be more complex than he or she can handle. Thus far, we have focused on the indications for such referral when treating the specific disorders discussed. This final section of the chapter will describe the broader indications for such referral. There are four main areas that should be investigated if one is to make a judicious decision regarding whether or not a child warrants psychiatric treatment (whether it be with the primary care physician or with someone else). Each will be discussed separately.

The Home

Although one should certainly inquire about the child's functioning in the home in order to learn about whether he or she is exhibiting abnormal behavior, it is important to appreciate that home behavior is the *least* valuable of the four areas in determing whether a child needs therapy. In the home, there is far greater tolerance for atypical behavior than in the neighborhood and at school (two of the other areas to be investigated). A child knows that he can "get away" with behavior at home that outsiders would never tolerate. In addition, parents tend to overvalue their children's assets and deny their liabilities. Accordingly, there is likely to be a certain amount of parental denial of deficits.

When a mother complains that Johnny does not want to take out the garbage, all this says is that Johnny is exhibiting normal behavior (at least in the area of taking out the garbage). In fact, when a child *wants* to take out the garbage, one cannot help wondering about a problem of abnormal compliance. When a mother complains that Sally dawdles in the morning, one may also consider that normal. It is the child who does not dawdle about whom one should wonder. When father complains that Billy and Mary fight a lot, the author would ask, "How many fights a day do they have?" If the number is less than 20 or 30 (there is no real cut-off point) it can be considered normal. It is only when significant physical harm has been done that one should consider the possiblity that the sibling rivalry has gone beyond its usual fierce level. Again, children who never (or hardly ever) fight are probably very inhibited; these are the children one might look at for possible psychopathology.

In short, the normal child exhibits a significant amount of disrespect for parents, "doesn't listen" when spoken to, dawdles, often fights with siblings, doesn't want to cooperate in doing household chores, and so on. Because such behavior is so extensive and commonplace in the normal, it is difficult to determine when pathological behavior in these areas is being exhibited. Accordingly, one does well to inquire into other areas to ascertain whether psychopathology is present.

The Neighborhood

The neighborhood is a far better place than the school to determine whether psychopathology is present. Friends and neighbors will not tolerate what a child's family will. Abuse a friend and he or she will quickly find another playmate. Abuse a younger sibling and there is little he or she can do. A younger sibling is captive prey. He or she cannot leave the home and, being smaller, is a safe target. Accordingly, most children will show more restraint regarding persecution of peers. The child who has not learned this, the child who is mistreating peers, is not only likely to be very lonely but to have psychological problems as well.

The healthy child knows that when visiting the homes of friends, there are different rules to be followed and that parents of friends will not tolerate the kinds of antics that his or her own parents might accept as a matter of routine. Talking back and being sassy to one's mother is normal (isn't that what mothers are for anyway?); being rude to the parent of a peer is another thing entirely. The child who has not clearly made this distinction is going to have few friends, will be very lonely, and is likely to have some psychiatric difficulties.

A good rule of thumb to follow in ascertaining whether a child is functioning adequately in the neighborhood is to find out whether the child seeks friends and if he or she is sought by friends as well. In addition, one wants to know the age of the friends. If the child seeks friends his or her age and is consistently sought by these children, then it is unlikely that there are problems in this area. A mother may complain that Robert has difficulties with other children, that he wants his own way, that he sometimes hits other children, and so on. However, if the other children are still seeking Robert as a friend and playmate it is unlikely that these traits are being exhibited to a pathological degree. Here the child's friends are more accurate determiners of psychopathology than a physician; they know far better than we what is sick and what is healthy in this area.

The School

Here, too, the physician has a most sensitive source of information about what is normal and what is sick. The teacher knows far better than we what is normal and what is abnormal for a particular age. Often she or he has been teaching the same grade level for years and can spot the atypical child the first day. In addition, not being the child's parent the teacher is not as likely to deny his or her difficulties. Furthermore, the child's problems might be a source of frustration and irritation in the classroom, and this makes it even more likely that the teacher will recognize the atypical behavior and bring it to the attention of the parents, the child study team, or the principal.

Accordingly, the school may be the first place where a child's problems are brought to the attention of the parents. One should inquire into both the behavioral and academic areas. There may be a problem, however, with regard to getting accurate information from the teacher. Although the teacher may be the one who referred the child in the first place, it may be particularly difficult to get accurate information from her or him regarding the exact nature of the child's difficulties. We are living at a time when there is a nationwide conspiracy of silence regarding giving children and their parents accurate information about deficits. A whole system of euphemisms have been contrived, under the misguided notion that it is psychologically detrimental to a child to confront him or her with deficiencies, no matter how benevolently stated. Accordingly, one does well to try to impress upon the teacher the importance of giving accurate information. In investigating the academic area one wants to know how the child's level of performance compares with that of other children in the class. To say that Nancy "is up to the three times table" gives no useful information. To say she is "now reading the Uncle Funny Bunny Book," is also a ploy. To say she is in the middle of the second grade and is at the mid-first grade level in reading is a clear statement of the child's performance level. In inquiring about behavior, one wants to know the specific nature of the behavioral abnormalities. Also, one wants to know how the child relates to peers in the classroom.

The author's experience has been that when a school refers a child for treatment he or she usually needs it. As mentioned, school personnel are quite good at differentiating age-appropriate behavior from the inappropriate. If the child is singled out for referral to therapy, he or she probably needs it—even though the referring people are not trained as mental health professionals. In addition, school personnel tend to be very cautious and hesitant when it comes to such referrals. They are ever defensive in their anticipation that aggressive parents will make trouble for them. Accordingly, they tend to let things ride rather than make an issue over a child's problems. When they do step forward and complain, there is a good chance that there is something significant to complain about.

Psychopathological Symptoms

If a child is functioning well in all of the above three areas, it is not likely that he or she will be suffering with significant psychopathology. However, a child occasionally exhibits traditional neurotic or personality problems yet continues to function adequately at home, with friends, and in school. Such problems are described in the American Psychiatric Association's *Diagnostic and Statistical Manual of Mental Disorders* (DSM-III), psychiatry's most widely used system of nomenclature.[18] For example, a boy may be very tense and have tics that are related to repressed hostile and/or sexual thoughts and feelings that he is too guilty to express. In spite of these difficulties, the parents describe no particular problems at home. On inquiry, however, we learn that parents never fight (and thereby serve as models for the suppression and repression of hostility) and the mother undresses in front of the patient (thereby titillating him sexually). But no "problems" are described because the boy is cooperative and obedient. In school, he is serious and gets good grades. In addition, his fear of anger expression lessens the likelihood of disruptive behavior. In fact, the tics notwithstanding, the teacher may consider him a good student and a good boy, "never any trouble." And in his neighborhood, he has friends whom he seeks and by whom he is sought. Although occasionally teased by peers because of his tics, the problem is not great enough to have interfered significantly with forming and maintaining friendships.

One last word of advice to the primary physician. There is not a child who does not occasionally exhibit difficulties in each of the areas of home, neighborhood, and school. Treatment is certainly not warranted for all these children. One must differentiate between transient symptoms and those that persist. The former generally do not require treatment, whereas the latter do. Accordingly, one does well to inquire how long the difficulties have been present before making a decision regarding treatment. Such an inquiry is especially important with anxious parents who are quick to see psychopathology in the most short-lived, atypical behavior. Also, there are parents who are deeply involved in psychotherapy and psychoanalysis (some of these may be psychotherapists themselves). Such parents are quick to bring their children into therapy and will tend to bring their children into treatment for the most frivolous reasons. It was because of this recognition of the frequent transiency of children's symptoms that the new third edition of the *Diagnostic and Statistical Manual* frequently includes a duration criterion for the justifiable diagnosis of many childhood disorders.[18]

REFERENCES

1. Wechsler D: Wechsler Intelligence Scale for Children–Revised. New York, The Psychological Corp, 1974
2. Gardner RA: The Objective Diagnosis of Minimal Brain Dysfunction. Cresskill, NJ, Creative Therapeutics, 1979
3. Gardner RA: The Reversals Frequency Test. Cresskill, NJ, Creative Therapeutics, 1978
4. Gardner RA, Broman M: Letter reversals frequency in normal and learning-disabled children. J Clin Child Psychol 8:146–152, 1979
5. Bender L: A Visual Motor Gestalt Test and Its Clinical Use, research monograph no 3. New York, American Orthopsychiatric Assocation, 1938
6. Bender L: Bender Motor Gestalt Test: Cards and Manual of Instructions. New York, American Orthopsychiatric Association, 1946
7. Koppitz EM: The Bender Gestalt Test for Young Children, vol 2. New York, Grune & Stratton, 1975
8. Purdue Pegboard, cat no 32020. Lafayette, Ind, Lafayette Instrument Co

9. Gardner RA, Broman M: The Purdue Pegboard: Normative data on 1334 school children. J Clin Child Psychol 8:156–162, 1979
10. Gardner RA: Throwing balls in a basket as a test of motor coordination: Normative data on 1350 school children. J Clin Child Psychol 8:152–155, 1979
11. Gardner RA, Gardner AK: The Gardner Steadiness Tester, cat no 32019. Lafayette, Ind, Lafayette Instrument Co, 1977
12. Gardner RA, Gardner AK, Caemmerer A, Broman M: An instrument for measuring hyperactivity and other signs of MBD. J Clin Child Psychol 8:173–179, 1979
13. Rappoport JL: Dextroamphetamine: Cognitive and behavioral effects in normal prepubertal boys. Science 199:560–563, 1978
14. Gardner RA: MBD: The Family Book About Minimal Brain Dysfunction. New York, Jason Aronson, 1973
15. Kronick D: A Word or Two About Learning Disabilities. San Rafeal, Calif, Academic Therapy Publications, 1973
16. Kronick D: What About Me? The LD Adolescent. San Rafael, Calif, Academic Therapy Publications, 1975
17. Gardner RA: Psychogenic learning disabilities. Acta Paedopsychiatr 42(5):188–209, 1977
18. Diagnostic and Satistical Manual of Mental Disorders, Ed 3 (DSM-III). Washington, DC, American Psychiatric Association, 1980
19. Johnson AM, Falstein EI, Szurek SA, et al: School phobia. Am J Orthopsychiatry 11:702–711, 1941
20. Johnson AM: School phobia workshop, discussion. Am Orthopsychiatry 27:307–309, 1957
21. Gittelmann-Klein R: Pharmacotherapy and management of pathological separation anxiety. Int J Ment Health 4:255–270, 1975
22. Gittelman-Klein R, Klein DF: School phobia: Diagnostic considerations in the light of imipramine effects. J Nerv Ment Dis 156(3):199–215, 1973
23. Coolidge JC: School phobia, in Noshpitz JD: Basic Handbook of Child Psychiatry. New York, Basic Books, 1979, pp. 453–463
24. Gardner RA: Psychotherapy with Children of Divorce. New York, Jason Aronson, 1976
25. Gardner RA: The Boys and Girls Book About Divorce. New York, Jason Aronson, 1970 (Paperback: New York, Bantam Books, 1971)
26. Gardner RA: The Parents Book About Divorce. Garden City, Doubleday, 1977 (Paperback: New York, Bantam Books, 1979)
27. Freud S: The interpretation of dreams, in The Complete Psychological Works of Sigmund Freud, vol 4. London, Hogarth Press, 1953, p. 254
28. Gardner RA: The Boys and Girls Book About One-Parent Families. New York, GP Putnam, 1978 (Paperback: New York, Bantam Books, 1982)
29. Gardner RA: Death of a Parent, in Noshpitz J (ed): Basic Handbook of Child Psychiatry, vol 4. New York, Basic Books, 1979, pp 270–283
30. Niebuhr R: From a sermon preached in Heath, Massachusetts, 1934
31. Redl F, Wineman D: Controls from Within. New York, Free Press, 1952
32. Bettelheim B: Truants from Life. Glencoe, Ill, Free Press, 1955
33. Holmes DJ: The Adolescent in Psychotherapy. Boston, Little, Brown, 1964
34. Bruch H: Eating Disorders. New York, Basic Books, 1973
35. Shaffer D, Stephenson JD, Thomas DS: Some effects of impramine on micturition and their relevance to its anti-enuretic activity. Neuropharmacology 18:33–37, 1979

Richard Wortman, M.D.

11

The Management of the Adolescent Patient

The adolescent can be a rewarding patient for the primary care physician who enjoys participating in the rapidly increasing physical, cognitive, emotional, and social maturity of young people. The adolescent patient will seek out, listen, and talk to the physician who is enthusiastic, interested, and non-judgmental. Adolescents must believe that their symptoms, behavior, and feelings, and not their parents', are the doctor's primary concern. The physician who knows about the major personal issues in the adolescent patient's life and encourages the patient to keep him or her informed of major developments will be able to assess developmental deviations and the significance of temporary crises.

Psychiatric impairment occurs in a minority of teenagers, and they can be differentiated from the normal majority by the presence of emotional and behavioral symptoms that persist over time or recur.[1–3] Inner turmoil, defined as feelings of misery and inadequacy, occurred in 20 percent of one sample population and were seen as distinct from clinical depression, which occurred much less frequently.[2] It is a great disservice to the adolescent to dismiss his or her distress or misbehavior as a developmental phase without looking at the adolescent individually, within the family constellation, and in a larger social context. Based on his recent study of a large sample of American teenagers, Daniel Offer states "Teenagers who need help don't grow out of it. They become adults who need help."[4]

A series of psychiatric referrals from parents who had listened to a Parent-Teacher Association (PTA) presentation on normal adolescent development reinforced the author's concern over the prevalence of benign neglect. The first boy referred had a several-month history of angry outbursts toward his mother, in which he would throw heavy objects about the house and punch walls. He was, otherwise, a quiet and pleasing youth, whom teachers found a delight because of his aptitude for learning. He was currently having mild academic difficulty because of his inability to concentrate. The friends he had had in previous years were slowly drifting away. His mother had been concerned about his behavior for a matter of months, but had intially dismissed the idea of professional consultation with the hope that he was just having a little more difficulty with adolescence than most boys and that things would improve with time and patience on her part. She eventually involved the boy's pediatrician who found him to be "quite nervous" but went no further. It was a couple of months later, after the PTA meeting about normal adolescence, that a psychiatric referral was made and the diagnosis of latent schizophrenia was made. By this time the patient had a marked thought disorder with bizarre mental content. Two additional referrals from parents followed this PTA presentation. In all three cases the problems had been progressive over a period of months and significant psychiatric illness, that had been written off as adolescent turmoil, was present.

BEHAVIORAL EVALUATION

Rather than attempt to determine the significance of individual symptoms, it is easier and more useful to assess a patient's level of functioning in the four major areas of his or her life: (1) family relations, (2) peer relations, (3) school performance, and (4) the use of leisure time. This assessment should be carried out using the parameters of (1) number of problems, (2) degree of severity, and (3) duration of problems. Table 11-1 describes six levels of functioning which comprise a useful framework for such assessment. If an adolescent's overall rating is below "good" over a period of weeks there is reason for closer scrutiny of the situation. To do so requires some knowledge of what is reasonably expected at varying ages.

Family Relations

At no age should an adolescent have a poor ongoing relationship with his or her parents. Adolescents must gain emotional distance from their parents, and this is most obvious in early adolescence when the pull toward the parents is greatest. The striving for separation may manifest itself in minor disagreements over matters of dress or curfew time, but young people continue to share common values with parents. Adolescents are, in general, trusting and respectful of their parents, though angry at times and not always emotionally close. The burden of respon-

Table 11-1.
Levels of Functioning in Family and Peer Relations, Academic Performance, and Use of Leisure Time

Level	Example
Superior: Extremely effective functioning in all four areas	A 13-year-old girl is getting excellent grades in school, is close to both parents, is extremely popular among her peers, and excels in tennis and swimming.
Very Good: Better than average functioning in all four areas	A 17-year-old boy is getting good grades, gets along well with parents, has several close friends, works part-time, and pursues astronomy enthusiastically.
Good: No more than slight impairment in one area of functioning	A 14-year-old boy argues with his parents over the clothes he must wear to school. He does well academically and has several good friends with whom he goes camping.
Fair: Moderate impairment in one area of functioning or some impairment in two or more	A 15-year-old girl is doing poorly in school, but has had adequate peer and family relations and likes to bike ride.
Poor: Marked impairment in one area of functioning or moderate impairment in two or more.	A 17-year-old girl has trouble getting along with peers and spends much of her free time in bed sleeping. She does adequately in school and gets along with parents.
Grossly Impaired: Marked impairment in all four areas.	A 12-year-old boy who has no friends, is almost failing in school and spends most of his free time wandering around the streets. He says his parents don't like him.

Adapted from Diagnostic and Statistical Manual of Mental Disorders (3rd ed). Washington, D.C., American Psychiatric Assoc., 1980.

sibility for discord may change when a parent has significant emotional problems. If an adolescent is experiencing difficulty in this area, an interview with the parents may be required to see where the problem lies.

Peer Relations

Peer relations are most significant in evaluating an adolescent, and comprise the most difficult area to assess. Most early adolescents have one or two close same-sex friends, usually a person who is "like me." The relationships are not exploitive and there is "collaboration in reciprocally meeting each others' needs."[5] By middle adolescence there should be heterosexual interest and active social contact among the sexes, though the boys may lag behind. Normal sexual experimentation is influenced by local custom. The physician's moral values may make assessment difficult. Adolescents are usually accurate when evaluating their peers' behavior in this regard, and a physician would do well to rely on their values of normal behavior. When a girl is seen as a "slut" by her peers, there is good reason to believe that the limits of normality have been transgressed. The midadolescent will quite often have a number of friends of both sexes as he or she continues to move away from his or her parents. A 15-year-old girl who has many boyfriends but no girlfriends because "they're jealous of me," is of concern. In late adolescence the need for group support diminishes, and a few serious relationships persist. The 18-year-old who tries to impress the interviewer with "how many friends he has" is unusual.

School Performance

The grading systems of most schools are constructed so that all students can do well. Chronic poor academic performance merits assessment. The presence of mental retardation or a specific learning disability must first be excluded. That an adolescent has passed grades one through six without notice by the school system does not guarantee that one of these disorders is not present. Academic demands often increase significantly in grades six through eight, and a low reading level may become an insurmountable obstacle for the first time. Once organicity is excluded, an emotional etiology can be entertained. The physician must be cautious when eliciting an account of his patient's school experience. The answer of "okay" by a patient or "terribly" by a parent when queried in regard to "grades" may mean anything from honor roll to barely passing. You must therefore ask the patient and/or the parents to be more specific. Discrepancies among the varying sources of information may provide valuable clues to understanding the problems. An obvious explanation for poor academic performance is chronic truancy from school or the cutting of classes. A limited amount of this behavior may not be significant, but if poor marks ensue, concern is warranted.

Leisure Time

Normal leisure time usage for adolescents covers a whole spectrum of activities. The patient should be involved in something outside of academic pursuits that excites him or her. This may be school associated, such as athletics or the school newspaper, or even academically related, such as special science projects. What is important is that some energy and interest is directed to something beside getting good grades. In attempting to assess this area, the physician should not be content with the frequent response of "I hang out." The physician needs to know that his or her patient is enthusiastically pursuing an activity and not merely avoiding boredom or anxiety through such means as drug-taking or aimless wandering.

TREATMENT AND REFERRAL

If the patient is experiencing difficulty that is more than transient and that is not improved by reassurance in a couple of weeks' time, the physician may want to set up a more formal counseling arrangement whereby the patient is seen weekly for the explicit purpose of bringing about change in the problem areas. A sensitive physician with the time and inclination can deal adequately with situational disturbances and the intermittent disruptions in life experienced by adolescents whose coping methods are not sufficiently developed. The most important component of this supportive therapy is listening and understanding. The physician is in the best position to motivate the patient toward therapy either with the physician himself or with a mental health worker. Having followed the major issues in the adolescent's life, the physician can place the current difficulties in historical perspective for the youth, persuading him or her of the need for change. However, if the patient's behavior has become a source of concern and irritation to family and school authorities, he or she may be feeling external pressure to change and the physician may be seen as the agent of these outside "intrusive" forces. For this reason it is especially important that the purpose of counseling or therapy be made clear to the adolescent and that it be presented in terms of what it can provide him or her. Jim may not want to do well in school because of father's expectations, but he might like to get father off his back and do well enough to eventually go away to college. In general, therapy is more acceptable to the adolescent if the purpose is clearly associated with the movement toward autonomy and independence.

Making a Psychiatric Referral

The physician's personal recommendation of a psychiatric consultant goes a long way in bridging the referral chasm. The referral should not be made until the patient is ready to accept it. After discussing the idea on several occasions and having had time to think about it, an adolescent will often come to the decision that therapy is desirable. A personal introduction to the psychiatric consultant is ideal. If your setting precludes this, a telephone conversation with the consultant while the patient listens to you explain the reason for your referral is a good second choice. The patient can then be put on the phone to set up an appointment time. The process has begun with the adolescent feeling some control over the situation.

Obstacles to Referral

It is not uncommon to be confronted by an adolescent with significant emotional problems who steadfastly refuses to acknowledge them, in spite of symptoms as obvious as severe anxiety, nightmares, paranoia, and social withdrawal. In some instances the patient will not even return to see you because of your failure to relieve the symptom with which he or she presented. An option available to the physician is to involve the parents, who can use their influence and authority to have their child go for a psychiatric evaluation. The youth will initially be resistant to the pyschiatrist, but this need not be an absolute barrier to successful treatment.

If the physician decides to undertake this course of action, he may be seen by his or her adolescent patient as breaching confidentiality. Where the indications for psychiatric intervention are clear and compelling, and it is your intention to involve the parents, you should explain this to the patient before contacting the parents. In most instances, though the young person is initially angry, the therapeutic relationship is maintained, as the youth is able eventually to accept the well-intentioned nature of his physician's action.

In other cases, it is the parents who resist the notion of the need for psychiatric intervention. A separate meeting with them may be needed so that they have the opportunity to voice the basis of their resistance to psychiatric referral and, quite likely, their fears about the idea of emotional illness. Frequently, the youth's problems are just part of a larger constellation of family problems. When presented as a broader family concern, with the onus of illness removed from any one individual, the idea of a family evaluation by an outside professional may be acceptable to all (see Chapter 8 on family and marital therapy).

PHYSICAL DEVELOPMENT AND BODY IMAGE

Physical development, with the acquisition of primary and secondary sexual characteristics, is probably the most striking aspect of adolescence. As a result, there is a heightened body consciousness. Schoenfeld has presented a detailed account of the bodily changes in adolescence and the effects that deviations from the norm have on body-image formation.[6] Basic to the understanding of the significance of these deviations is that for adolescents, "to be different is to be inferior." Being different will be a particular problem for the late developing boy with a small penis and minimal pubic hair compared to peers. He may even skip school on the days of gym class so as to avoid his embarrassment in the shower room. Similar avoidance patterns may develop in boys with even minimal gynecomastia. Withdrawal from these situations may lead to further stigmatization as a "sissy" or "faggot." Late developing girls may be kidded about the absence of breasts and may worry or have mothers who worry about an "overdue" menarche. It is usually the early developing girl, though, who must bear the heaviest burden. The awkward and rather insensitive attention her male peers pay to her developing breasts and the assumptions that older boys will make about sexual availability, along with the frantic sexual prohibitions of well meaning but threatened parents, may be more than an eleven-year-old can comfortably handle. She may see herself as a little girl with a woman's body, which may become a source of discomfort and possibly shame.

As part of the history, the physician should ask if the patient is comfortable and happy with his or her body and the way he or she looks and functions. A surprising number of patients, more girls than boys, will say no. Most of the complaints will be nothing more than discomfort over normal variation. A discussion by the doctor of the range of normal growth and development, possibly augmented by Tanner's photographs and graphs, will go a long way to assuage the normal adolescent's discomfort.[7] Some adolescents with no gross abnormalities may still not be satisfied as they are, wishing to change their appearance. Their proposed methods of change may range from cosmetic surgery to diets and exercise.

Two surgical procedures often sought by adolescent girls are breast reduction and rhinoplasty. These procedures will not improve the patient's body image if no abnormalities exist. Even without a distorted body image, an adolescent may project his or her inadequacies onto a normal physical characteristic. Parents may support an adolescent's request for surgery because they believe it will make a significant difference or because they can't bear up any longer to the patient's constant badgering.

If the physician believes that a request for cosmetic surgery is based on either a distorted body image or the projection of emotional inadequacies, surgery should be postponed and further psychological assessment obtained. It may be possible to help such patients understand that they are attributing their problems to this physical feature but that its modification will probably not really make a significant difference in their lives. Some patients will respond to such an observation, and this may begin a meaningful dialogue between patient and physician. For some patients, referral to a psychiatrist will be indicated to complete the task of dealing with the underlying problems.

Acne

If an adolescent patient has acne beyond minimal severity, the physician should mention it when the patient fails to do so. You can assume that the patient is not only aware of it but also concerned about it. Acne is an obvious physical "defect" which can undermine a patient's self-esteem and lead to social uncertainty and withdrawal, especially from heterosexual relationships. Appropriate medical treatment, including consultation with a dermatologist where indicated, should be undertaken. The medical regimen should be generously supplemented with optimistic encouragement and support.

Dieting

Because of a heightened body awareness and increased interest in heterosexual relations, adolescence is often a time when an interest in dieting occurs in the obese patient. Such an interest should certainly not be discouraged, and the physician can assist by providing reasonable diets and exercise regimes and by encouraging the patient to maintain records of food intake. However, it is important that the physician not pressure the patient to do so. Failure to maintain a diet is guaranteed if the motivation is more the physician's than the patient's, and this will only serve to undermine the teenager's self-respect and confidence.

In some instances, it is the parents who refer their unmotivated child for weight reduction. The physician who can help these well-intentioned parents decrease their pressure on the adolescent can relieve a source of potential family conflict. The situation changes somewhat if there are specific medical indications for weight loss, such as a prediabetic condition or hypertension. It is then the physician's responsibility to discuss the advisability of weight reduction, though the outcome will still be determined wholly by the patient's motivation. Even if the physician is frustrated by the patient's inability to lose weight, it is important that he or she not respond judgmentally to the situation. The patient already feels guilt and this needs no reinforcement.

A striking condition, which often begins insidiously with a reasonable weight-reducing diet, is anorexia nervosa. The condition is most common from mid-adolescence through early adulthood, though it may occur in 11-year-olds. The physician should have a high index of suspicion when assessing the thin, dieting, adolescent girl. He will often be the first person to raise serious concern over the state of nutrition because parents frequently allow the situation to progress to an amazing degree before requesting professional help. If the slender patient continues to see herself as overweight and expresses an intense fear of obesity, then the diagnosis of anorexia nervosa is very likely appropriate. An electrolyte imbalance with hypokalemia may be the result of induced vomiting and should raise the physician's suspicions in a patient with weight loss. The condition has a high mortality rate, treatment is difficult, and psychiatric evaluation is indicated when the diagnosis is suspected. Chapter 10 deals with the management of this condition in more detail.

Sexual Maturation Disorders and Pregnancy

Associated with the physical development of adolescence is a change in sexual feelings and behavior. The adolescent patient should feel that you are available to discuss sexual matters. You can begin to establish that atmosphere by routinely asking each patient, in a matter-of-fact way, if they have any questions about sex that you might be able to answer. As with patients' concerns about their bodies' appearance, factual information regarding the range of normality will allay much anxiety. Masturbation remains a source of discomfort for some adolescents, and reassurance that masturbation is part of the normal adolescent's progress toward maturity is helpful.[8] The limited homosexual behavior of early adolescence is another source of discomfort. Again, reassurance as to the normality of such activity can be of value to the guilt-ridden adolescent.

Many adult patients who engage in atypical sexual behavior (homosexuality, transsexualism, exhibitionism, and so forth) are not interested in changing and do not volunteer information about such behavior when seeking medical care. Adolescents, however, are more likely to experience anxiety, shame, and guilt, and often, after acknowledging their behavior, may state their desire to change. Psychotherapy can be helpful in treating such patients. For example, some patients with homosexual impulses may be able to overcome these conflicts and develop a heterosexual orientation. It is therefore essential that the adolescent not assume that homosexual impulses or fantasies represent a fixed sexual orientation.[9] These patients should be referred for psychiatric consultation. For other patients their goals may change during therapy, with guilt-free acceptance of homosexuality replacing the goal of heterosexuality.

Like drug use, sexual behavior may be a manifestation of psychiatric illness. For instance, there is a relationship between sexual promiscuity among college students seeking psychiatric help and the presence of severe emotional conflict.[10] When such behavior is the expression of serious psychopathology, it is not an isolated symptom. Obsessive masturbation may be present in an impending schizophrenic break, but it is then only one of the many pieces of the puzzle. The physician can establish the significance of this symptom by inquiring briefly into related areas of sexual behavior and into peer and family relationships.

With the rapid increase in the prevalence of sexual activity among never-married U.S. teenage women (30 percent between 1971 and 1976), and with few teenagers beginning the use of contraception at the time they initiate intercourse,[11] teenage pregnancy is becoming much more common. This situation is a tremendous public health problem of unclear and multifactorial etiology. Though the individual physician cannot solve the national public health problem, it may be within his power to help a limited number of his patients avoid unwanted pregnancy. The patient most vulnerable to an unwanted pregnancy is a young and relatively inexperienced adolescent. Though fertile and sexually active, she may not have had time to integrate into her image of herself either her fertility or her sexuality. During the physical examination or review of systems, the physician should plan a discussion of physical differences, physiology, and sexual activity. Questions regarding menstruation can be followed by a discussion regarding such things as sexual activity, and birth control.

Knowledge about contraception, among teenagers, is sparse. For example, a high proportion of adolescent women believe that the safest period of time to have intercourse is half-way between two menstrual periods. Others believe that they will not become pregnant if they "do it" only once.[12] This points to the necessity of adequate physiologic and contraceptive information, which can be provided at the time of the examination and followed up with outside reading, such as *Our Bodies Ourselves*.[13]

Many young unmarried women unconsciously want to become pregnant regardless of the impracticality. No amount of integration of one's sexuality or information will prevent pregnancy if the unconscious urge is too strong. When your patient's behavior consistently contradicts her stated intention of avoiding pregnancy, it may be useful to explore these areas of discrepancy. If she is able to accept the validity of your observations and wants to resolve the dilemma, psychotherapy should be recommended.

GENERAL PRINCIPLES OF MEDICATION

Adolescent psychopharmacology is quite similar to that of adults. Specific psychotropic medications will be discussed in connection with the problems for which they are recommended. Following are a few helpful general principles to keep in mind when you are considering medication.

Young people fluctuating between feeling indestructible and feeling frighteningly vulnerable have difficulty accepting themselves as "sick" and needing medication, psychotropic or otherwise. Adolescents are afraid of being different and will hide such treatment from peers, thus increasing resistance to treatment. The potential for unreliability in taking medication is, therefore, great. One way of avoiding this problem is to make the parent responsible for the administration of the medication.

If either parent or patient significantly resists taking the prescribed medication, the attempt will surely fail. It is, therefore, important that both be included in this decision and that negative feelings be elicited and discussed. The responsibility for taking the medication must be shared between parent and patient. The physician must try to involve the adolescent as actively as the latter's maturity permits.

The adolescent's concern over peers' attitudes can be made less of a problem by prescribing medication to be taken in the morning and before sleep, thus avoiding the necessity of carrying medication around and taking it in front of their friends. A once-daily drug regimen is preferable. Try also to use a single drug. Both techniques decrease the possibility of drug defaulting.

Adolescents live more in the here and now, much less in the future. This poses specific problems when medications that have no immediate clinical effect are prescribed, such as tricyclic antidepressants. One depressed adolescent finished his first week's supply of antidepressants during the first day, because the initial dose "had not worked." Thus one needs to speak directly of the anticipated therapeutic effects of medication in a realistic and hopeful fashion but to make clear the time lag before drug effects will be felt. Providing such information is especially important with adolescents who have a relatively high potential for suicidal gestures.

Maintenance drug therapy can also become a victim of the adolescent's existential approach to life. The patient who is feeling fine and would just as soon forget a past depressive or schizophrenic episode has trouble anticipating a future disturbance with sufficient intensity to motivate current, conscientious drug taking. The same is true for the young diabetic who is asymptomatic and finds the daily insulin regimen an unwanted reminder of illness.

It is best to avoid prescribing minor tranquilizers. These drugs are often a poor substitute for the supportive counseling that can either help patients resolve the dilemmas in which they find themselves or sustain them until the crisis has passed. Minor tranquilizers will not alleviate an underlying depression. On the other hand, these drugs have a high potential for abuse because they make troubled people "feel so good."

They are also potentially physically addictive. Their effects are potentiated by alcohol, which raises the probability of accidental or intentional overdose. Given all of the above contraindications to using minor tranquilizers with adolescents, a physician may justify their use when an individual patient is relatively mature and responsible, and has a low potential for drug abuse. If, after weighing the potential risks involved, a physician believes that a minor tranquilizer is indicated on a short-term basis for disabling anxiety or insomnia, the benzodiazepines are preferable. They are safer in terms of suicidel potential than are such drugs as the barbiturates, and they have minimal effect on REM sleep.

DRUG ABUSE

Most of the adolescent drug and alcohol users seen by a physician come for treatment for problems unrelated to drug use. Unless the patient is questioned about drugs, this behavior will not be apparent. Of course the answers to your questions may be unreliable unless the patient has been actively looking for an opportunity to get help. The questioning of all patients is necessary to find those who are hoping that you will ask about drug use. Adolescents' dissembling about drug usage stems from ambivalence and conflict over their behavior and their concern that the physician will think badly of them or report the behavior to their parents. It is often helpful to ask "What drugs have you tried?" rather than "Do you take drugs?" It is often initially easier for the patient to acknowledge having tried something as opposed to being a current user, especially if the question is phrased as though an affirmative response is anticipated. If a patient responds that he has never tried any drugs, it is a good idea to mention marijuana and alcohol, since some adolescents do not consider these drugs. If a patient answers in the negative, you can drop the subject and consider reopening it in future, if other signs or symptoms point to drug usage.

After a patient acknowledges trying drugs, it is less difficult for him or her to talk about this experience and continuing usage. Much drug experimentation and social usage is motivated by curiosity, peer pressure, and the assertion of independence from parental values, and it is not indicative of serious emotional illness. When the drug usage does not infringe on the four basic areas of functioning previously outlined, there is little to be gained by pursuing the subject. Sermons on the evils of drugs may have only a negative effect, undermining the physician's credibility as a provider of objective information. However, the patient is entitled to have all current information on the hazards of such substances as marijuana.[14] For example, they should know that marijuana contains a high concentration of carcinogenic hydrocarbons.

Outside of such immediately dangerous drugs such as carbon tetrachloride, most of the drug hazard information sounds about as compelling to the teenager as the argument, "You should not drink a beer because you may become an alcoholic." Adolescents, as well as most adults, continue to regard their own experience as the most reliable indicator for future decisions. Some teenagers will ask physicians about the dangerousness of certain drugs, usually to reinforce their own beliefs that their parents and teachers are overracting to the situation. However, an adolescent sometimes looks for outside authoritative support to refrain from using drugs. Rather than issue a blanket condemnation of "drugs," it is often helpful to speak to some particularly high risks. The idea of being addicted, needing increasingly higher doses, and facing the possibility of physical withdrawal is distressing to most adolescents and is associated in their minds with street, heroin addicts. The fact that barbiturates and some minor tranquilizers are addictive with potentially serious withdrawal syndromes has, in the author's experience, caused some adolescents to reevaluate their usage. The use of inhalants such as glue and paint thinner is looked upon by most older adolescents as indicating immaturity, stupidity, and/or craziness because of the toxic effects and because the "high" is contaminated by nausea and dizziness. This information may dissuade a younger adolescent from experimentation.

To many adolescents, the possibility of a psychotic break appears too foreign or unlikely for a warning to deter them from trying a major hallucinogen such as LSD, mescaline, or psilocybin. PCP ("angel dust"), however, is different from those other agents since in addition to its hallucinogenic effect, it can have depressant, stimulant, analgesic, anesthetic, and convulsant activity. An acute toxic pcychosis with an agitated delirium and violent outbursts can occur. An overdose can produce convulsions and coma. It is, therefore, a much more dangerous agent[16] and adolescents should be made aware of these potential consequences of its use.

Even though a real risk to health is present, it is close to impossible to convince any adolescent of personal danger in the use of alcohol or cigarettes. They have been exposed to lectures and films in school and probably know all the facts. However, it is worth trying to reinforce this information with your personal advice. The teenager's parents' use of these substances will probably play an important role in his or her action. An occasional parent has given up tobacco to set a good example for a teenage child. Physicians who smoke cigarettes in the presence of their patients lose credibility in all areas of preventive medicine.

Perhaps the most subtle danger of drug usage of any kind is the psychological dependency that insidiously develops. While some adolescents and young adults stop because they tire of the expense and side effects, others continue to the point where to listen to music, to walk in the park, to be with friends, or to be alone and enjoy it, they must be "high." When you can make your patients realize that they have reached a point where their zest for life needs constant augumentation with drugs, they may become ready to accept the idea of counseling. Once a pervasive pattern of drug usage has been established, the patient's environment, including drug-using friends and drug-associated activities, continues to reinforce this behavior and make change difficult. If such a situation exists, then a residential setting that removes the patient from this environment may be necessary.

In some cases drug usage is an attempt at self-medication for diagnosable and treatable psychiatric disturbances. This may occur in depression, mania, and schizophrenia. A careful drug and psychosocial history is important, so that the preexisting emotional conditions can be separated from the effects of the drugs. This is not always easy to accomplish, and a drug-free period of time may be required before a definitive determination can be made as to what is schizophrenia as opposed to LSD-induced psychosis or what is depression as opposed to chronic barbiturate intoxication. Hospitalization is indicated in both cases to assure the safe discontinuation of drugs as well as a comprehensive evaluation and the initiation of psychiatric treatment.

THE THREAT OF VIOLENCE

Acute Management

The primary care physician may be the first person called by the frightened parents of an adolescent exhibiting or threatening violence. The immediate priority is the prevention of injury to all concerned. If the parents do not have sufficient control of the situation to assure safety, reinforcements, including the police, may be necessary. Once a youth has assaulted another person, legal and emotional complications may become obstacles to ideal treatment. The most effective way of preventing violent behavior is to have enough manpower to subdue the patient easily. By his or her presence, the physician can often restore calm to the situation. If the patient remains agitated in spite of reassurance and physical restraint, diazepam (Valium) 5–10 mg IM will usually have a calming effect.

Violence may be seen in a functional psychosis (schizophrenia or manic–depressive disorder) or in a drug-induced psychosis following the use of amphetamines, LSD, or PCP. Often the initial clinical pictures of the above states cannot be differentiated, but the acute management of agitation and violence in psychosis requires chlorpromazine 25 mg IM, followed by another 25 mg in an hour, when indicated, and possible hospitalization. Blood pressure needs to be monitored for hypotension. (See Chapter 7, The Management of Psychosis.)

Short-Term Management

For the majority of individuals who regain control of their violent impulses without medication or hospitalization, a determination of etiology must be made. If the violent behavior is just part of a larger picture of progressive intimidation and delinquency over which the patient experiences minimal regret, medicine, including psychiatry, may have little to offer. Still, psychiatric evaluation is indicated, and some residential treatment programs report success with recalcitrant delinquents.

Episodic assaultive behavior may, on rare occasions, have an organic etiology, as in the case of temporal lobe epilepsy (complex partial seizures—psychomotor seizures). Although purposeful aggressive acts are uncommon in the course of a psychomotor seizure, when assaultive behavior is preceded by an aura of intense anxiety and initiated by minor motor acts, such as chewing and smacking movements, purposeless fumbling or patting of the hands and picking at clothes, an organic etiology must be entertained. A psychomotor seizure will be followed by postictal drowsiness or clouding of consciousness and complete amnesia for the attack. Menkes' *Textbook of Child Neurology* provides a more complete presentation of diagnosis and treatment of temporal lobe epilepsy.[15]

In the majority of cases, the etiology of an episode of violent behavior is something far less serious than psychosis, sociopathy, or a seizure disorder. With frustration tolerance not fully developed and a tendency to turn passive into active, the adolescent is more likely than an adult to respond to pressure by striking out impulsively at his or her environment. If a specific precipitating cause is found, such as excessive parental punishment or a ridiculing teacher, an attempt should be made to diminish or remove this factor. The youth has most likely been frightened by his or her own loss of control, which will help prevent future episodes. Short-term supportive counseling may go a long way in reassuring the adolescent of his or her future control and competence. The continuation of episodic violent oubursts, without obvious precipitants, may indicate a deficiency in impulse control as part of a broader picture of generally poor coping mechanisms and low self-esteem. Psychotherapy is indicated. In the presence of an underlying depressive state, such behavior may respond well to antidepressant medication (see Chapter 6, on depression).

In all cases, the patient and his parents should be informed as to your understanding of the situation and of the treatment plan, so that they can raise any questions or doubts before returning home. With this assurance, everyone is much more likely to feel that the situation is under control. Thus the likelihood of recurrence is reduced.

PCP and Violence

Phencyclidine (PCP)[16] produces a state of agitated delirium that is clinically distinct from the schizophrenic-like picture alluded to above, and its management requires special comment.

An accurate history of PCP usage is not assured because the drug is sometimes sold as LSD or amphetamines or it may be added surreptitiously to marijuana. In their confused state, patients may be amnesic with respect to having taken the drug. In this state of agitated delirium, they may experience paranoid delusions and hallucinations of a threatening nature. There can be gross ataxia, rigidity, motor restlessness, repetitive movements, nystagmus, drooling, sweating, grimacing, and disorientation.

Management of the acute toxic reaction includes diazepam (Valium), a quiet environment, and seclusion. It may be possible to avoid violence by reducing sensory stimulation and maintaining a calm, reassuring relationship with the patient. When necessary, sufficient assistance should be available to apply physical restraints. The strength of a PCP-intoxicated person can be very impressive. In a medical setting, the use of intravenous diazepam (Valium) can be considered with extremely violent patients to prevent them from injuring themselves. Phenothiazines should be avoided in this acute phase. The toxic delirium may last from 24 hours to one week and requires hospitalization and close medical supervision for its duration.

DEPRESSION

Diagnosis

Adolescents do experience pathological depression that is distinct from the mood fluctuation inherent in this developmental period. A depressed mood affects one's perception of the world and of one's self. At a time in life when a stable identification is being established, a sustained depression can lead to a changed sense of self. This highlights the importance of diagnosing and treating this illness.[17] If there is a sustained reduction in the level of functioning associated with a depressed mood, and the additional vegetative signs and symptoms outlined in Chapter 6 are present, the diagnosis is clear. Therefore, questions must be asked to elicit this information, since it may not be offered spontaneously.

Features that may point the examiner in this direction are: (1) pervasive boredom, with loss of interest and pleasure; (2) the inability to concentrate, with diminished school performance; (3) hypersensitivity and irritability, with consequent social withdrawal, running away, and attacks on authority; (4) somatization and hypochondriacal concerns, with tiredness, insomnia, and anorexia; and (5) self-depreciation, with suicidal ideation or behavior. With the presence of any of the foregoing symptomatology, the physician should explore the adolescent's feelings. A flood of tears may quickly replace the expression of apathy, angry defiance, or superficial smiling.

It is extremely important to diagnose and treat this illness. The term "illness" is used purposely to help the physician avoid a seductive trap. It is all too easy to note such symptoms as headaches and intermittent crying, explain them on the basis of life stress, prescribe a sleeping medication for symptomatic relief, and fail to address the core problem. Most serious depressions in adolescents are preceded by an objectively serious stress.[1] Instead of resolving spontaneously within a few weeks, however, these depressions persist and worsen.

Treatment

In choosing the type of treatment, the level of functioning at school and at home must be considered, in addition to the extent of family support available. If a patient's functioning is severely impaired or if he or she is suicidal, both hospitalization and psychiatric consultation are indicated. If a patient appears bizarre, paranoid, psychotic, or in a confused mental state, in addition to being depressed, the presence of other psychiatric illness such as manic depressive psychosis, schizophrenia, or drug toxicity should be suspected. Diagnosis and treatment in these cases are best handled by a psychiatrist, though with psychiatric assessment and supervision some nonpsychiatrists may wish to follow their own patients.

Many depressions are short-lived and can be treated effectively by a nonpsychiatrist on an outpatient basis. A majority of first time depressions remit in one to two months so that the physician can be realistically optimistic in his communication with the patient. The physician must be a compassionate listener who does not attempt to avoid or minimize the patient's discomfort. If family and/or close friends are available, the physician can facilitate the patient's sharing some of his feelings with them. This approach will further reduce the separateness often experienced in depression. The patient should be encouraged to continue all activities that are not directly contributing to his or her depression. Major decisions, such as dropping out of school permanently, should not be made.

It is too easy to attribute etiological significance to the demands of school when the school difficulty may be secondary to the depression and its accompanying symptoms of fatigue and inability to concentrate.

If the adolescent's tension prevents adequate sleep or interferes with school or work functioning, medication should be considered. Frequently, the initial meeting between patient and physician, in which support is provided, will go a long way to alleviate such distressing symptoms. It is often helpful to mention the possibility of medication, because it is usually on the patient's mind, even though he or she does not mention it. The adolescent patient is particularly aware of adult apprehensions about drug usage and may be fearful that a request for medication will be misinterpreted by the physician. When symptoms are only mildy disabling and may subside substantially in a few days to a week, medication is not justifiable in either the physician's or the patient's eyes. Weathering this brief period of discomfort without medication can only add to the patient's own self-respect and sense of autonomy. If insomnia and tension remain a serious source of concern on a return visit, the physician should not withhold medication that will alleviate this distress. The benzodiazepines (diazepam [Valium], oxazepam [Serax]) are relatively free of side effects and have a relatively low potential for suicidal overdose when taken alone. They have a high potential for abuse, however, since they make the user feel "good." The patient should be seen at least weekly which will preclude the need to prescribe more than a week's supply of medication at a time. If the need for medication does not decrease within two to four weeks, then the entire situation should be reassessed. The patient may be developing an unhealthy reliance on a medication that cannot adequately treat a more serious, endogenous depression or persistent depression.

In such a situation one of the tricyclic antidepressants is the first choice of treatment in adolescents as well as in adults. These are lethal drugs, especially when combined with alcohol or other depressants, and should be approached with caution in this suicide-prone population. An overdose of 2.5 grams may be fatal unless expertly managed. Thus, no one prescription should be written for more than 1.25 grams total.

The choice of a particular tricyclic can usually be determined by the desirability of sedation, which is present in amitryptyline (Elavil) and absent in imipramine (Tofranil) and desipramine (Norpramin). The agitated adolescent with insomnia should be given amitriptyline in divided doses, with the major portion at bedtime or in a single bedtime dosage. The dosage can begin at 50 mg/day with a rapid increase to 150 mg/day at the end of seven days. Possible side effects secondary to the anticholinergic activity are dry mouth, blurry vision, and constipation. This is not usually a serious problem. Up to 300 mg/day may be necessary to achieve therapeutic effect with either amitryptyline or imipramine or 200 mg with desipramine. Desipramine is somewhat less anticholinergic. None of the tricyclics should be considered ineffective until they have been given for 3 weeks at a dose of 300 mg/day. This time factor must be explained to the patient and family at the outset so that the initial absence of improvement is not misinterpreted, causing disenchantment with both the medication and the physician.

The return of a normal sleep pattern is the first objective indication of improvement. The physician can point out improvement in such areas as mood, relatedness, and activity level to the patient, who can use all the realistic encouragement available. Patients should continue to be reassured that they will improve and that their current feelings and situations are not their fault. They should be told that while psychological factors may have triggered their depression, the illness itself is physical and therefore not within their control. Although deep and stressful exploration of psychological conflicts should not be undertaken at this time, the patients may benefit from a clarification of what has caused their current dilemma if the stress or conflict is apparent.

After improvement has been achieved, antidepressant medication can be tapered to one-half the effective dosage and should be continued for at least eight months to prevent a relapse.[18]

The majority of patients will respond to the above treatments; if a patient does not, a psychiatric consultation is indicated. More intense psychotherapy may be required to bring about complete recovery. Monoamine oxidase inhibitors and electric shock treatment can be used in those cases where the tricyclic antidepressants have failed. These treatments are discussed in more detail in Chapter 6.

SUICIDAL COMMUNICATIONS

Suicide attempts and serious suicidal communications are not specifically features of adolescence but are manifestations of serious psychiatric disorders. Physicians who find depressive features in their patients must pursue the possibility of suicidal intent. Because a large majority of adolescents who attempt suicide have seen a physician within a few months of the act, complaining of such problems as headaches, stomach aches, and fatigue, the primary care physician holds a key position in the prevention of this third greatest killer of adolescents.[19]

It is not easy for many physicians to ask patients if they want to kill themselves. In the first place, the physician fears "putting the idea into the mind" of a patient who has not already thought of it. Second, there is concern that a patient who is not thinking of suicide will be insulted by the question and not return. Third, if the patient acknowledges thoughts of suicide, the practitioner is faced with managing a difficult, anxiety-producing situation. All of these concerns can be dealt with.

The physician can begin by saying "Many patients who are depressed will often think that life is no longer worth living. Have you had such thoughts?" Most patients who are noticeably depressed have had suicidal thoughts, so that you take no risk of initiating the idea. It can also come as a relief to the patient to know that such thoughts occur commonly with depression and that they will disappear as the mood lifts. If the question is asked out of sincere concern, and the answer is no, the patient will welcome this opportunity to assure you and himself or herself that things are not so bad as to warrant suicide and will appreciate your frankness in broaching the awkward subject. If the patient acknowledges a desire to kill himself or herself, you must then determine the seriousness of the intent.

Although the specific circumstances preceding the thoughts of suicide—such as receiving poor grades in school, not being invited to a party, or being refused permission by parents to go out—may appear trivial, this does not indicate that the patient is not at serious risk. There is most likely a longstanding history of dissension within the family so that an apparently trivial event may be experienced as a serious loss of love and may precipitate a suicidal attempt.

Once the patient has communicated suicidal intent, the physician should determine whether specific plans have been thought out. If such plans have been made and the patient, even with encouragement from the physician, is unable to acknowledge any viable alternatives for life, then the patient should be hospitalized or have arrangements made that assure adequate supervision.

There are some adolescents who will intimate suicidal intent but will then shut the physician out of their thoughts and feelings, so that it becomes impossible to pursue the seriousness of the situation. If this withdrawal from the physician is part of a more extensive isolation from family and friends, the patient should not leave the office until the doctor is satisfied that someone has made real emotional contact with him or her. It is important that the patient not feel alone and that he or she know that there will be someone available if thoughts of suicide become more intense. Frequent appointments during this period of time are necessary, and support from the youth's school counselors, friends, and family can be extremely useful. Obviously, underlying emotional disturbances such as schizophrenia must be evaluated and treated, since this very significantly increases the risk of suicide, however, an adolescent need not be psychotic to make a suicide attempt. A psychiatric consultation should be obtained in order to help in planning a treatment program for all patients who express suicidal ideation.

CONCLUSION

The primary care physician has much to contribute to the care of adolescent patients. These patients are less accessible to the psychiatrist than any other patient population, yet much in need of adult support and guidance. Having given the doctor access to their personal behavior in the medical history and to their bodies in the physical examination, adolescents have acknowledged an implicit trust. The physician can make use of this relationship to explore concerns, to teach, and to comfort, thus becoming a healer in the broadest sense.

References

1. Hudgens RW: Psychiatric Disorders in Adolescents. Baltimore, Williams & Wilkins, 1974
2. Rutter M, Graham P, Chadwick O, et al.: Adolescent turmoil: Fact or fiction. J Child Psychol Psychiatry 17:35–56, 1976
3. Offer D, Ostrov E, Howard KI: The Adolescent: A Psychological Self-Portrait. New York, Basic Books, 1981
4. Offer D: Adolescence appears far happier than adults usually imagine. The New York Times, Science Times, pp 1–2, July 7, 1981
5. Sullivan HS: The Collected Works of Harry Stack Sullivan, Vol. 1. New York, Norton, 1953
6. Schoenfeld W: The Body and the Body Image, in, Caplan G, Lobovici; NY (eds): Adolescence, Psychosocial Perspectives. New York, Basic Books, 1969
7. Marshall WA, Tanner JM: Variations in pattern of pubertal changes in girls. Arch Dis Child 45:13–23, 1970
8. Borowitz G: The capacity to masturbate alone, in Feinstein SC, Giovacchini P (eds): Adolescent Psychiatry, Vol. 2. New York, Basic Books, 1973 pp. 130–143
9. Ovesey L: Homosexuality and Pseudohomosexuality. New York, Science House, 1969
10. Halleck S: Psychiatric treatment of the alienated college student. Am Psychiatry 124:5:642–650, 1967
11. Kantner JF, Zelnik M: Sexual experiences of young unmarried women in the United States. Fam Plann Perspect 4:9–18, 1972
12. Zelnik MF, Kantner JF: Sexual and contraceptive experience of young unmarried women. Fam Plann Perspect 9:55–71, March/April, 1977
13. Bell R: Changing Bodies, Changing Lives. New York, Random House, 1980
14. Secretary of Health and Human Services: Marijuana and Health. Eighth Annual Report to the Congress. Washington, D.C., 1980
15. Menkes JH: Textbook of Child Neurology, ed 2. Philadelphia, Lea & Febiger, 1980
16. Cohen S (ed): PCP (Angel Dust) New Trends in Treatment. Drug Abuse and Alcohol 7:6, July 1978
17. Malmquist CP: Depressions in childhood and adolescence. N Engl J Med 284:957–961, April, 1971
18. Coppen A, Ghose K, Montgomery S, et al.: Continuation therapy with amitriptyline in depression. Br J Psychiatry 133:28–33, 1978
19. Teicher J: "Children Who Choose Death." Emergency Med, 7:137–141, August 1975

Richard J. Glavin, M.D.
Paul F. Califano, M.D.

12

The Management of Geriatric Patients

That the primary care physician plays a crucial role in the aged individual's life is evident. The aged become increasingly prone to serious degenerative diseases as well as to the normal physiological losses of the aging process itself. There is no denying that these losses and others associated with aging can be staggering and can strongly test a person's ability to cope, both physically and emotionally. The usual mental mechanism of denying illness and death becomes less available to the aged person, who is often surrounded by illness and death in friends and family. As a consequence, physical symptoms—which are more common among the aged than among younger people—can be more frightening and threatening than they might have been earlier in the person's life. The aged thus become increasingly dependent on their physicians. Not only are physicians expected to provide the usual comfort and caring; in addition, there is the hope that they can stave off the expected ravages of aging. This can place a great strain on physicians, who traditionally feel they must "cure" their patients. However, with a shift in goals, so that "caring" is the important focus, treating this group of patients can be very rewarding. These are responsive patients who can be greatly helped, both physically and emotionally.

Obviously, the doctor who has not examined or dealt with his own fears of aging and death cannot be comfortable and effective with this group. Until recently, undergraduate and specialty medical training have generally ignored this phase of life. Society has also conspired either to ignore the aged or to see them as unproductive and burdensome. The sensitive physician can do much to help the aged patient deal with these persistent prejudices and sterotypes. Aging does not necessarily lead to serious debilitation, and the physician can help by communicating his expectations that the individual can and should be well and active. (No aged individual should ever hear from his or her doctor, "What do you expect at your age?" as an explanation for some symptom). The expectation of health can become a potent force in the patient's life.

In this chapter we will deal with the management of a wide range of problems. The focus is always on an attempt to remove or reduce a disability or, if that is not possible, to help the patient and his or her family deal more effectively with the disability and its consequences.

PSYCHOTHERAPY IN THE AGED

Psychiatrists report that work with older patients can be among the most gratifying work they do. That should not be surprising. After all, such patients have survived, many of them in spite of great adversity. They have a lifetime of experience to draw upon. The strengths that have carried them through in the past are probably still there. The skilled therapist learns how to tap these strengths. As Abraham has said, "It is the age of the neurosis, not the age of the patient which determines how amenable it is to treatment[1]"

As in any type of psychotherapy, with patients of any age, one must establish realistic goals. Significant behavior change can be even more difficult for some younger patients who still have a need to do things their way. Older patients who have found that their way has not worked may be more willing to explore alternatives.

> In response to a question from his doctor about his family, a 71-year-old man told his physician that he was still troubled by his daughter's way of life. A bright, well-educated 35-year-old woman, she had ten years ago married a man who was obviously—to this man and to many others—a poor choice. The marriage ended in divorce. She was now dating a similar kind of person. The patient feared a repetition of the previous disastrous marriage. He wanted to do a better job this time of advising her.
>
> The physician knew that this man ran his family in the old world tradition in which father's word is law. He brooked no deviation and admitted he would lose his temper on those rare occasions when a child dared to defy him. When his daughter's first relationship threatened to become serious, he had (1) laid down the law forbidding it and (2) reminded her what a devastating effect if would have on her mother. She married the man and was soon divorced. Although she had remained unmarried, she had continued to form inapropriate, self-destructive relationships.
>
> The physician asked his patient why he thought his daughter had made such a choice. The patient speculated, "Perhaps it was an act of rebellion. I was pretty strict in those days and had a violent temper. I've mellowed though." He was tempted, however, to warn her that another such marriage

would mean disinheritance. The physician pointed out that his daughter had a fine job that she enjoyed and that she had made it clear that money was not really important to her.

What did seem important to her was that she maintain some relationship with her parents. The problems usually began when she would disagree with her father on political matters or on what should be done about the "misbehavior" of her younger sister. However, even these arguments were becoming less common as the father, now more "mellow," was learning to listen and to treat her opinions with more respect. He came to realize that his "mellowing" represented a diminished need to demonstrate his power and a greater need for family closeness. The physician praised him for that, pointing out that one difficult but essential task for all parents was to be able to shift the nature of the parent–child relationship as the child grows. His 35-year-old daughter was very much an adult and he was learning to treat her with appropriate respect, something she probably felt was missing in her teens and twenties. He could understand that and acknowledged that she had much more education and did more reading than he and could probably teach him some things. He was reminded that he could take much pride in those very accomplishments that he had worked so hard to finance. If having her get an education was so important to him, he could not then behave as though it had had no effect.

The physician also pointed out that the patient's strategy regarding the daughter's new relationship was a replay of the old one, which had failed. What made him think it would work this time? The patient himself had acknowledged that her first marriage may have been an act of rebellion. Why not avoid that possibility again, and shift his position from "Don't do it because I say so and I will punish you if you do," to "Don't do it because it's bad for *you.*" He felt that very strongly and that was why he had "forbidden" these relationships in the first place. He was urged to talk to her only in those terms and to avoid any statement that would suggest punishment or invoke guilt. The patient began to understand that in this way they could develop a relationship in which the daughter need not continue to act out her adolescent rebellion.

In this case, the physician took a relatively active role, asking questions and offering possible courses of action. In other situations, more passive listening is indicated. Physicians tend to be action-oriented and too readily dismiss the value of a passive activity. They feel guilty if they have not given a patient something concrete in exchange for his or her fee. Such an attitude is most unfortunate in the management of patients at any age, but it is especially so in dealing with the aged.

Listening to the aged can serve many purposes. For example, Butler believes that the tendency of old people to relive their past in conversation, is a necessary concomitant of this stage of life. This *life review* process not only serves as a means of countering loneliness through conversation but may serve other purposes as well.[2] For some patients, it can provide a means of expiating guilt: you may have to hear a confession and then simply acknowledge that the patient truly regrets some act of omission or commission. It can provide the patient with an opportunity to talk out an old family conflict that perhaps can still be resolved. The process can thus serve a variety of inner needs and our job is often merely to listen, with the knowledge that to do so is therapeutic.

This "life review" of past experiences may also revive earlier unresolved conflicts. Chapter 6, on the management of depression, tells of a 65-year-old man who became depressed upon retirement because he had not resolved conflicts regarding competition, achievement, and self-worth. His physician, although almost 20 years his junior, was able, by virtue of his role as a symbolic parental substitute, to provide some understanding of the basis for the patient's persistent discontent and to give him permission to acknowledge his successes as real.

The interesting thing about members of this age group is that they will assign you different roles. At one moment you are the all-knowing parent to whom they turn for advice. Later you become the child who can be lectured to about "life." They can give advice about your children's rearing, vacation spots, good books, or tell you what it was like growing up in the ghettos of Europe or the inner cities of America. Our listening to them with the respect their experience merits is therapeutic. If necessary, charge the patient a little more for the visit but allow time for talk and listening.

One word of caution regarding the role of *countertransference* in your treatment of aged patients. Countertransferences is the emotional response a patient may elicit in you—a response that reflects your own personal experiences with the aged, with your parents, with chronic illness, and with death. The physician whose experiences with his own parents are laden with conflict will find his relationships with his older patients colored by feelings that are the product more of internal than of external stimuli. If you find that you are not really as comfortable or understanding as you would like to be with your older patients, you might stop and review the role of these unconscious factors.

SEX

Of course there is sex after 65. But for unconscious reasons many of us have assumed that our parents were without sexual lives. Not surprisingly, there is a tendency to minimize the role of sex in the geriatric patient. Most surveys, however, show that sexual interest can persist until death. In a Duke University study of men and women, age 60 or over, 80 percent of men whose health, intellectual status, and social functioning were not significantly impaired reported continued sexual interest, and 70 percent were sexually active. Ten years later 25 percent were sexually active[3]. The best determinant of continued sexual functioning in older age is regular pleasurable sexual activity earlier in life. The Duke longitudinal studies also found that among men and women asked to give reasons for having ceased sexual activity, men tended to place the responsibility on themselves, and women tended to place the responsibility on their husbands.[4] Having no spouse or having a sexually inactive spouse would appear to be major determinants of diminution of sexual interest in females.

While drive may diminish with diminished frequency and longer periods required for full arousal, interest in sex and the capacity to enjoy it persist. Men of 50–75 may find it easier to control ejaculation than when they were younger and so enjoy sex more. Although a woman's physiological responses to sexual stimulation may be reduced, there need be little change in her capacity for sexual pleasure. Occasionally, hormonal insufficiency can produce local vaginal changes such as dryness and cracking, but these symptoms respond to hormonal treatment.

The assumption that the elderly no longer care about sex can prevent a physician from discussing the sexual implications of surgery or serious illness. This can produce unnecessary disability. For example, the fearful patient who, after myocardial infarction, discontinues all sexual activity should have been given special advice regarding what activity is acceptable at each stage of convalescence. The angry surgical patient who was unprepared for the impotence produced by his abdominal-perineal resection should have been prepared for this and helped to find alternative sexual techniques for satisfying himself and his partner.

Chapter 9 deals with the management of these and other sexual problems in more detail. Masters and Johnson report a 50-percent success rate in therapy with older patients, even when sexual problems have been present for more than 25 years.[5]

RETIREMENT

Recent congressional action raising the mandatory retirement age to 70 years reflects the recognition that for many people, forced inactivity may have dire consequences. Of course, there are many people who happily anticipate the end of a work career in a dull, deadend job. They have been planning for that day for years and are ready when it arrives with an active retirement plan. They have included their spouses in the planning process and the marriage can prosper from it.

On the other hand, there are those who do not want to retire. They have no outside interests and dread the day when they will no longer have jobs. Their self-esteem is wrapped up in proving to the world and to themselves, each day, that they are worthwhile. Retirement deprives them of that compulsive act. It may shut them off from the most meaningful social interaction in their lives. For men, it may mean spending 24 hours a day with a wife who has functioned independently for many years. It may mean days without purpose or structure.

Ideally you should be helping your patients deal with this problem in the years that precede it. You cannot allow your patients in their 60s to pretend that it will not happen. Your forcing husbands and wives to face the problems early can be a most significant therapeutic intervention. Try to get them to plan early. They may benefit from some joint sessions with you to iron out conflicts regarding their plans. Subsequent sessions may be needed if their plans go awry. They must realize that successful retirement is a difficult task. It takes planning, and one should not be ashamed to ask for help with it. If the problems do not resolve themselves easily, a referral to a psychiatrist or psychologist is indicated.

Mrs. W, a 56-year-old woman, told her doctor that she was becoming increasingly tense and depressed. Her 65-year-old husband had just retired from his job and was now eager to move south. She had a job she enjoyed and did not want to become a full-time homemaker. She was also disturbed by her husband's lack of planning for their move. They had never spent more than two weeks in the South; thus, neither of them really knew what it would be like to live there. She was confident that she could find a job there, given enough time, but did not want to move into an area without doing some groundwork. She had initially indicated her reservations about his plans, but when he quickly put her concerns aside, she decided there was nothing more she could do.

The problem now was her fear of repeating any of these reservations about the move. She felt her job as a loyal wife was to go along with her husband's plans, but that decision created great conflict within her. She had been brought up to believe that a wife's role was to defer to her husband's wishes. However, times had changed, and her late-blooming career was a manifestation of that change. However, these two perceptions of a woman's role existed side by side, creating great tension.

The physician suggested a joint session with her husband. The physician related the severity of the tension the wife was experiencing regarding their retirement plans. He explained that she was in great conflict about what her role should be and that he had encouraged her to be more forthright in her discussions with her husband. He added that he believed that Mr. W would understand her conflict and that the problem had probably been her unwillingness to make her point more forcefully. Mrs. W was then encouraged to spell out her reservations.

Mr. W listened quietly. He indicated that he had no idea she felt this strongly. He could understand the wisdom of taking more time to research the South. He had been a successful executive who could appreciate the value of that. He speculated that his own uncharacteristic impulsivity had probably been a manifestation of his emotional reaction to retirement.

SLEEP DISORDERS

Patients often complain about their insomnia while their spouses complain about the patients' daytime naps. Both phenomena are manifestations of the changes in sleep patterns that do occur with aging.

Most older patients have difficulty falling off to sleep and experience some loss of stages 3 and 4, the deep sleep phases. Sleep is, therefore, generally lighter. Older patients will awaken more frequently during the night and, therefore, total sleep time is diminished. These normal changes in sleep pattern can become a cause for concern for some patients who complain of insomnia. For most of these patients reassurance that their bodies now require less sleep is adequate. However, some patients will persist in this complaint.

Chapter 14, which deals in detail with the complaint of insomnia, emphasizes that this symptom is best treated without drugs. The hypnotic drugs produce more problems than they relieve. This is particularly true in the aged, in whom drug accumulation can produce serious problems. For older patients with organic brain disease who are complaining of serious insomnia, consider the possibility that the diminished sensory input at night may be making them anxious and that this may be the basis of the insomnia. In such a case a night light or a radio may be able to provide enough stimulation and orientation to reduce anxiety and allow sleep. For such a patient the quiet, rear bedroom may be, paradoxically, contributing to the problem.

If it is felt necessary to use medication, it should be used for a limited time only. To do otherwise is to run the risk of compounding the problems as these drugs begin to accumulate. Barbiturates are likely to increase nighttime confusion as they can impair cerebral function. There are older patients who have taken these drugs for years without difficulty; however, these are usually patients who were started on the drug in middle age. Chloral hydrate (0.5–1.5 gm) or small doses of an antihistamine such as diphenhydramine (Benadryl) (25–50 mg) can be safely used. Remember that the antihistamines can produce anticholinergic effects. Flurazepam (Dalmane), a commonly used hypnotic, like many benzodiazepines has a long half-life and can, therefore, accumulate. The shorter-acting, oxazepam (Serax) or lorazepam (Ativan) are theoretically preferable, but good clinical reports on their effectiveness are not yet available. The chapter on sleep disorders should be reviewed for methods of treating insomnia without using medication.

Daytime napping may be due to intrinsic central nervous system change, diminished stimulation and activity, or excessive sedation. For example, the accumulation of drugs used for the treatment of insomnia can produce daytime somnolence. Such napping can interfere with normal nighttime sleep; otherwise it is a benign phenomenon. Providing more daytime stimulation may reduce the napping time. Should the patient complain of feeling tired despite the naps, you should seek a specific explanation—such as depression or a variety of physical causes—since these patients are usually quite alert between their naps.

NONCOMPLIANT BEHAVIOR

Noncompliant behavior in the elderly can become a world of endless controversy and misery. Although others may consider certain behavior to be self-destructive, or a risk to good health, the patient usually does not see it that way. It is important not to interpret all noncompliant behavior as either hostile, defiant, or suicidal. It is almost always quite the opposite, that is, a patient's fear of death or illness produces behavior that he believes can control or mitigate this dread. The usual reason people overeat, drink excessively, or fail to take prescribed medication is not their wish to die or destroy their bodies. It is more likely that they are using food or alcohol to neutralize anxiety or depression. The failure to take pills is often an unconscious denial of illness. Of course, it is also possible that the forgetting is related to dementia.

It is especially hazardous to interpret this kind of behavior as suicidal. The patient may then feel both totally misunderstood and accused of "sinful" behavior. Such an interpretation may itself lead to true hostile and oppositional behavior. If you can accept that the patient has the right to refuse our good medical advice, then you are well on your way to a better handling of the problem. Second, if the purpose of the behavior in question is to reduce anxiety regarding fear of death or loss of control, our efforts to deal with the behavior should not be designed merely to frighten the patient further. Anything that increases that anxiety may only lead to increasing the behavior in question. Most people do not drink too much, overeat, or forget their medication out of ignorance of the consequences. Anyone who does not "know" these basic principles for good health by three score and ten is not about to be enlightened.

Unless the patient is delirious, psychotic or grossly demented, he or she should still retain freedom of choice and of self-determination. However, with better understanding, perhaps we can help ease the conflict that such behavior engenders.

In a nursing home, the psychiatrist was asked to write an order restricting a patient to the home. The patient was losing his vision and his daily need to walk in a heavily trafficked street led the staff to feel that he either wanted to be run over to end his life or was unable to understand the risk he was taking with this behavior. The patient was interviewed. He explained that he had no desire to die, but he was unable to accept a life that curtailed his daily walks outside of the home. He was well aware of the risks involved but felt it was worth it. "If I can't get out a little, I may as well be dead." In his very restricted world, this was one of his few remaining pleasures. It provided a sense of some independence. He stated that if the staff restricted him, he would have to break the locked doors. With the staff's better understanding of the patient's motivation and rights, and their acceptance of the risk/benefit ratio involved, the problem was resolved. It was interesting to note that it was later learned that this man had been doing this for over a year without incident but without the staff's awareness.

HYPOCHONDRIASIS

This disorder is a common and vexing problem best treated by the primary care physician. These patients need not and usually should not, in most cases, be referred to a psychiatrist. Such a referral will generally result in an angry patient who moves on to yet another doctor.

That this disorder should be more prevalent in the aged is understandable. Although they are concerned with prolonging healthy and active living, the elderly also are confronted with physical symptoms and illnesses that are debilitating and immobilizing more frequently than are younger people. Thus a certain amount of bodily concern is natural and useful. The hypochondriac, however, goes beyond the limits of protective concern and makes illness the prime concern of his or her life. For some patients the absence of outside interests also heightens their awareness of bodily function.

The aged do frequently present themselves to their doctors with hypochondriacal complaints as a mechanism for coping with the many stresses of aging. Altman has said that hypochondriasis at all ages is often an attempt to deal with either anxiety or anger.[6] That is, these emotions are associated with physical symptoms that, otherwise might have been treated more lightly. Since the doctor is viewed as a potential source of strength and support, he or she is the "logical" helper for all problems. The physical symptoms are the ticket of admission to the doctor's office. Of course, this view of the doctor is held on an unconsious level, but the symptoms and the accompanying anxiety are very real to the patient.

The diagnosis of depression must be ruled out in all patients with hypochondriacal complaints, since depression is often accompanied by increased somatic concerns. The depressed patient, however, will usually have a more discrete illness pattern than the purely hypochondriacal patient, that is, the anxious preoccupation with bodily sensations will usually reflect a distinct change in the patient's behavior or a marked intensification of a milder tendency. The patient will also display sad affect, and it is likely that specific vegetative signs of depression such as early morning awakening or diurnal mood variation will also be present (Chapter 6 deals with depression in more detail).

After the doctor convinces himself that there is no significant organic pathology or depression and that any existing diseases are being adequately treated, the hypochondriacal complaints still must be handled. They can be most effectively treated if the doctor can recognize that the goal should not be to get the patient to stop complaining about physical ills. Our goal should be to allow the patient to function without the disabling effects of untreated hypochondriasis. This is a chronic illness with acute exacerbations. If we are able to provide the patient with a friendly, understanding, nonrejecting source of support, he or she should be able to function reasonably well between episodes. To do this the patient must be reassured of the doctor's ongoing concern.

Almost by definition, simple reassurance will fail. Patients feel the doctor will reject them unless they are truly ill. Therefore, physicians must learn how to address patients' anxiety regarding their physical symptoms without raising patients' anxiety about their relationship with their doctors. One should avoid telling patients that there is is nothing wrong and then censoring or lecturing them about becoming hypochondriacal. Performing more and more laboratory tests to "prove there is nothing wrong" will also not work. The last thing these patients want to hear is "There is nothing wrong," which implies neuroticism and potential rejection. However, "There is nothing to be worried about" is quite acceptable since it allows for the continuation of the relationship and does not suggest the complaint is not real. The patient is told he has symptoms of a benign illness with which he will have to live and that you will do what you can to help minimize the symptoms. Trying to explain in psychiatric terms how anxiety can be transformed into physical complaints usually does not work. Patients may appear to understand but they will quickly be off for more "doctor-shopping," an expensive and inefficient complication of this condition.

Follow-up visits should be scheduled on a regular basis, not too far apart. This will reduce the likelihood of numerous telephone calls or requests for "urgent" appointments. These patients may be very conscious of the time interval between visits; therefore, do not change the pattern without an explanation. It will be important at each visit to allow time for the patients to talk about other aspects of their lives. The doctor's interest is invaluable for its effect upon the individual's self-esteem.

It may be necessary for the physician to prescribe medication as symbolic recognition that the patient is indeed suffering and that the physician will take care of him. Patients should be told that we doubt that any medication can totally alleviate their symptoms, but we will try to minimize their discomfort. The placebo effect can be very powerful. The medication should be chosen, if possible, to deal with the target symptom but the drugs chosen and doses given should, of course, be designed to do no harm. Medication with anticholinergic properties, which includes most psychotropic medication, should be used cautiously, if at all. Tranquilizers should be used with great caution since they can be abused, and agents with a long half-life can quickly accumulate. Chapter 5 deals with their use in more detail.

Most hypochondriacal patients complain fairly constantly to their families, who usually gradually lose sympathy and patience. The family may turn to the doctor for relief, but even where they do not seek your help directly it can be very useful to include them in your treatment program. It is important not to imply to them that the patient's complaints are psychogenic or imaginary. The emphasis should instead be on the benign nature of the problem. The family should receive sympathy for the frustration they must feel at their inability to reassure the patient and they should be encouraged to have the patient continue his program of contact with the doctor. They should also be made to feel free to maintain this contact. Their ready access to you for reassurance can reduce the anger and guilt that the complaints induce, and in that way the patient will benefit from his or her family's enhanced ability to listen to him.

When dealing with hypochondriacal patients, there is always the fear that a serious illness is being missed or ignored. Some of these patients, indeed, may at times withhold symptoms from their physicians since they truly fear the worst and may, therefore, be in conflict about revealing a symptom that they sense is potentially serious. After all, what many really want is reassurance that all is well and that you will continue to care for them. With a program of short but regular and frequent office visits as evidence of the physician's concern they can be helped considerably with their hypochondriasis, and simultaneously their physical state can be carefully monitored.

ANXIETY STATES

Old age can be a time of life filled with anxiety-provoking events. Losses due to the death of friends or of a spouse and especially the loss of children who move away or are otherwise inaccessible can be severely trying, as can sudden changes in the environment or loss of security due to financial problems. At these times, the patient may seek out the physician and ask for "something for my nerves." Before reaching for the prescription pad, it is useful to remember that the most potent therapeutic agent may well be the physician–patient relationship. A few sessions set aside for brief psychotherapy can be most helpful in lowering anxiety by allowing patients to ventilate their concerns to a trusted person who shows real interest. For the widowed patient with grown children living at a distance "with enough problems of their own," the doctor may be the only important person to whom she can turn. At the unconscious level, the physician can be as reassuring to a patient as any parent can be to an anxious child. The fact that the patient may be 35 years the physician's senior means nothing to his or her unconscious perception of the doctor as a parent-substitute.

At a more conscious level, patients may need some realistic advice regarding nonmedical problems. In fact, it is generally a good thing to be much more active with this group than with others in such matters and, in a sense, to foster a dependence on the doctor that would not be desirable for a younger patient. Many of your older patients, by virtue of loss and illness, are very dependent, and some recognition of this can be very therapeutic. This does not mean that these patients should be infantilized. For example, too often we automatically assume we can call elderly patients by their first names, as we do children. This is an unconscious act, often in response to our perception of patients' dependence on us. However, you can allow a patient to be dependent on you without resorting to a device that can lower self-esteem. Other patients are reluctant to acknowledge any loss of independence. For them it is essential that you limit your role to those areas that they delegate to you. To do otherwise can damage self-esteem.

Short-term use of minor tranquilizers can be useful if the anxiety is very severe and is interfering with functioning or if the initial response to the psychotherapeutic approach is not completely successful. The reduction in extreme anxiety is helpful in restoring the patient's sense of control. However, since these drugs can accumulate and produce toxic effects (Chapter 5), judicious use is advised in the elderly. Diazepam (Valium) in small doses (2 mg) can be given initially 3 to 4 times a day but within 5 days should be reduced to a bid schedule to prevent the development of toxicity. Oxazepam (Serax) or lorazepam (Ativan) are short-acting drugs and are less likely to accumulate. They may, therefore, be preferable in older patients. The chronic use of these drugs in the aged is contraindicated. Only small supplies should be given, and prescriptions should indicate no refills without the physician's permission.

Before you do write a prescription for a tranquilizer, be sure to ask yourself, "Am I sure this patient isn't really depressed?" The agitation that often accompanies depression can cause you to miss the true diagnosis. A sedating antidepressant, e.g., doxepin (Sinequan) would then be the appropriate treatment (see Chapter 6).

PARANOID REACTIONS

Paranoid reactions are common in the aged. In some cases this may be related to diminished hearing and eyesight, since those factors that tend to reduce discriminatory faculties and the ability to cope with environmental stress are likely to foster paranoid reactions. Paranoid disorders in the elderly have a wide range of symptoms, from moderate suspiciousness to possesion of a well-organized delusional system. The suspicions frequently center on feelings of neglect and mistreatment by a hostile environment. The delusional systems usually involve family, friends, or other people close at hand rather than the global or national conspiracies more typical of the younger, paranoid schizophrenic.

The paranoid disorder can best be understood as an adaptive mechanism using projection and denial as major mechanisms of defense. The person denies his or her own deficiencies and makes the environment responsible for them; for example, the man who misplaces his wallet complains that he has been robbed; the woman whose hearing is diminished attributes her difficulty to people purposefully speaking softly and then saying insulting things. The formula becomes, "There is nothing wrong with me, it's them." The mistrust may be mild and may not interfere with functioning or it may be severe enough to lead to disruptive behavior and further isolation. For example, a 78-year-old woman in a home for the aged began to feel that her next-door neighbor was deliberatly moving furniture around at night to disturb her. She would misinterpret any normal noise coming through the wall as harassment solely directed at her. At first she only grumbled about this to staff members, but eventually she would bang loudly on the wall or her neighbor's door with a cane, at one point even denting the door. This finally brought some staff intervention. In this same home was another woman who reported that her dead husband visited her every night but that he couldn't be seen during the day because of staff interference. This latter case is an example of a reparative delusion that appears to help the patient, leads to no difficulty, and does not need to be treated.

Patients with paranoid ideation can be most difficult to manage. Most seldom seek out treatment for the very reason that they see the problems as outside themselves. They bitterly resent and vigorously resist referral to a physician, let alone a psychiatrist. Though these traits tend to put off and discourage the physician and other potential helpers, such patients can be successfully treated. This can be done if the goals are limited to improving the behavior by reducing the anxiety and the anger but without directly attacking the delusions. A sympathetic and open attitude should be assumed and such supportive and neutral remarks as "That must be very upsetting" or "You sound quite frightened" can be made in discussing the delusions. This can be done without in any way appearing to confirm the delusional system. You can say, "Of course, I can't tell you I know for a fact that your neighbor is not plotting against you, but I do know those thoughts are upsetting you and I would like to give you some medicine for that."

The doctor should try to help the patient deal with the problem as the patient perceives it. The doctor's interest and attention can help diminish the patient's sense of helplessness and loss of mastery. (The lady who pounded on the wall, for example, was seen a number of times, and the situation was discussed without any suggestion that she was really misinterpreting benign noises. She was soon able to talk about her feelings of loneliness as a childless widow who knew that her nieghbor had a devoted and attentive family.) It is striking how many paranoid patients come to physicians with their complaints of infidelities, plots, voices and the like. Although they loudly insist that they are correct in their beliefs, they still choose to go to a physician and not an attorney or a policeman. Apparently at some level there is an awareness that they are ill. If we deal with them properly they will remain motivated and will return to us for talk and medicine.

Initially, any physical problem, particularly those involving hearing and visual impairment or impaired mobility should be attended to. In this way, perceptual distortions are minimized and some autonomy restored. Should this fail to eliminate the paranoia, drug treatment should be considered.

Antipsychotic medications are most useful and can mute or at times eliminate the delusions or hallucinations. The patient can be told that it must be difficult to live with these kinds of feelings and that there are medications that can help deal with the fear. Elderly patients are more sensitive to both the therapeutic effect and the side-effects of most drugs. Haloperidol (Haldol) is an effective agent with few sedating properties and minimal anticholinergic and cardiovascular side-effects. Elderly patients should be started on as little as 0.5 mg bid. Thioridazine (Mellaril) can be used if a sedating effect is desired. Small doses such as 10 mg during the day and 25 mg at bedtime should be used initially.

Orthostatic hypotension and anticholinergic effect are the most common side-effects of these phenothiazine compounds. The hypotension can be especially dangerous in the aged. Therefore, blood pressures should be taken sitting and standing before doses are increased. Patients should be cautioned to get out of bed in stages, sitting on the edge for a minute before arising. If orthostatic hypotension remains a problem, support stockings may help.

Electrocardiographic changes have been reported with phenothiazines. These changes usually comprise an increased QR interval and a flattening of T waves and are most likely to occur with doses above 300 mg. These changes are not thought to have any clinical significance.

The anticholinergic effects of drugs such as chlorpromazine or thioridazine can produce dryness of the mouth, constipation, diminished bladder contractility, and difficulty with visual accommodation. These effects can usually be handled with time and dose adjustments. The intensity of this effect varies within this group of drugs; for example, haloperidol has minimal anticholinergic effects. (Table 7-3 in Chapter 7 contains a table outlining the strength of these side-effects in antipsychotic agents). Should these side-effects prove troublesome, laxatives can be used for the constipation and bethanechol (Urecholine) for the relative bladder atony. As a rule, however, try to use agents or doses that do not require additional medication to deal with side-effects.

These drugs can also affect the extrapyramidal system, producing a parkinsonian syndrome. This is a dose-related phenomenon. High-potency drugs such as haloperiodol and fluphenazine are more likely to produce this effect than the more sedating drugs, such as chlorpromazine. Generally, the more anticholinergic a drug the less likely it is to produce these neurological effects. Dyskinesias, peculiar movements of the head or neck, and akathisia, a restlessness especially of the lower extremities can also occur. The akathisia is sometimes mistaken for agitation and the drug dose is increased instead of decreased. Although these neurological effects can be neutralized with antiparkinsonian medication, in this age group it is preferable to try to find a dose of a drug that is effective and free of side-effects.

Tardive dyskinesia is a syndrome characterized by abnormal movements of the face and tongue. It can occur after prolonged use (more than a year) of relatively high doses of these drugs. The elderly are more vulnerable. Therefore, these patients should be checked regularly (at least every two months) for abnormal movements. Involuntary chewing movements may be the first indication of toxicity. Although there is no specific treatment, discontinuation of the drug usually brings relief.

When patients' symptoms have been brought under control patients can be maintained on a single nighttime dose, since the drugs are long-lasting. However, patients should be reminded about the hypotensive effect if they are likely to get up during the night. Paranoid patients are, of course, often reluctant to take any medication but they may be willing to take something to help them sleep at night or for their "nervousness." In some cases, where disruptive behavior has to be controlled, it may be necessary to administer these medications without the patient's knowledge in juice or coffee. Both haloperidol and thioridazine come in liquid form and are practically tasteless. However, this type of administration can be accomplished only if the patient is in a skilled nursing setting or if there is a reliable person available to administer it. Often, after a few such covert doses, the patient is willing to take the medication in regular form.

Environmental manipulation can be an important treatment modality. A person who feels persecuted by a roommate in a nursing home sometimes can benefit by a transfer to another floor. While this does not always leave the delusional system behind, at least the patient is made to feel that he is in some control of the situation, and that he is being supported by a significant individual, his doctor.

Attempts to reduce isolation and withdrawal through visits by visiting nurses and referral to senior citizen centers can be very helpful. Counseling the family (and sometimes staff members) is almost always required, since they are frequently the focus of delusional ideas. Family and staff members may react with anger, guilt, and extreme anxiety and defensiveness, and they may engage in repeated and elaborate attempts to prove their innocence. By helping them understand the underlying mechanisms, this reaction can be minimized and they can remain more supportive and concerned. This is what the patient needs most of all.

DEPRESSION

Depression is a common and too frequently missed diagnosis. There is an unfortunate tendency to assume that depression is an inevitable accompaniment of old age. The unhappiness and frustration created by the losses and disabilities of this period are best treated psychotherapeutically. However, clinical depression is a medical diagnosis that calls for specific treatment. Unhappiness and depression share overlapping symptoms such as feelings of sadness, feelings of tiredness and weakness, intense fears of poverty, incapacity, sickness, and death and a loss of pleasure and interest in many aspects of living. However, the "unhappy" patient retains the capacity for enjoyment should some special positive event take place in his life. The depressed patient loses all capacity for pleasure. The presence of vegetative signs and symptoms in the depressed patient are another important differentiating point. The clinically depressed individual usually manifests psychomotor retardation or agitation, anorexia, and insomnia (particularly in company with early morning awakening) and experiences diurnal variation, with mood and appettite improvement by the end of the day.

The depressed patient often presents initially with physical complaints, such as fatigability, insomnia, nausea upon awakening, constipation, or difficulty with memory or concentration. Some patients will complain of persistent pain that is often unrelated to an underlying illness. These patients may also abuse alcohol, analgesics, and tranquilizers in a desperate attempt to gain relief from their emotional pain and insomnia. These symptoms and the dysphoric mood are all reversible with appropriate use of antidepressant medication or electric shock treatment. The lifting of the depression may not produce a completely happy patient since the aged person may, of course, have much good reason to be unhappy. However, without the symptoms of depression which so completely interfere with coping the person can begin to find more effective ways of dealing with those factors that have contributed to the unhappiness. An important aspect of depressive illness is that it tends to feed upon itself. Family and friends find the depressed person frustrating and irritating to deal with. Efforts to cheer the person up or to help him or her usually fail and lead to further withdrawal and isolation.

It is useful to try to find a precipitating cause for the depression, but this is not always possible. At times the cause can appear to be a minor event that has strong symbolic meaning; for example, a delayed or lost Social Security check or a lost keepsake or phone number. Other times there may be a significant loss, such as the death of a loved one or the development of a debilitating illness. However, depression must be distinguished from mourning and grief reactions. These normal reactions to significant loss are usually not associated with diminished self-esteem, severe guilt, or self-contempt. They are limited to a mood of sadness over the specific loss and, in time, the mood lifts. Such patients should be permitted to mourn, to discuss their loss, to weep. The use of antidepressants is inappropriate. However, if there is a past history of affective illness, vegetative signs appear, or if the syndrome is particularly severe and persistent, a diagnosis of treatable depression should be considered.

Another precipitant of depression can be a patient's awareness of early signs of organic brain syndrome, such as difficulties with recall, calculation, and learning. The management of dementia is dealt with later.

The diagnostic work-up for depression should include a careful review of all medications the individual is currently taking. Certain drugs, such as reserpine, can produce clinical depression, and chronic use of minor tranquilizers can be a contributing factor (this problem is discussed in more detail in Chapter 6).

The depressed patient should always be questioned about the presence of suicidal ideas. Suicide is a great danger in the depressed aged individual. The aged, who make up 10 percent of our population, account for 25 percent of suicides. The aged man who lives alone and has an alcohol problem is particularly at risk. Aged individuals will frequently express the feeling that they would welcome death as a relief: "I wish I wouldn't wake up in the morning" or "I wish the Lord would take me." These expressions are quite different from those of the persons who tell you that they have actually formulated a plan and a method to kill themselves. Any sudden change in behavior that could be interpreted as preparing for death, such as giving away money, property, or cherished objects should be a signal to inquire into suicidal ideas. If any suspicion exists, you should request a psychiatric consultation and consider the possibility of psychiatric hospitalization or some other form of continuous supervision.

Once the diagnosis of clinical depression has been made the patient should be told he has a treatable, medical illness for which effective medication is available. Whereas the patient presents a picture of incapacity, helplessness, and hopelessness, the physician should counter with hopefulness, resourcefulness, and the expectation that this very treatable condition will be ameliorated. One must understand depressive symtomatology as a communication, that is, a cry for help. The patient will be relieved to find that his cry of anguish has been heard and that help is at hand.

The tricyclics are the drugs of choice in the aged. Amitryptiline (Elavil) has sedating properties and should be used if the patient is anxious or if insomnia is a prominent complaint. Imipramine (Tofranil) is very much less sedating and should be used for the patient with psychomotor retardation. Desipramine (Norpramin) has fewer anticholinergic side-effects. (Chapter 6 discusses anti-depressant drugs in more detail).

In the aged, it is very important to "start low and go slow." This means starting, for example, with 10 mg tid or qid and then gradually increasing doses if there are no serious side-effects. These medications generally do not produce noticeable improvement in the depression for 10 days to 2 weeks or more (though insomnia may improve earlier), so sufficient time must be allowed for them to work. The dose can be increased by 20–25 mg week. While younger patients are more likely to respond in the 150–300-mg range, the geriatric patients tend to respond in the 50–150-mg range. Doses need to be increased until an effective blood level is achieved, but side-effects should be carefully monitored.

The most potentially harmful side-effect is probably orthostatic hypotension, since a fall can be so dangerous in the elderly. Blood pressures should be taken sitting and standing with each office visit. It is usually found that most patients have fewer anticholinergic side-effects if the bulk of the drug is given at bedtime. However, this can pose serious problems with the aged patient who may awaken during the night to void, get up too quickly, and then perhaps have a large blood pressure drop. Patients should be told to change positions slowly and carefully and to report any signs of dizziness immediately. They should be cautioned to arise from bed in two stages, sitting on the edge of the bed for one minute before standing up.

The tricyclics have a quinidine-like effect on the heart and therefore, should not be used in the presence of heart block. Premature beats are usually not a contraindication and it has been suggested that these drugs might even prove to be therapeutic.[7] The cardiac effects are discussed in more detail in the chapter on the management of depression.

The anticholinergic side-effects can be annoying. Dryness of the mouth may gradually diminish but generally responds to frequent sips of water and the use of lozenges, lemon drops, and the like. Constipation may require laxatives. Bladder tone may have to be augmented with bethanecol (Urecholine) (10 mg tid to start). Amitryptiline is the most potent anticholinergic agent, desipramine the least.

Occasionally, an elderly patient on a tricyclic will develop a severe delirium with agitation, disorientation, and hallucinations. This condition may result from the central anticholinergic property of the drug. In any event, the medication must be stopped immediately. A lower dose may prove to be safe, but a trial of such a dose should be carried out in the hospital.

When the depression is severe, the threat of suicide is present, or the patient does not seem to be responding to antidepressants, the use of electroshock therapy (EST) must be considered. EST is a very effective and safe treatment, and there are few contraindications even in the very old. The transitory memory loss it produces, however, can be quite disturbing to an aged individual whose memory is already somewhat borderline. To overcome this, fewer treatments are given and those that are needed are spaced further apart. Some experts believe that unilateral EST to the non-dominant hemisphere is less likely to produce memory loss. The memory difficulty rarely persists.[8]

Psychotherapy for these patients must be supportive. It is never helpful to lecture depressed patients. Friends and family have generally already told them such things as "pull yourself together," or "things aren't really that bad." Such remarks only serve to make them feel more guilty, as does any premature pressure to get involved in social activities. Instead the depressed must be helped to understand that their symptoms are manifestations of an organic illness. Their sole obligation should be to take their medication and keep their appointments with you. The visits can allow patients to communicate their suffering to you, but they can also be used to review some of the events in their lives that may have triggered the depression. This may help in planning to prevent a recurrence.

Once medication begins to take effect it is useful to encourage a return to socialization. You want to prevent a curtailment in social, emotional, or intellectual life that can ultimately lead to another depression. Consider the use of special agencies, such as senior citizen centers. You can use the patient's faith in you to encourage an activity even if the patient is not convinced it will be useful. You should be well aware of those facilities that might be available and prepared to give specific recommendations to meet the aged person's needs. It is always better to say, "Call Mrs. Jones at the Golden Age Club and find out when the next Bridge Club meeting will be," than to say, "You like to play cards; why not join a club?"

As in any serious medical conditions, the family should not be ignored since they may be part of the problem or part of the solution, and they certainly share the suffering. The depressed, hostile, agitated patient usually involves the family in the illness, and family members soon experience anxiety, discouragement, guilt, and hostility. Old family disappointments and resentments can be rekindled. The family often has something to offer in the diagnostic work-up and evaluation, since the depressed individual may be quite unable to give an effective history. Family members can also be helpful in the development and facilitation of a treatment program. They should be informed that while the patient's illness may have begun as a psychological reaction to an event, it is now a biological illness even though symptoms may appear to be behavioral or emotional. They must understand, for example, that the patient's pessimism is a symptom and will not respond to their encouragment or urgings to "cheer up" until the illness itself begins to improve. They and the patient must be helped to wait the weeks it will take for the antidepressant to work.

Patients should be maintained on the therapeutic dose for at least three months after the depression lifts. The dose can then be gradually reduced over the next 6–9 months. (Chapter 6 discusses this in more detail).

ORGANIC BRAIN SYNDROMES

Organic brain syndromes can be either reversible (acute brain syndrome, delirium) or irreversible (chronic brain syndrome, dementia). The clinical distinction is often impossible to make on initial mental examination unless one has adequate test results and a reliable history at hand. In some situations delirium can be superimposed on dementia. Perhaps the most common error made in their managment is the assumption that they are a necessary, and perhaps acceptable, untreatable concomitant of old age. The discussion that follows emphasizes the need for active treatment in these disorders.

Delirium

Delirium is a more common problem in the aged, especially when they are hospitalized. These patients, because of reduced cerebral reserve, are more vulnerable to the physical and environmental stresses of hospitalization. Thus an acute delirium can be superimposed on a chronic dementia to which the patient has made a satisfactory adaptation. A wide variety of medications can adversely affect a patient's nervous system—anesthetic agents, narcotics, hypnotics, anticholinergic agents. Cimetidine (Tagamet) is currently widely used for the treatment of peptic ulcer and has been reported to produce delirium, especially in the aged.[9] Reduction in dosage may be all that is necessary to successfully treat a delirium. The patient who develops a delirium on reasonable doses of medication may also be suffering from a previously undetected dementia.

The shift to an unfamiliar environment can cause difficulty, especially at night when familiarizing cues are diminished. A night light will help and, if needed, a sedating antipsychotic agent such as chlorpromazine, 25 mg, can be given at sleep. Other management measures will be found in Chapter 7.

It is important to keep in mind that the aged patient who has been hosptialized with delirium but has been functioning well at home should be able to return home after successful treatment of the delirium. In some cases, complete clearing of the confusion may not occur until after the patient returns to a familiar environment. An occasional patient may not clear completely at home and may require additional help or even transfer to a nursing facility. However, most of them will do well. An anxious family will need reassurance from you that there is little to lose in making this effort and much to gain.

Dementia

Dementia is best defined as a deterioration of mental function due to organic disease of the cerebral hemispheres. It is generally assumed that this is an irreversible process, particularly when it occurs in the aged. Such an assumption is most regrettable, since reversible and treatable problems are common. In one study of "dementia" in a group of patients with the average age of 66, 30 percent were found to have potentially treatable illness.[10] The physician's responsibility is therefore to: (1) make the diagnosis, (2) determine if the etiology indicates a treatable disorder, and (3) provide treatment for the emotional and behavioral problems that can accompany the illness.

The usual criteria for the diagnosis of dementia are

- a deterioration of intellectual function, significant enough to interfere with social or occupational functioning
- memory impairment
- impairment of judgment
- lability or shallowness of affect
- impairment of abstract thinking as manifested by reduced capacity for such activities as generalization and synthesizing

In the early stages, changes are usually quite subtle, detectible only by those who know the patient well. For example, typical early signs are a diminution of energy, drive or creativity; difficulty in concentrating; and increased distractibility. Old psychological defense mechanisms are still used, but they are exaggerated and less effective.

The diagnosis therefore, is, established on the basis of history, mental status exam, and physical and laboratory findings.

Mental Status Exam

A good portion of the mental status exam is actually carried out during the process of history taking and physical exam. The essential components should include an evaluation of appearance and behavior, orientation, language, memory, intellectual functioning, and, mood.[10]

The findings of a formal mental status exam are often difficult to interpret, since anxiety or depression can produce apparent deficits. Therefore, weaving your questions into the medical history is preferable. A negative mental status exam does not rule out dementia, since subtle changes may not be detectible.

Appearance and behavior. Is the patient appropriately groomed? Grooming can become sloppy or bizarre; for example, the patient may wear layers of sweaters or dresses. Is the patient alert? Is his or her speech appropriate? In retrospect, has there been a significant change in the patient's appearance or behavior over the last year or two?

Orientation. Orientation can usually be established in the history taking. You want to be sure the patient knows where he or she is, the day of the week, the date, the year, and who you are.

Intellectual functioning. Such functioning is obviously dependent on both the patient's basic intellectual level and his or her education. Therefore, for some patients simple tests of arithmetic, history, or current events are not going to pick up any deficiencies. You will have to use your own judgment as to what test will best measure deterioration.

Mood. Mood is a most important variable, since depression in the aged can produce a "pseudodementia." Be particularly alert for the signs and symptoms of depression. A history of unstable or rapidly shifting moods can be an indication of dementia.

Language. Does the patient have difficulty finding the specific words he or she wants to use? Does the patient tend to ramble? Does his or her speech lack abstractions?

Memory. Specific tests of recent memory can be utilized; for example, patients can be asked to repeat a series of three nonconsecutive digits. Additional digits are added until the patient fails. They are then asked to repeat the task after first reversing the digits. Most patients can repeat at least six digits forward and four in reverse. However, this test can be influenced by anxiety or depression. Perhaps the best tests of memory are woven into the clinical history as the patient presents his or her story and responds to your specific questions about recent and remote events. This is often more valuable than the formal mental status examination, since the latter can produce errors related to the patient's "test anxiety."

Neuropsychological tests can be performed by a psychologist to supplement the clinical exam. They can be helpful in localizing a lesion. The test can also provide a baseline against which future functioning can be compared and also serve as a method for quantifying the extent of the deficit.

It is worth repeating the earlier warning not to assume that dementia in an older patient is necessarily a product of the aging process. A variety of physical and emotional etiologies should be considered. A complete list of the causes of reversible dementia is to be found in Table 1.[11] These causes should be considered before assuming that a patient has a relatively untreatable illness, such as senile dementia (Alzheimer's disease).

All patients with signs and symptoms of dementia should have the following laboratory tests:

- Complete blood count
- Metabolic screening, for example, SMAC or SMA 12/60
- Thyroid function (T3/T4)
- Vitamin B12 and folate levels
- Urinanalysis
- Chest X-ray
- Computerized axial tomography (CAT scan)

Depression and pseudodementia. A pseudodementia related to depression is common. Often the assumption is made that depressed mood is a reaction to the apparent loss of intellectual function and not

Table 12-1
Causes of Reversible Dementia

INTRACRANIAL CONDITIONS
- Meningiomas
- Subdural hematomas
- Hydrocephalus
  - Communicating
  - Noncommunicating
- Epilepsy
- Multiple sclerosis
- Wilson's disease

SYSTEMIC ILLNESSES
- Pulmonary insufficiency
- Cardiac arrhythmia
- Severe anemia
- Polycythemia vera
- Uremia
- Hyponatremia
- Portosystemic encephalopathy
- Porphyria
- Hyperlipidemia

DEFICIENCY STATES
- B_{12} deficiency
- Pellegra
- Folate deficiency

ENDOCRINOPATHIES
- Addison's disease
- Panhypopituitarism
- Myxedema
- Hypoparathyroidism
- Hyperparathyroidism
- Recurrent hypoglycemia
- Cushing's disease and steroid therapy
- Hyperthyroidism

DRUGS
- Methyldopa and haloperidol
- Clonidine and fluphenazine
- Disulfiram
- Lithium carbonate
- Phenothiazines
- Haloperidol and lithium carbonate
- Bromides
- Phenytoin

DRUGS (*continued*)
- Mephenytoin
- Barbiturates
- Clonidine
- Methyldopa
- Propranolol hydrochloride
- Atropine and related compounds

HEAVY METALS
- Mercury
- Arsenic
- Lead
- Thallium

EXOGENOUS TOXINS AND INDUSTRIAL AGENTS
- Trichloroethylene
- Toluene
- Carbon disulfide
- Organophosphates
- Carbon monoxide
- Alcohol

INFECTIONS
- General paresis
- Chronic meningitis
- Cerebral abscess
- Cysticercosis
- Whipple's disease
- Progressive multifocal leukoencephalopathy

COLLAGEN-VASCULAR AND VASCULAR DISORDERS
- Systemic lupus erythematosus
- Temporal arteritis
- Sarcoidosis
- Cogan's syndrome
- Behçet's syndrome
- Carotid artery stenosis (?)

"POTENTIALLY RECOVERABLE DEMENTIA"
- Cerebral anoxia
- Trauma
- Excessive electroconvulsive therapy
- Encephalitis

Reproduced from Cummings J, Benson F, Leverme S: Reversible dementia. JAMA 243:2434, 1980. With permission. © 1980, American Medical Association.

vice versa. Table 12-2 outlines the important features that differentiate pseudodementia from depression. For example, depressed patients are more likely to complain of their memory deficits, while it is the families of patients with dementia who are most aware of it. The onset of the pseudodementia is also more clearly delimited with depression and usually associated with a shift in mood, often related to a traumatic event. On mental status examination, the depressed patient is more likely to have deficits in both recent and remote events and to say, "I don't know" rather than attempt to offer answers.[12]

Adequate treatment with antidepressants will provide a marked improvement in the symptoms of pseudodementia. Those patients with an underlying true dementia will, of course, continue to manifest these deficits, but they should be able to function more effectively.

Drugs as Etiological Agents in Dementia

A review of all medications and an inquiry into the use of any over-the-counter drugs may uncover a causative agent for an organic syndrome. The aged are particularly sensitive to the toxic effects of medication and since they are often on a fairly large number of drugs, a careful initial review is always in order. Among the most common causes of cognitive deficits are sedatives, narcotics, and any drugs with anticholinergic properties such as over-the-counter medications for sleep or anxiety. The antiparkinsonian drugs, which have anticholinergic properties, can produce both delirium and psychosis. These symptoms can often be reversed by lowering the dose. The tricyclic antidepressant drugs can produce an acute organic brain syndrome, and, on very rare occasions, the central anticholinergic effect of some antipsychotic agents, pushed too vigorously, can also increase delirium. It is the altered patterns of drug absorption, metabolism, and excretion in the aged that produce these toxic effects.

> A previously alert 90-year-old woman was seen for the rather sudden onset of confusion and paranoid delusions. It was discovered that she had been on hydroxyzine HCL (Atarax) 25 mg qid for pruritis for over 2 weeks. This dosage was too high for this aged and petite lady. Her mental status cleared within a few days after the drug was discontinued.

Do not overlook the chronic effects of alcohol on cerebral function. Significant improvement is possible with discontinuation of the alcohol, and with adequate nutrition and vitamin supplements.

Malnutrition

Malnutrition with vitamin deficiencies should be considered, since eating habits in the aged may be seriously disordered by economic or

Table 12-2.
Major Differentiating Clinical Features of Pseudodementia and Dementia

Pseudodementia	Dementia
Clinical course and history	
Family is always aware of dysfunction and its severity.	Family is often unaware of dysfunction and its severity.
Onset can be dated with some precision.	Onset can be dated only within broad limits.
Symptoms are of short duration before medical help is sought.	Symptoms are usually of long duration before medical help is sought.
Rapid progression of symptoms after onset.	
History of previous psychiatric dysfunction is common.	History of previous psychiatric dysfunction is unusual.
Complaints and clinical behavior	
Patients usually complain a great deal of cognitive loss.	Patients usually complain little of cognitive loss.
Patients' complaints of cognitive dysfunction are usually detailed.	Patients' complaints of cognitive dysfunction are usually vague.
Patients emphasize disability.	Patients conceal disability.
Patients highlight failures.	Patients delight in accomplishments, however trivial.
Patients make little effort to perform even simple tasks.	Patients struggle to perform tasks.
Patients do not try to keep up.	Patients rely on notes, calendars, etc. to keep up.
Patients usually communicate a strong sense of distress.	Patients often appear unconcerned.
Affective change is often pervasive.	Affect is labile and shallow.
Loss of social skills often occurs early and is prominent.	Social skills are often retained.
Behavior is often incongruent with severity of cognitive dysfunction.	Behavior is usually compatible with severity of cognitive dysfunction.
Nocturnal accentuation of dysfunction is uncommon.	Nocturnal accentuation of dysfunction is common.

Clinical features related to memory, cognitive, and intellectual dysfunctions	
Attention and concentration are often well preserved.	Attention and concentration are usually faulty.
"Don't know" answers are typical.	Near-miss answers are frequent.
On tests of orientation, patients often give "don't know" answers.	On tests of orientation, patients often mistake the unusual for the usual.
Memory loss for recent and remote events is usually equally severe.	Memory loss for recent events is usually more severe than loss for remote events.
Memory gaps for specific periods or events are common.	Memory gaps for specific periods are unusual. *
There is marked variability in performance on tasks of similar difficulty.	Performance is consistently poor on tasks of similar difficulty.

* Except when due to such phenomena as delirium, trauma, or seizures.

Reproduced from Wells CE: Pseudodementia. Am J Psychiatry 136:895–900, 1979. With permission, the American Psychiatric Association.

social factors. B-12 deficiency may produce psychiatric changes before abnormalities appear in the blood, motor, or sensory systems. Patients on diphenylhydantoin (Dilantin) may be more likely to develop B-12 deficiencies.

> A prominent social worker who had been professionally active until her early eighties finally retired. She lived frugally in a small apartment and doted on her one companion, a small dog, whom she would feed regularly, while neglecting herself. Within a year she was grossly organic but with hospitaliztion, a normal diet, and vitamin supplements she was back to a clear and alert mental status within a week.

Normal Pressure Hydrocephalus

Normal pressure hydrocephalus[13] is a progressive dementia associated with a communicating hydrocephalus and essentially normal cerebrospinal fluid pressure. It has been reported to be a potentially treatable but rare form of dementia. The condition may develop without any apparent antecedent, or it may be associated with a history of subarachnoid hemorrhage, trauma, meningitis, or tumor. The patients usually present with a triad of dementia, ataxia, and urinary incontinence. CAT scan and other neurological diagnostic aids are needed to confirm the diagnosis. The effectiveness of shunting procedures is still not clear. The low improvement rate may be related to the possibility that some of these patients also have Alzheimer's disease.

Thyroid Disease

Both hypo- and hyperthyroidism can produce signs and symptoms of dementia, although the latter is a more common finding in hypothyroidism. Very mild abnormalities can produce detectible illness.

Carcinoma

Dementia has been reported in patients with carcinoma when there was no evidence of metastases to the brain.[14] Pulmonary cancer seems most likely to produce this effect, but the exact mechanism of the effect is unknown.

Cerebral Vascular Disease

Traditionally, this was the diagnosis assigned to older patients with dementia. Actually it represents a small fraction of this population compared to the group that exhibit Alzheimer's disease. The differentiation is important since it has therapeutic and prognostic implications.

Dementia with vascular disease usually has an abrupt onset that is often associated with a cerebrovascular accident. Focal neurological signs and symptoms are often present. There may be a history of hypertension. This form of dementia tends to have a fluctuating course, with stepwise deterioration.[15] Treatment of the hypertension or vascular disease may slow the progression of the dementia.

Alzheimer's Disease (Senile Dementia)

The term Alzheimer's disease was formerly reserved for the presenile dementias. However, the neuropathology is the same in both the presenile and senile forms of the disease. In recent years, the term Alzheimer's disease has been used for this syndrome regardless of the age of onset. The disease is characterized by neurofibrillary degeneration of cerebral neurons, the presence of argyrophilic plaques, and diffuse cerebral atrophy. Clinically, the diagnosis is made when there are: (1) chronic symptoms of dementia, (2) diffuse cerebral dysfunction, (3) diffuse cerebral atrophy on CAT scan, and (4) when other specific diagnoses have been ruled out.[16] In the early stages, the EEG usually shows an absence or reduction in alpha rhythm; in later stages theta and delta activity may occur in bursts.[17] The absence of major atrophy on CAT scan should alert the physician to the possibility of a treatable reversible dementia, although the amount of atrophy and severity of the dementia are not always correlated.[18] The presence of dementia has also been found to be associated with reduced survival time, independent of the presence of coexisting illnesses.[19] Close relatives of patients with senile dementia have a risk four times that of the general population of developing the disease.[20] There is no known cause for this disorder and no effective treatment. Vasodilators, stimulants, and most recently, lecithin, have not been found to be consistently effective.

Treatment of Irreversible Dementia

Obviously, where treatable dementia is present it should be treated, but what of the patients with Alzheimer's disease? Wells suggests we divide our treatment efforts into three categories: (1) Restitution of those functions that can be restored, (2) Reduction of the patient's need to employ functions that have been lost, and (3) Maximal utilization of residual function.[12] We would add two more categories: (4) Treatment of behavioral symptoms that result from the illness, and (5) Support for the family and friends.

Restitution of lost functions. It is important to correct such complicating factors as hearing and visual deficits, inadequate nutrition, and cardiac or pulmonary failure, all conditions that can add to the severity of the dementia.

Reduction of need for lost functions and optimal utilization of residual function. The physician must use his or her psychotherapeutic skills to help the patient give up the need to do "business as usual." Patients must be helped to use reminder lists so that they need not struggle to get along on their memories alone. A night light can help patients to orient themselves. Medicine bottles can be labeled with symbols—for exmple, a heart—for the patient with failing vision who cannot read small print. Patients can be encouraged to put out their entire dose of each of their medications every morning, so that they will always know if a particular dose has been taken. Some nursing homes have found that using different colors on each floor or in particular areas can help in orientation. This technique can be extended to the patient's home.

Treatment of behavioral symptoms. Dementia is not necessarily associated with psychiatric disorders. However, some patients will become anxious, paranoid, or depressed as a reaction to the awareness of their failing cognitive capacities or perhaps as a direct effect of the central nervous system damage itself. Restlessness, agitation, wandering, and verbal and physical abusiveness are all treatable.

The treatment of anxiety, paranoia, and depression were described earlier. The confused, agitated, or potentially assaultive patient should be treated with an antipsychotic agent starting with very small doses; for example, chlorpromazine (Thorazine) 25 mg bid, or haloperidol (Haldol) 0.5 mg bid. The more sedating phenothiazines can be helpful in patients who are agitated during the night. The bulk of the dose can be used at sleep.

Helping the family. The doctor can help the family by explaining the nature of the deficits. Family members frequently become exasperated with the individual who seems to remember details of his or her youth quite clearly but who forgets appointments and recent family visits. It may help if they understand that there is a specific deficit in recent memory. They will appreciate your acknowledging the frustrations in dealing with such patients. Your specific suggestions as outlined above can be helpful.

The family may have to be helped to learn to live with a certain amount of anxiety regarding a parent's physical well-being in order to allow the patient to enjoy the better psychological climate of his or her own home. If the organicity, however, leads to the possiblility of serious errors in judgment or dangerous activities such as leaving on gas jets, then a live-in companion obviously is needed.

Home care programs are available in many communities to provide assistance for the elderly. These programs may be hospital based or may offer services through departments of health and visiting nurse associations where skilled nursing supervision and other ancillary services usually are provided. These services may be paid for through Medicare and/or Medicaid if the patient meets eligibility requirements. Some private insurance carriers also offer home care benefits. In addition, homemaker/home health aide services increasingly are becoming available in many communities through voluntary, nonprofit organizations and proprietary services. A homemaker can help the elderly remain in the household by doing shopping, cooking, laundry, and errands. The home health aide receives some training and usually is able to provide personal care such as bathing, supervision of an exercise regimen, and preparation of therapeutic diets. Other services that may be available are "chore services"—in which volunteers help the elderly with home maintenance including minor carpentry, plumbing, and yardwork—and visitor services—in which volunteers either call or visit the elderly on a regular basis. The local government office that handles funds for the elderly should be able to give you a list of services available in your community.

Alternatives to Independent Living

Failing physical and/or mental abilities may make it necessary for a patient to have more supervised care than can be provided in his own home even with additional home nursing care. One indication for placing a patient in a nursing home is that specific people have become less important to the patient than the service they provide.[21] For the patient with severe dementia this is often the case. The decision can come as a relief to the family and even to the patient, but more often it is a potentiallly devastating threat. It is frequently the doctor who is called upon to make such a decision and to take the "responsibility" for the recommendation, since the family may be too guilt ridden to acknowledge it as their decision.

This is usually a very difficult time for everyone involved. The individual must generally give up most of the material goods (furniture, memorabilia, souvenirs, pictures, and so on) that make up a lifetime identity. The person also gives up considerable autonomy in day-to-day living. The family generally reacts with considerable guilt, and frequently old wounds are opened and old quarrels reignited. The doctor may be the one stable figure the group can turn to. We know that many people see such a move as the final one, the final step toward total disability and death. By encouraging the ventilation of such feelings we can help smooth the transition. Of course, the physician must emphasize the advantages of the move over the existing situation. However, too often, in our zeal to convince the patient to accept the nursing home placement, we oversell the placement and fail to indicate to the patient our understanding of the enormity of the patient's loss. The latter must be acknowledged if the patient is to believe we understand him or her and are offering intelligent advice.

It is important to know the specifics of the alternative living arrangements because they range so widely. There are "adult homes" (domiciling care), where meals and a few amenities are provided. There are "health-related facilities" (intermediate care facilities), where considerable amounts of medical and nursing care are provided but where the individual is expected basically to be responsible for his or her daily activities. Finally, there are "skilled-nursing facilities" where there is a much larger component of nursing help in order to care for more severe physical or mental deficiencies.

It is essential to know specifically what is available in the community and what available placements cost. It is especially beneficial if you can tell the family that you are familiar with particular facilities and have visited them. Since many facilities have their own medical staffs, it may be necessary to prepare the person for a change of physician. This can be very traumatic when the patient–doctor relationship has been long and good. It can symbolize to the individual all his losses rolled into one. This needs to be dealt with directly. If at all possible, the doctor should be in touch with the staff at any institution to which his or her patient may be going. Frequently, the doctor alone has the insight into the needs, personalities, family relationships, and the like that would make the transition easier for all concerned. The patient and his or her family should be told that these conversations will be held. Since this is an exceedingly traumatic time for the patient, he or she needs all the help the physician can provide. If possible, personal visits and phone calls should be made until the patient has shifted his or her trust to the nursing home staff. This will pay off in lessened depression and confusion and a quicker adjustment to the new environment.

REFERENCES

1. Abraham K: The applicability of psychoanalytic treatment to patients of advanced age, in Glover E (ed): Selected Papers in Psychotherapy. London, Hogart Press, 1949
2. Butler RN: The life review: An interpretation of reminiscence in the aged. Psychiatry 26:65–76, 1963
3. Pfeiffer E, Verwoerdt A, Wang HS: The natural history of sexual behavior in a biologically advanced group of aged individuals. J Gerontol 24:193–198, 1969
4. Pfeiffer E: Sexual behavior in the psychiatry of old age, in Howells JG (ed): Modern Perspectives in the Psychiatry of Old Age. New York, Brunner/Mazel, 1975, pp 313–325

5. Masters WH, Johnson VE: Human Sexual Inadequacy. Boston, Little, Brown, 1970
6. Altman N: Hypochondriasis, in Strain JJ, Grossman S (eds): Psychological Care of the Mentally Ill: A Primer in Liaison Psychiatry. New York, Appleton-Century-Crofts, 1975, pp 76–92
7. Bigger TJ, Giardin EA, Perel J, et al: Cardiac anti-arrythmic effects of imipramine hydrochloride. New Eng J Med 296:206–207, 1977
8. Weiner, RD: The psychiatric use of electrically induced seizures. Am J Psychiatry 136:1507–1517, 1979
9. Basavaraju NJ, Wolf-Klein G, Silverstone FA, Libow LS: Cimetidine-induced mental confusion in elderly, NY State J Med 80:1287–1288, 1980
10. Freeman FR: Evaluation of patients with progressive intellectual deterioration. Arch Neurol 33:658–659, 1976
11. Cummings J, Benson F, Leverme S: Reversible dementia. JAMA 243:2434–2439, 1980
12. Wells, CE: Pseudodementia. Am J Psychiatry 136:895–900, 1979
13. Katzman R: Normal pressure hypocephalus, in Wells CE (ed): Dementia, ed 2. Philadelphia, FA Davis, 1977, pp 69–92.
14. Brain R, Henson RA: Neurological syndromes associated with carcinoma. Lancet 2:971–974, 1958
15. Hachinski VC, Lriff LD, Zihka E, et al: Cerebral blood flow in dementia. Arch Neurol 32:632–637, 1975
16. Wells CE: Diagnostic evaluation and treatment, in Wells CE (Ed): Dementia, ed 2. Philadelphia, FA Davis, 1977, pp
17. Wilson WP, Musella L, Short MS: The electroencephalogram in dementia, in Wells CE (Ed): Dementia, ed 2. Philadelphia, FA Davis, 1977, pp 205–221
18. Huckman MS, Fox J, Topel J: The validity of criteria for the evaluation of cerebral atrophy by computerized tomography. Radiology 116:85–92, 1975
19. Jarvik LF, Ruth VR, Matsuyama SS: Organic brain syndromes and aging. Arch Gen Psychiatry 37:280–286, 1980
20. Pratt, RTC: The Genetics of Neurological Disorders. Oxford Monographs on Medical Genetics. New York, Oxford University Press, 1967
21. Haycox JA: Late care of the demented patient. N Eng J Med 303:165–166, 1980

BIBLIOGRAPHY

Bellak L, Karasu T: *Geriatric Psychiatry*. New York, Grune and Stratton, 1976

Busse EW, Pfeiffer E: *Behavior and Adaptation in Late Life*, ed 2. Boston, Little, Brown, 1977

Busse EW, Pfeiffer E: *Mental Illenss in Later Life*. Washington, D.C., American Psychiatric Association, 1973

Butler RN: *Why Survive? Being Old in America*. New York, Harper and Row, 1975

Butler RN, Lewis M: *Aging and Mental Health*. ed 2. St. Louis, Mosby, 1977

Eisdorfer C, Fann W: *Psychopharmacology and Aging*. New York, Plenum, 1973

Post F: Dementia, depression and pseudo-dementia, in Benson DF, Blumer D (Eds): Psychiatric Aspects of Neurological Disease. New York, Grune & Stratton, 1975

Smith L, Kinsbourne M (Eds): *Aging and Dementia*. New York, Spectrum Publications, 1977

Wells CE: *Dementia*, ed 2. Philadelphia, FA Davis, 1977

Sheldon Zimberg, M.D.

13

The Management of the Patient Who Abuses Alcohol

Alcoholism is a major public health problem in this country. There are at least 9–10 million alcoholics, including people in all walks of life, men and women, the aged and, increasingly, adolescents.

Every primary care physician encounters in his or her office a significant number of patients who have some problem with alcohol. It is unusual, however, for physicians to make the diagnosis of alcoholism, confront the patient with the diagnosis, and offer appropriate treatment or referral for treatment. Only when the patient has experienced significant physical consequences of excessive drinking are most doctors able to establish the diagnosis. Even when patients are diagnosed, physicians are often frustrated in their efforts to deal with the problem. This is because of their own lack of knowledge about alcoholism and its treatment, their consequent feelings of hopelessness, and the patient's denial of the illness.

This chapter will present information to assist primary care physicians in diagnosing alcoholism and in understanding the various clinical manifestations and psychological aspects of alcoholism. It will also provide guidelines regarding the treatment of alcoholism and indications for referral.

DIAGNOSIS OF ALCOHOLISM

Since a significant number of patients who appear in a physician's office are alcoholic, but very few will openly acknowledge a problem with alcohol, it is necessary for the physician to take a thorough history of drinking and sedative-drug usage as part of the medical history that is obtained. The physical examination should also be done with a high index of suspicion for possible physical effects of alcohol.

Criteria for Diagnosing Alcoholism

The National Council on Alcoholism has established a set of major and minor criteria for the diagnosis of alcoholism. These criteria can be found in Tables 13–1 and 13–2. They are divided into two tracks: Track I concerns physiological and clinical manifestations of alcoholism: Track II includes behavioral, psychological, and attitudinal manifestations. Each criterion is assigned a diagnostic level of from 1 to 3. Level 1 represents a definitive diagnosis of alcoholism; level 2 represents probable alcoholism and requires several other criteria for diagnosis; and level 3 is a possible diagnosis requiring considerably more evidence than several level 3 criteria. These criteria can provide a structured basis for establishing the diagnosis and providing the physician with information to substantiate the diagnosis to the many patients who are resistant to accepting alcoholism as a problem.

Some recent work on establishing a laboratory test for alcoholism indicated that the plasma alpha-amino-n-butyric acid/leucine ratio may be a biochemical marker for chronic alcoholism.[1] This approach is currently undergoing intensive validation. Recent reports have suggested that the mean corpuscular volume of red blood cells is elevated in alcoholics. This is a test that is readily available as part of a complete blood count. The macrocytic condition of the red blood cells is due to folic acid deficiency or to a direct toxic effect of alcohol on the bone marrow. It is likely that these or other laboratory tests that measure specifically physiological aberrations resulting from long-term chronic alcohol abuse will be established in the near future to assist physicians in making the diagnosis of alcoholism.

Currently, the best approach to the establishment of the diagnosis of alcoholism is to determine that the continued abuse of alcohol has caused problems in the individual's social and family relationships, physical health, or employment situation, or has produced financial or legal problems (drunk-driving arrests, for example). It should be understood that alcoholism is not an all-or-none phenomenon but one of degree, and that the severity of alcoholism can vary in the individual over time. The expression of "going on the wagon" is as much a part of alcoholism as "falling-off the wagon." Alcoholics often try to modify the effects of alcohol on themselves by "cutting down" for periods of time, maintaining short periods of sobriety, restricting drinking to weekends or evenings, or changing from spirits to wine or beer. These efforts of control in the face of evidence of loss of control over the impulse to drink are characteristic of the disorder.

Table 13-1.
Major Criteria for the Diagnosis of Alcoholism

Criterion	Diagnostic Level	Criterion	Diagnostic Level
Track I. Physiological and Clinical			
A			
Physiological Dependency			
1. Physiological dependence as manifested by evidence of a withdrawal syndrome when the intake of alcohol is interrupted or decreased without substitution of other sedation. It must be remembered that overuse of other sedative drugs can produce a similar withdrawal state, which should be differentiated from withdrawal from alcohol.		2. Evidence of tolerance to the effects of alcohol. (There may be a decrease in previously high levels of tolerance late in the course). Although the degree of tolerance to alcohol in no way matches the degree of tolerance to other drugs, the behavioral effects of a given amount of alcohol vary greatly between alcoholic and nonalcoholic subjects.	
a. Gross tremor (differentiated from other causes of tremor).	1	a. A blood alcohol level of more than 150 mg without gross evidence of intoxication.	1
b. Hallucinosis (differentiated from schizophrenic hallucinations or other psychoses).	1	b. The consumption of one-fifth of a gallon of whiskey or an equivalent amount of wine or beer daily, for more than one day, by a 180-lb. individual.	1
c. Withdrawal seizures (differentiated from epilepsy and other seizure disorders).	1	3. Alcoholic "blackout" periods. (Differential diagnosis from purely psychological fugue states and psychomotor seizures).	1
d. Delirium tremens. Usually starts between the first and third day after withdrawal and minimally includes tremors, disorientation, and hallucinations.	1	B. Clinical: major alcohol-associated illnesses. Alcoholism can be assumed to exist if ma-	

Table 13-1. *(continued)*

Criterion	Diagnostic Level
jor alcohol-associated illnesses develop in a person who drinks regularly. In such individuals, evidence of physiological and psychological dependence should be searched for.	
Fatty degeneration in absence of other known cause	2
Alcoholic hepatitis	1
Laennec's cirrhosis	2
Pancreatitis in the absence of cholelithiasis	2
Chronic gastritis	3
Hematological disorders:	
Anemia: hypochromic, normocytic, macrocytic, hemolytic with stomatocytosis, low folic acid.	3
Clotting disorders: prothrombin elevation, thrombocytopenia.	3
Wernicke-Korsakoff syndrome	2
Alcoholic cerebellar degeneration.	1
Cerebral degeneration in absence of Alzheimer's disease or arteriosclerosis.	2
Central pontine myelinolysis: Diagnosis only possible postmortem.	2
Marchiafava-Bignami's disease: Diagnosis only possible postmortem.	2
B. Peripheral neuropathy (see also beriberi)	2
Toxic amblyopia	3
Alcohol myopathy	2
Alcoholic cardiomyopathy	2
Beriberi	3
Pellagra	3

Track II. Behavioral, Psychological, and Attitudinal

All chronic conditions of psychological dependence occur in dynamic equilibrium with intrapsychic and interpersonal consequences. In alcoholism, similarly, there are varied effects on character and family. Like other chronic relapsing diseases, alcoholism produces vocational, social, and physical impairments. Therefore, the implications of these disruptions must be evaluated and related to the individual and his pattern of alcoholism. The following behavior patterns show psychological dependence on alcohol in alcoholism:

A Drinking despite strong medical contraindication known to patient	1	(arrest for intoxication, driving while intoxicated)	1
B. Drinking despite strong, identified, social contraindication (job loss for intoxication, marriage disruption because of drinking,		C. Patient's subjective complaint of loss of control of alcohol consumption.	2

From Criteria Committee, National Council of Alcoholism: Criteria for the Diagnosis of Alcoholism, Am J Psychiatry 129:127–135, 1972. Reprinted with permission.

Table 13-2.
Minor Criteria for the Diagnosis of Alcoholism

Criterion	Diagnostic Level	Criterion	Diagnostic Level
	Track I. Physiological and Clinical		
A. Direct Effects (ascertained by examination)		B. Indirect Effects	
1. Early		1. Early	
Odor of alcohol on breath at time of medical appointment	2	Tachycardia	3
2. Middle		Flushed face	3
Alcoholic facies	2	Nocturnal diaphoresis	3
Vascular engorgement of face	2	2. Middle	
Toxic amblyopia	3	Ecchymoses on lower extremities, arms, or chest	3
Increased incidence of infections	3	Cigarette or other burns on hands or chest	3
Cardiac arrhythmias	3	Hyperreflexia, or if drinking heavily, hyporeflexia (permanent hyporeflexia may be a residuum of alcoholic polyneuritis)	3
Peripheral neuropathy (see also Table 12-1, Major Criteria, Track I, B)	2		
3. Late (see Major Criteria, Track I, B)			

Table 13-2. *(continued)*

Criterion	Diagnostic Level
3. Late	
Decreased tolerance	3
C. Laboratory Tests	
1. Major—Direct	
Blood alcohol level at any time of more than 300 mg/100 ml	1
Level of more than 100 mg/100 ml in routine examination	1
2. Major—Indirect	
Serum osmolality (reflects blood alcohol levels): every 22.4 increase over 200 mOsm/L reflects 50 mg/100 ml. alcohol	2
Track II. Behavioral, Psychological, and Attitudinal	
A. Behavioral	
1. Direct effects	
Early	
Gulping drinks	3
Surreptitious drinking	2
Morning drinking (assess nature of peer group behavior	2
Middle	
Repeated conscious attempts at abstinence	2
Late	
Blatant indiscriminate use of alcohol	1
Skid Row or equivalent social level	2
2. Indirect effects	
Early	
Medical excuses from work for variety of reasons	2
Shifting from one alcoholic beverage to another	2
Preference for drinking companions, bars, and taverns	2
Late	
Chooses employment that facilitates drinking	3
Frequent automobile accidents	3
History of family members undergoing psychiatric treatment; school and behavioral problems in children	3
Frequent change of residence for poorly defined reasons	3
Anxiety-relieving mechanisms, such as telephone calls inappropriate in time, distance, person, and motive (telephonitis)	2

Outbursts of rage and suicidal gestures while drinking	2
3. Minor—Indirect	
Results of alcohol ingestion	
Hypoglycemia	3
Hypochloremic alkalosis	3
Low magnesium level	2
Lactic acid elevation	3
Transient uric acid elevation	3
Potassium depletion	3
Indications of liver abnormality	
SGPT elevation	2
SGOT elevation	3
BSP elevation	2
Bilirubin elevation	2
Urinary urobilinogen elevation	2
Serum A/G ration reversal	2
Blood and blood clotting	
Anemia: hypochromic, normocytic, macrocytic, hemolytic with stomatocytosis, low folic acid	3
Clotting disorders: prothrombin elevation, thrombocytopenia	3
ECG abnormalities	
Cardiac arrhythmias; tachycardia; T waves dimpled, cloven, or spinous; atrial fibrillation; ventricular premature contractions; abnormal P waves	2
EEG abnormalities	
Decreased or increased REM sleep, depending on phase	3
Loss of delta sleep	3
Other reported findings	3
Decreased immune response	3
Decreased response to Synacthen test	3
Chromosomal damage from alcoholism	3
B. Psychological and Attitudinal	
1. Direct effects	
Early	
When talking freely, making frequent reference to drinking alcohol, people being "bombed," "stoned," etc., or admits drinking more than peer group	2
Middle	
Drinking to relieve anger, insomnia, fatigue, depression, social discomfort	2
Late	
Psychological symptoms consistent with permanent organic brain syndrome (see also Table 12-1, Major Criteria, Track I, B)	2
2. Indirect effects	
Early	
Unexplained changes in family, social, and business relationships;	

Table 13-2. *(continued)*

Criterion	Diagnostic Level	Criterion	Diagnostic Level
complaints about wife, job, and friends	3	Late	
Spouse makes complaints about drinking behavior, reported by patient or spouse	2	Overt expression of more regressive defense mechanisms: denial, projection, etc.	3
Major family disruptions, separation, divorce, threats of divorce	3	Resentment, jealousy, paranoid attitudes	3
Job loss (due to increasing interpersonal difficulties), frequent job changes, financial difficulties	3	Symptoms of depression, isolation, crying, suicidal preoccupation	3
		Feelings that he is ''losing his mind''	2

From Criteria Committee, National Council of Alcoholism: Criteria for the Diagnosis of Alcoholism, Am J Psychiatry 129:127–135, 1972. Reprinted with permission.

Table 13–3 presents an alcohol abuse scale developed by the author that approximates various levels of severity of alcohol abuse, from none to extreme. It is easy to establish the diagnosis of alcoholism at the extreme level (skid row alcoholics) or the severe level. However, alcoholism is more readily treatable when diagnosed at the mild or moderate levels of severity. The mild stage of severity can be considered a pre-addictive stage in which the individual is psychologically dependent on the use of alcohol. The moderate stage is the stage of physiological addiction as evidenced by the presence of withdrawal signs (tremors) and

Table 13-3
Scale of Alcohol Abuse

Level of Severity	Signs and Symptons
None	Drinks only on occasion, if at all.
Minimal	Drinking is not conspicuous; occasional intoxications (up to four per year). No social, family, occupational, health, or legal problems related to drinking.
Mild	Intoxications occur up to once a month, although generally limited to evenings or weekends. Some impairment in social, family relations, or occupational functioning related to drinking. No physical or legal problems related to drinking.
Moderate	Frequent intoxications, up to one or two times per week and/or significant impairment in social, family, or occupational functioning. Some suggestive evidence of physical impairment related to drinking, such as tremors, frequent accide ts, epigastric distress, occasional loss of appetite. No history of DTs, cirrhosis, nutritional deficiency, hospitalizations related to drinking, or arrests related to drinking.
Severe	Almost constant drinking, practically every day, History of DTs, cirrhosis, chronic brain syndrome, neuritis, or nutritional deficiency. Severe disruption in social or family relations. Unable to hold a steady job but able to maintain himself on public assistance. One or more arrests related to drinking (drunk or disorderly). One or more hospitalizations related to drinking.
Extreme	All of the characteristics of severe impairment plus homelessness and/or inability to maintain self on public assistance.

the beginning of physical consequences and disability as well as significant social impairment.

The Drinking History

In obtaining the drinking history, one should ask about the frequency of use of alcoholic beverages and about when and where they are used and for what purpose. If the patient drinks repeatedly to reduce anxiety or for fatigue or to get through stressful situations, there is evidence of psychological dependence on alcohol. You should ask about areas of potential problems associated with drinking and about what family members say of patients' drinking. Have there been efforts to cut down or modify drinking by switching to other alcoholic beverages? Have they ever been told by a physician to stop drinking, and if so what has been their reaction? Do they have tremors in the morning or a history of blackouts or seizures? Information regarding the quantity of alcohol consumed, however, is usually unreliable. It should be remembered that the use of sedative drugs and minor tranquilizers—e.g., chlordiazepoxide (Librium), diazepam (Valium), or meprobamate (Miltown)—often coexists with alcohol abuse and that information concerning use of such drugs should be sought as well.

When information regarding the use of alcohol and its impact on the person's life has been determined to indicate that there is a drinking problem, the patient should be confronted with the information and told he or she has a drinking problem. The diagnosis of alcoholism must be presented to the patient as you would present the diagnosis of any other chronic disorder (e.g., diabetes), along with the necessary treatment approaches. Most patients will resist and will deny the diagnosis at first. However, it should be pointed out that denial is a basic part of the illness and that patients' very resistance to giving up the use of alcohol is further evidence of their dependence on it.

Most physicians are reluctant to proceed in this straightforward professional approach because they are unwilling to stigmatize the patient and/or believe that alcoholism cannot be treated. However, there is currently much more acceptance of alcoholism as an illness by the health care professions and general public. The diagnosing of this illness is the first step in the provision of treatment for an illness that has a high mortality. The balance of this chapter will be involved in the discussion of the treatment of alcoholism in its various manifestations. This author's experience as well as the experience of the management of alcoholism in industry have indicated that up to 80 percent of alcoholics can achieve recovery.

PSYCHOLOGICAL ASPECTS OF ALCOHOLISM

The major psychological conflict in many alcoholics centers around dependency needs due to childhood deprivations. These dependency needs are not conscious. In fact, they are denied and they lead many alcoholics to develop efforts to compensate for their feelings of loss of self-esteem by developing a need for power and control and a tendency toward grandiosity. Alcoholics are often overachievers whose "reach exceeds their grasp." They are often driven, perfectionistic people who need to maintain control over their lives. When they realize that they are not going to be able to achieve their goals, their latent dependency needs are reawakened, causing them to seek alternate methods of recovering their self-esteem. The passive and dependent traits of alcoholics become apparent only when they are under the influence of alcohol, which tranquilizes their anxiety over their failures and serves pharmacologically to produce feelings of omnipotence and control.

Thus, alcohol usage serves as a principal reinforcer of the need to compensate for feelings of worthlessness and inadequacy. If the alcohol is consumed long enough, they become psychologically dependent upon its euphoria-producing effects and eventually become physically addicted.

Alcoholics have an expectation that they will be rejected, and often provoke rejection. An accepting, supportive, and nonjudgmental attitude therefore is necessary to engage the alcoholic in treatment.

The reasons for the success of Alcoholics Anonymous (AA) have been the supportive environment and the availability of recovered alcoholics as role models who can meet the active alcoholic's dependent needs. In addition, the needs for power and for compensation for their lack of self-esteem are achieved by recovered alcoholics by being involved in the rescuing of other alcoholics. Thus, AA has intuitively responded to the psychological needs of alcoholics by its very approach. However, not all alcoholics are willing or able to utilize AA effectively.

CLINICAL PRESENTATIONS OF ACUTE AND CHRONIC ALCOHOLISM

Most alcoholics who appear in a physician's office are suffering from long-term chronic alcoholism rather than presenting acute manifestation of the illness. In many cases, alcoholics may have reduced their alcoholic intake or appear sober. Therefore, the thorough medical evaluation and drinking history indicated will be necessary to diagnose these less obvious alcoholics. Once the diagnosis is established and the patient is confronted with the diagnosis, the treatment plan should be outlined for the patient in terms of the approaches to be described later in this chapter.

Problems exist, however, with some alcoholics regarding differential diagnosis from alcoholic psychosis, related psychotic disorders, uncomplicated alcohol intoxication, and alcohol withdrawal syndromes.

Differential Diagnosis of Alcoholism, Alcoholic Psychoses, and Related Psychiatric Disorders

Psychiatric disorders occur frequently enough in individuals who abuse alcohol that their occurrence should always be considered when evaluating possible physical disorders. Alcoholism can occur along with any other psychiatric disorders, including schizophrenia, mood disorders, severe anxiety, neurotic disorders, and personality disorders. Individuals suffering from functional psychoses may use alcohol as self-medication to tranquilize severe anxiety and depression. Alcoholics have a high rate of suicide and conversely, suicide-prone individuals often resort to combinations of drugs and alcohol in suicidal attempts.

Alcohol produces both acute and chronic toxic effects on the brain that result in organic psychoses. Acute toxic reactions include alcohol intoxication and alcohol idiosyncratic intoxication. Chronic toxic effects on the brain include alcohol amnestic disorder, Korsakoff's psychosis, and dementia associated with alcoholism.

The syndromes of alcohol withdrawal, which involve the acute and chronic toxic effects of alcohol on the brain, include delirium tremens, alcoholic hallucinosis, tremulousness, and seizures. These withdrawal syndromes are discussed in detail later in this section.

In order to make a differential diagnosis between primary alcoholism and alcoholism secondary to a functional psychosis it is necessary to observe and evaluate the individual in an alcohol-free state. If the history or examination of the patient reveals evidence of psychosis including hallucinations, delusions, suicidal intent, severe depression, and severe agitation or excitement, it is best to carry out this evaluation in an inpatient psychiatric setting. When the individual is free of alcohol, the primary functional disorder can be distinguished. Effective psychiatric treatment of the functional disorder can often eliminate alcohol abuse as a problem, and such individuals may be treated in a psychiatric program. Consultation provided by specialists in the field of alcoholism may be helpful in the management of such patients.

In contrast, individuals with coexisting neurotic and personality disorders can be treated by the primary physician in an effort to educate them about their alcoholism and to help them achieve sobriety. Psychotherapy for their neurotic or personality disorders can best be provided after sobriety has been well established. It is clear that psychotherapy is not an effective treatment for an actively drinking patient because the therapeutic process itself produces anxiety that can lead to drinking. Therefore, it is necessary to treat the alcoholism first and to help the patient establish a firm internalized set of controls over the impulse to drink through the use of disulfiram (Antabuse), counseling, and/or Alcoholics Anonymous. Once these controls have been established, psychotherapy can be effective in dealing with the neurotic or personality problems.

Alcohol idiosyncratic intoxication is a rare phenomenon. It occurs in individuals who develop a severe change in mental state and behavior after the consumption of a small amount of alcohol. The intoxication is characterized by confusion, transitory delusions, visual hallucinations, and impairment in consciousness. These symptoms may be accompanied by increased activity, rage, aggression and destructive behavior, or by depression and suicidal behavior. Such a state can last from a few hours to a few days. It is best treated with sedation in a hospital setting because the individuals affected can be a serious danger to themselves or others. After a period of sleep the condition clears and the individual has no memory of the episode.

Other alcohol-related psychoses include alcohol amnestic disorder and dementia associated with alcoholism. Alcohol amnestic disorder is an organic mental syndrome consisting of disorientation, confusion, confabulation, suggestibility, and the inability to recall and retain immediate information. This mental picture is frequently accompanied by polyneuropathy and Wernicke's syndrome. Wernicke's syndrome consists of ataxia, nystagmus, and ocular muscle palsies. This syndrome results from necrotic and hemorrhagic lesions of the brain stem; its mental and neurological signs and symptoms result primarily from a thiamine deficiency. The treatment involves immediate admission to a hospital and parenteral administration of 50–100 mg of thiamine daily, supplemented by oral B complex and ascorbic acid.

Dementia associated with alcoholism occurs in individuals with longstanding alcoholism. The clinical picture is one of emotional instability, personality and social disintegration, and subtle signs of dementia. This syndrome was previously thought to be associated with avitaminosis. However, recent evidence of the direct toxic effects of alcohol on the brain indicate that alcohol ingestion alone may be the primary cause. Computerized axial tomographic studies (CAT scans) have found a significant percentage of chronic alcoholics with cerebral atrophy.[2] Such individuals require hospitalization to treat coexisting medical problems, to improve their nutritional status and to remove them from access to alcohol. Significant improvement can be expected only with treatment of their alcoholism in a long-term residential program.

Acute Alcohol Reactions

If the individual is suffering primarily from the effects of alcohol, without evidence of psychosis, a determination must be made of the type of reaction—whether it is alcohol intoxication, alcohol stupor or coma, or alcohol withdrawal. Alcohol intoxication of a mild or moderate degree can usually be managed by having the individual sleep it off. This is the usual method of self-detoxification for individuals who become intoxicated, whether or not they are alcoholics. In uncomplicated cases the patient can be sent home in the company of a responsible person.

Individuals who are stuporous or in coma as a result of alcohol ingestion should be sent to an emergency room where they can be carefully evaluated to rule out other causes. These individuals should be observed and blood alcohol, blood barbiturate, blood urea nitrogen, and blood sugar levels should be measured. Efforts should be directed at maintaining blood pressure and adequate respiration. There should be careful observation for 24–48 hours before a disposition is made. The use of sedatives or tranquilizers should be avoided in such cases because they can potentiate the stupor and lead to respiratory arrest. Stupor should be considered a medical emergency and managed accordingly.

Alcohol Withdrawal Syndromes

An alcoholic may appear in a physician's office experiencing any one of the several manifestations of the syndromes of alcohol withdrawal. Alcohol withdrawal syndromes occur in persons addicted to alcohol who have stopped drinking abruptly or begun reducing alcohol consumption so that there is a significant reduction in the blood alcohol level. The severity of the withdrawal cannot be predicted, and thus caution should be exercised wtih anyone manifesting symptoms of alcohol withdrawal. The etiology of withdrawal syndromes is not yet fully understood.

Characteristics

Several levels of alcohol withdrawal have been observed and reported by Victor and Adams.[3] The mildest form is termed tremulousness and is characterized by tremors, vomiting, flushed face, injected conjunctivae, tachycardia, and occasionally agitation. Tremulousness is a common condition among alcoholics, who note that they have the "shakes" upon awakening. This condition will subside with mild sedation, a small amount of alcohol, or eventually with complete abstinence.

However, in some cases if untreated, the shakes will progress to delirium tremens.

Hallucinosis is a form of alcohol withdrawal syndrome that can occur with or without tremulousness. It is characterized by visual, auditory, or tactile hallucinations. The hallucinations are usually threatening and unpleasant. They are often transitory but can persist for months in some cases. Hallucinations that continue for weeks to months after withdrawal from alcohol and without the resumption of drinking should lead to the suspicion of schizophrenia. Hallucinosis in a chronic alcoholic is most likely an alcohol withdrawal phenomenon and should not be considered a functional psychosis. Alcoholics experiencing acute hallucinosis have often been inappropriately admitted to psychiatric hospitals. Such individuals risk the danger of developing delirium tremens in an inappropriate setting; it must be remembered that alcohol withdrawal syndromes are primarily medical disorders and require medical treatment.

Seizures, called "rum fits" in alcoholics, can be a manifestation of alcohol withdrawal. Individuals who experience seizures related to alcohol withdrawal primarily require medical detoxification from alcohol. The effectiveness of anticonvulsants is somewhat controversial. Some authorities believe they are not of value, except for barbiturates, which have a cross-tolerance with alcohol. However, as a practical matter, most alcohol detoxification units use diphenylhydantoin (Dilantin), 100 mg tid, for alcoholics who have experienced seizures.

Any of these syndromes of alcohol withdrawal can be self-limiting or lead to delirium tremens. Delirium tremens is clearly a medical emergency and has a mortality rate of from 5–30 percent. Delirium tremens consists of tremulousness, hallucinations, disorientation, and a delirious state. Other signs include fever, profuse perspiration, tachycardia, tachypnea, and severe agitation.

Treatment

Treatment of withdrawal syndromes consists primarily of sedation. Chlordiazepoxide (Librium) has been found to be the most useful drug in this regard because of the lack of seizure potentiation and the minimum risk of oversedation and adverse effects on the liver. The dosage for the first day consists of 150–200 mg in four doses by mouth, or intramuscularly if the patient is unable to take medication orally. The Librium is gradually reduced over a 5-day period. It should be noted that chloradiazepoxide (Librium) is erratically absorbed intramuscularly. Lorazepam (Ativan) is said to be more reliably absorbed intramuscularly, but no clinical trials of its use for alcohol withdrawal have yet been published. In an acute situation with a patient who cannot take medication by mouth, diazepam (Valium) can be used intravenously, giving it very slowly—10 mg over a 60-second period.

In addition to the benzodiazepine, 2 cc of magnesium sulfate, 50 percent, can be given intramuscularly three times a day for the first day and twice daily for the next 2 days, since low serum magnesium may be an etiologic factor in alcohol withdrawal syndromes, and magnesium sulfate's anticonvulsant properties are well known. Chloral hydrate, 0.5–1.0 g, also can be given for sleep. Serious sleep disturbances are characteristic of alcohol withdrawal syndromes.

In addition to sedation, thiamine (100 mg IM), B-complex, and multivitamins should be given because vitamin deficiencies are often found in alcoholics secondary to their poor dietary habits. Intravenous 50-percent glucose and water can be administered if there is a suspicion of hypoglycemia. Because recent evidence indicates that during withdrawal alcoholics are often overhydrated rather than dehydrated, large amounts of intravenous fluids should be avoided unless there is clear evidence of dehydration and the individual is unable to tolerate fluids by mouth.

A number of patients who are experiencing mild to moderate alcohol withdrawal symptoms (mild to moderate tremulousness) can benefit from ambulatory detoxification carried out under close medical supervision. Such patients can be treated with oral doses of chlorodiazepoxide (Librium), 100–150 mg/day or diazepam (Valium), 20–30 mg/day, with a decreasing dosage over 5–7 days. Diphenylhydantoin (Dilantin) can be administered in doses of 100 mg tid if there is a history of seizures. During ambulatory detoxification the patient should be seen daily or at least two to three times per week by medical personnel and should be engaged in supportive counseling. The patient should be given no more than a one-week supply of medication.

The final stage of alcohol detoxification in an inpatient setting or in a doctor's office should be cessation of all sedative–hypnotic and minor tranquilizing medication. Alcoholics should not, in general, be maintained on sedatives or minor tranquilizers because there is abundant evidence that these drugs become subject to abuse.

The treatment of alcohol withdrawal syndromes in moderate to severe stages (severe tremulousness, seizures, hallucinations, agitation, delirium) is best carried out in an alcohol detoxification unit or a medical service in a general hospital.

A *protracted withdrawal syndrome* occurs in some alcoholics after withdrawal from alcohol and can persist for months. The condition includes a fine tremor of the hands, feelings of anxiety and depression, insomnia, irritability, feelings of fatigue, memory impairment, distractability, and difficulty in concentrating. This is believed due to the prolonged effects of alcohol on the central nervous system. If major clinical depression is present for at least 6 weeks after detoxification, then the patient should be treated with antidepressant medication. The insomnia can be treated with small doses of the antihistamine diphenhydramine (Benadryl), 50 mg hs. The patient should not be treated or maintained on minor tranquilizers, since this can easily lead to a new addiction. The signs and symptoms of protracted withdrawal will gradually subside with prolonged abstinence from alcohol.

THE TREATMENT PROCESS OF ALCOHOLISM

Alcoholism is a chronic illness with a high potential for relapse. As in other chronic disorders, continuous care is required, sometimes for life. Alcoholics Anonymous is particularly well-suited to provide this supportive treatment for an indefinite duration. However, professional intervention during the early stages of treatment is necessary to provide detoxification from alcohol, a thorough medical evaluation, and continued support for alcoholics unwilling or unable to make effective use of AA.

Patients with serious depression, psychoses, or severe anxiety states along with alcoholism should be treated for these conditions as well as the alcoholism and should be referred to psychiatrists for this evaluation and treatment. It has often been found that alcoholism that is secondary to these major psychiatric disorders clears up when the primary disorder is effectively treated. A period of observation in a hospital setting may be required to make a differential diagnosis among such patients.

Directive counseling by the physician during the process of detoxification can enhance an alcoholic's motivation to continue the treatment. Acquainting the alcoholic with the physical effects of alcohol on his body and the effects of his ability to perform his necessary functions should be part of this effort.

The Use Of Disulfiram

The deterrent use of disulfiram (Antabuse) is also effective. The usual maintenance dose is 250 mg/day but as little as 125 mg/day may be adequate. The only contraindications for the use of Antabuse are the presence of serious cardiac disorders; decompensating liver disease; psychosis; or brain damage, with significant impairment in judgment. Patients should be educated about what to avoid when taking disulfiram and should be given an Antabuse identification card. Few patients will drink on disulfiram. The disulfiram effect lasts about 5–7 days after the last dose. Those who do drink and have a disulfiram-alcohol reaction can be treated with oral Benadryl. Or the reaction will remit, without treatment, after the patient sleeps for a while. More serious disulfiram–alcohol reactions require the use of oxygen, vasopressors, and intravenous Benadryl.

Disulfiram acts by interfering with the enzymatic breakdown of alcohol at the step of acetaldehyde production. When alcohol is consumed, acetaldehyde is produced in a dose-related amount that produces the toxic reaction consisting of flushing, nausea, vomiting, anxiety, hyperventilation, and hypotension. This is very rarely a fatal reaction.

Disulfiram can itself occasionally produce a toxic psychosis. Anyone experiencing such a toxic psychosis should be admitted to a hospital, and the disulfiram should be discontinued. Minor tranquilizers can be used to control the anxiety. Phenothiazines may be used cautiously if there is severe agitation and overt psychotic symptoms. The reaction usually subsides within a few days.

A history of other medications must be secured from all patients on disulfiram because a number of toxic psychotic reactions have been reported when disulfiram has been used in conjunction with isoniazid, and similar reports have been made about the combination of disulfiram and metronidazole (Flagyl). Disulfiram potentiates the effect of diphenylhydantoin (Dilantin), barbiturates, and coumarin anticoagulants. Individuals on amitriptyline (Elavil) and disulfiram may experience an enhanced alcohol–disulfiram reaction if alcohol is ingested.

Principles of Treatment

Several principles are important in the treatment of an alcoholic individual.[4] These principles apply whether the alcoholic is involved in a therapeutic relationship with a physician, with a mental health professional, or with a paraprofessional alcoholism counselor. First, the drinking itself must be terminated if therapy is to be effective in achieving rehabilitation. A common mistake of mental health professionals who consider alcoholism a symptom of an underlying personality disorder is to attempt to treat this underlying disorder without dealing directly with the alcoholism. Psychological conflict does exist as indicated, but efforts must first be directed to achieve sobriety for the patient through detoxification and the maintenance of sobriety through intensive directive counseling and the use of disulfiram. A patient who continues to drink will not respond to counseling, and a power struggle will develop between the physician and the drinking patient.

The second principle is the necessity to understand the feelings that the alcoholic will develop toward the physician. These feelings are very intense and are characterized by a considerable amount of dependence coupled with hostile, manipulative, and testing behavior. Thus, a great deal of ambivalence will be noted in the patient–doctor relationship. Alcoholics will be dependent, but at other times grandiose, believing they can control their drinking as well as their lives when the evidence is obviously to the contrary.

The third principle is that one must understand the feelings that may develop in the physician in response to the patient's provocative behavior and drinking designed to test the physician's continued interest. Because of this type of testing behavior, the treatment of an alcoholic can seem frustrating and unrewarding. The physician must recognize, however, that he or she is not omnipotent in regard to the alcoholic's drinking. The physician cannot—no one can—stop an alcoholic who is determined to drink. A physician can only provide the means to assist the alcoholic in achieving sobriety; the physician cannot force the alcoholic, for long, to refrain from drinking. Only patients, by their own conscious efforts, can achieve this for themselves. Recognizing this reality, the doctor must impose limits on the behavior of the patient and conditions under which treatment can continue. If the patient cannot meet these conditions, treatment should be discontinued. The door, however, should be left open to renew the efforts to achieve sobriety as the first step in the treatment process.

Stages of Treatment

The treatment has been observed to progress through several stages. Stage I involves the situation in which the alcoholic "cannot drink." This situation exists when there is external pressure on the patient to stop drinking such as the threat of loss of job or a spouse's leaving, or when the patient is taking disulfiram. Under such conditions alcoholics are, in a sense, forced to stop drinking, at least for a short time. Their attitudes toward drinking and their denial of drinking as a serious problem have not changed. They have stopped drinking not because they see abstinence as necessary, but because someone else does. They must be helped, by directive counseling, to face problems and stress without resorting to alcohol. These sessions do not have to be long; 15–20 minutes is usually adequate. Involvement of the family in joint discussions with the patient and referral of the family to Al-Anon (the offshoot organization of AA designed to help alcoholics' families) are helpful in changing family attitudes about the alcoholic family member and in giving the family greater understanding of the illness of alcoholism. During this stage patients should be taught to recognize cues that might lead to drinking so that they can develop alternative coping mechanisms. Forgetting to take a disulfiram tablet can be such a cue, and therefore the use of disulfiram can serve as an early-warning system.

Often when patients have stopped drinking early in treatment, they feel extremely confident about their newly acquired sobriety and experience a feeling of euphoria. This feeling is a reaction formation to their unconscious lack of control over their drinking, which they now experience as a certainty of control over not drinking as well as control over other aspects of their lives. Patients should be warned to expect such inappropriate feelings. This situation is by its nature very unstable since there has been no significant change in attitude about drinking. The situation can easily lead to a return to drinking or, through counseling and/or Alcoholics Anonymous involvement, to a stage where the alcoholic "won't drink."

The stage in which alcoholics are able to refrain from drinking is reached when the controls on the compulsion to drink have become internalized and there is no longer a serious conscious conflict about whether or not to drink. In this stage II, the individual's attitude toward the necessity of drinking and the deleterious consequences of resuming drinking are apparent; he or she has experienced a considerable attitudinal change toward drinking. The conflict about drinking is still present, but at an unconscious level. This stage is the level many Alcoholics Anonymous members have achieved. Discontinuation or the intermittent use of disulfiram in stressful situations can be considered. Further help in developing alternative coping mechanisms for stress and unpleasant feelings should be provided. This stage represents a reasonably good stage of recovery and is fairly stable, only occasionally leading to a "slip" after years of sobriety. The grandiosity has now been sublimated (redirected) in the ego-enhancing feelings of control over a previously uncontrollable problem. For active AA members, their work with other alcoholics serves as an additional outlet for the unconscious need for grandiosity. At least six months to one year of directive counseling is required to achieve this stage of recovery.

The third stage of recovery involves the situation in which the alcoholic "does not have to drink." Stage III can be achieved only through insight into the individual's personality problems and conflicts and their resolution to a major degree. At this stage the patient understands that the habitual use of alcohol was a way of dealing with his or her conflicts. With the resolution of the conflicts, the patient can achieve more adaptive ways of coping with problems, internal and external. This stage can be achieved only through psychoanalytically oriented psychotherapy and self-understanding. It is a stable stage as long as the alcoholic refrains from drinking, and it is relatively easy to maintain.

After reaching stage II or III, some patients enter a situation in which they believe, "I can return to social drinking." It may be that a small percentage of alcoholics can achieve such a stage, but at our present level of knowledge it is impossible to predict which patients they may be. All alcoholics believe, during the initial stages of treatment, that they can return to controlled drinking. Alcoholics who have achieved recovery (stage II or III) in most cases do not desire to resume social drinking, because of the risk involved. Recent publicity regarding this issue has raised the question in some recovered alcoholics, but generally they have been persuaded not to take the chance of resuming social drinking. For all practical purposes at the present time, abstinence should be the goal in the treatment of all alcoholics. Alcohol is not necessary to life, and it is quite possible to live and be happy without consuming alcohol. This fact should be part of the attitudinal change an alcoholic experiences during the process of recovery.

Termination of Treatment

The termination of treatment with an alcoholic is critical. If the treatment process has been successful, the alcoholic will have established a dependent, trusting relationship with the physician and therefore termination will produce anxiety and the possibility of return to drinking. This termination should be based on mutual agreement between the doctor and patient, a termination date should be determined, and the final period of therapy should deal with the issue of termination.

Termination can occur at stage II or III since both are relatively stable stages regarding control of drinking. A decision has to be made, however, when a patient reaches stage II, as to whether further treatment should continue on to stage III to achieve insight into the psychological conflict related to the patient's drinking problem. This option should be left to the patient. Nonpsychiatric physicians can provide the directive counseling and the use of disulfiram, where indicated, to help alcoholics reach stage II. More traditional psychotherapy is required to reach stage III, and physicians might consider referral of such patients to psychotherapists.

This approach to counseling of alcoholics, presented in terms of stages of progression of treatment in relation to varying abilities to control the impulse to drink, provides a framework for a complex and often amorphous treatment process. It provides a goal-directed approach to achievable levels of improvement. Complex therapeutic decisions regarding involvement of the family in treatment, starting or stopping of disulfiram, attendance at AA meetings, use of uncovering techniques, discontinuation of therapy, and other matters can be considered in relation to these fairly predictable stages in the recovery process. It is possible to make predictions of outcome of therapeutic intervention or lack of intervention based on knowledge of the stage of recovery the patient has entered. Therefore, such an awareness can make the complex treatment process with alcoholics potentially understandable and subject to a certain degree of predictability.

REFERRALS TO ALCOHOLISM SPECIALISTS

In general, primary physicians should refer alcoholics with coexisting major psychiatric disorders to psychiatrists who are knowledgeable about alcoholism. Alcoholics who do not respond to directive counseling, disulfiram, and AA should be referred to specialized alcoholism treatment programs or alcoholism specialists. Local chapters of the National Council of Alcoholism usually have referral and information services and/or directories. Such information sources should be sought to facilitate the referral of alcoholics who have not responded to initial treatment efforts.

Patients who do not respond easily and quickly should not be a source of discouragement to the primary physician. Many patients, in the author's experience, require several efforts at treatment before a therapeutic impact is made. At times, the most reluctant alcoholic will respond when the right approach is applied. Patients desiring insight into their underlying psychological conflicts should be referred to psychotherapists after they have achieved at least a year of sobriety. Psychiatrists who are experienced with alcoholics are probably best equipped to treat such patients since they can reinstitute disulfiram if a "slip" should occur and can diagnose possibly underlying severe psychiatric disorders that might require the use of major tranquilizers or antidepressants.

Helping alcoholics recover can be a very satisfying experience, if the clinician recognizes his or her own limitations as well as the tools that are available to assist the alcoholic in treatment.

REFERENCES

1. Shaw S, Stimmel B, Lieber C S: Plasma alpha-amino-n-butyric acid/leucine ratio: An empirical biochemical marker of alcoholism. Science 194:1057–1058, 1976
2. Lusins J, Zimberg S, Smokler H, et al: Alcoholism and cerebral atrophy: A study of 50 patients with CT scan and psychologic testing. Alcoholism [Clin Exp Res] 4:406–411, 1980
3. Victor M, Adams R D: Alcohol, in Harrison T R, Wintrobe M M, Thorn G W, Adams R D, et al [eds]:Principles of Internal Medicine. New York, McGraw-Hill, 1974
4. Zimberg S: Principles of alcoholism psychotherapy, in Practical Approaches to Alcoholism Psychotherapy Zimberg S, Wallace J, Blume S B [eds]: New York, Plenum, 1978

Neil B. Kavey, M.D.
Kenneth Z. Altshuler, M.D.

14

The Management of Sleep Disorders

Few clinicians can go through their day without meeting at least one patient with a sleep complaint. If time allows for questions about sleep, the incidence of difficulties mushrooms. Inpatients, outpatients, and non-patients in the general population all show such a high incidence of disorders of sleep that it has become essential for clinicians to keep abreast of the constantly changing and developing diagnostic and treatment measures. Yet, an aura of mystery surrounds sleep and despite rapid growth in our scientific understanding of both normal sleep and disorders of sleep, physicians remain poorly informed.

Issues of sleep touch even those physicians who rarely are confronted with sleep complaints, for normal sleep is not a quiet, physiologically passive state of repose, as we once thought. It is a complex, physiologically active state with broad fluctuations that may even be stressful. As sleep progresses in the night, normal sleep physiology may profoundly affect the patient's disease state and the course of events during both night and day.

This chapter will present a brief review of those areas of normal sleep physiology that are pertinent to medical practice and will discuss the commonly seen sleep disorders.

Polygraphic recordings of normal sleep reveal a continuous flow of five distinct patterns, called the stages of sleep, that cycle, one into another, over the course of a night as shown in Figure 14-1. Stage 1, considered dozing by some investigators and the earliest and lightest stage of sleep by others, is the transition from awake to sleep in the beginning of the night and after arousals during the night. Stage 2, a definite sleep state, follows Stage 1 in the beginning of the night and thereafter occurs periodically throughout the entire night. Stages 3 and 4, because of their high arousal threshold, are considered deep sleep. They typically occur early in the night and are often referred to in combination as delta sleep or slow-wave sleep, because of the appearance of large, slow delta waves.[1]

The fifth stage of sleep, called REM sleep, is dramatically different from the other four stages, which are commonly classified together as nonREM sleep (stages 1, 2, 3, 4). REM refers to periods of sleep during which rapid eye movements and dreaming occur.[2] By contrast, in nonREM sleep the eyes are quiet and few dreams occur. In further contrast to the quiescence of stages 2, 3 and 4, REM sleep is characterized by autonomic excitement, physiologically similar to active wakefulness. Men have penile erections and in both men and women heart rate, cardiac output, respiratory rate, and blood pressure are highly variable and can undergo dramatic changes within seconds or minutes, making REM sleep potentially stressful.

Figure 14-1 shows the normal sleep of young healthy adults. Beginning with a short period of Stage 1, they descend into variable amounts of stages 2, 3 and 4. There is then an ascent to an EEG pattern that resembles stage 1 but which at this point is a true sleep accompanied by rapid eye movements and dreaming.[3] Following REM sleep there is a second descent to stages 2, 3 and 4. This alternation between REM and nonREM sleep occurs throughout the night in a cycle length of 7–120 minutes, with REM sleep equal to about 25 percent of total sleep. REM periods typically get longer as the night goes on, at first lasting only a few minutes and later enduring as long as 20–45 minutes. Therefore, most of one's REM time occurs in the early morning hours. Children spend more time in REM sleep and delta sleep than do young adults. In the mid-20s and 30s one begins to spend less time in stages 3 and 4. Over the ensuing years, stages 3 and 4 may almost totally disappear, REM time decreases slightly, and one experiences more awakenings, more total time awake, more time in stages 1 and 2 and less total time asleep.[4]

The maintenance of sleep or wakefulness and the cycling from one stage to another are controlled mainly by brain stem systems. Serotonergic, noradrenergic, cholinergic and dopaminergic systems are proba-

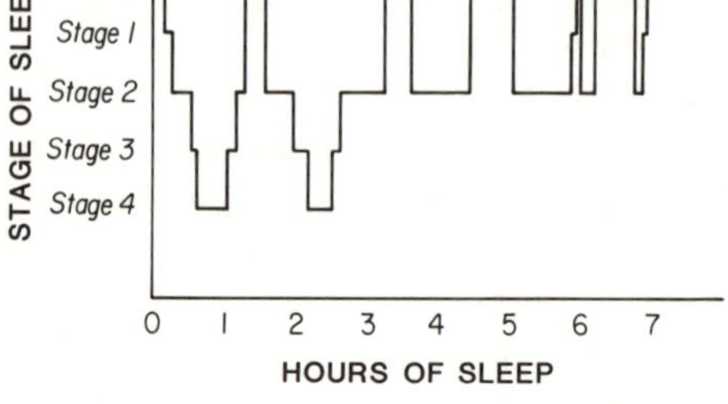

Sleep pattern of a young adult.

bly all involved. Drugs affecting neurotransmitter balances will, therefore, influence the sleep–awake or REM–nonREM periodicities.[5]

DISORDERS OF INITIATING AND MAINTAINING SLEEP: THE INSOMNIAS

Insomnia is one of the most common complaints in medicine. It refers to the patient's persistent inability to obtain sleep adequate in quality or quantity to leave him feeling comfortably rested during the usual waking hours. The diagnosis is a subjective one since normals show wide variation in sleep requirements. A "short sleeper" may require only 5–6 hours of broken sleep to feel rested while a "long sleeper" may require as much as 9–10 hours and may feel tired and drowsy during the day if he or she repeatedly gets only 7–8 hours of sleep. Findings that commonly typify insomniac sleep include a longer time to fall asleep, decreased total amount of sleep, increased number of awakenings, and lowered amounts of stages REM, 3, and 4. However, it is not at all rare for polygraphic studies of insomniacs to show no abnormalities. Even in such cases one must consider the possibility that there exist physiological factors that cannot be measured or as yet understood but that may play a role in the sense of not sleeping restfully. For example, increased nonREM mentation or generally higher levels of physiologic arousal throughout the night could contribute to a sense of not sleeping well.

As with any area of medicine, the most crucial aspect of evaluation is the history taking. Therefore, a thorough knowledge of possible etiology is needed (see Table 14-1). This section includes a brief discussion of the various causes of insomnia and the treatment possibilities for each.

Table 14-1.
Origins of Sleep Disorders

Insomnias	Hypersomnolence
1. Medical Illness	1. Medical Illness
2. Psychological Conflicts and Disorders	2. Psychological Conflicts and Disorders
3. Medications, Drugs	3. Medications, Drugs
4. Sleep Apnea	4. Sleep Apnea
5. Nocturnal Myoclonus	5. Nocturnal Myoclonus
6. Gastroesophageal Reflex	6. Narcolepsy
7. REM Interruption Insomnia	7. Subjective Complaint Without Presence of Objective Findings
8. Subjective Complaints Without Presence of Objective Findings	8. Disorders of the 24 Hour Sleep–Wake Cycle
9. Disorders of the 24-Hour Sleep–Wake Cycle	9. Ideopathic

Insomnia Secondary to Medical Illness

Cardiovascular, pulmonary, renal, hepatic, pancreatic, and other gastrointestinal diseases, nutritional and endocrine disorders, infectious or other toxic states, and intracranial disturbances are only some of the medical problems associated with disordered sleep. A partial list of specific disorders would include: nocturnal angina, nocturnal palpitations, congestive heart failure, anemia, nocturnal dyspnea, asthma, Cheyne-Stokes respirations, renal failure, hepatic failure, pancreatitis, cholecystitis, alcoholic liver disease, Wernicke's encephalopathy, Korsakoff's psychosis, Addison's disease, Cushing's syndrome, diabetes mellitus, hyperthyroidism, hypothyroidism, gross obesity, nutritional disorders, tuberculosis, syphilis, arthritis and rheumatoid disease, Lafora's disease, gastroesophageal reflux, neoplasms of the central nervous system (CNS), cluster headaches, migranous neuralgia, brain abscess, tetanus, kuru, other infections of the CNS, Wilson's disease, heavy metal poisoning, carbon monoxide poisoning, radiation poisoning, other toxic encephalopathies, multiple sclerosis, Parkinson's disease, Shy-Drager's syndrome, senile dementia, Alzheimer's disease, amyotrophic lateral sclerosis, trauma to the CNS, myotonic dystrophy, peripheral neuritis, and night cramps. Surgery, both minor and major, is almost always associated with at least temporary sleep disturbances. Ill patients commonly show a breakdown of the normal sleep cycling, decreases in REM and delta sleep, and increases in stage 1 and awake time.[6] Furthermore, in states of severe illness the sleep stages may lose their specificity, diffusing into each other. Alterations in a patient's sleep pattern may presage, accompany, or follow changes in medical status and in fact, the status of a subject's sleep may be an indication of the patient's state of health.[7] Treatment of these "secondary insomnias" is effected through treatment of the primary disease. Sleep medications are often helpful on a short term basis.

Psychological or Psychophysiological Causes of Insomnia

The psychological causes of insomnia range from "normal" tension states to psychotic disturbances. Strong and yet normal affects such as anxiety, tension, or excitement about work, home, or social life can disrupt sleep temporarily in even the healthiest of subjects. Disturbed sleep is a common symptom of almost all true psychological disorders whether they be acute and reactive to light or major stresses, or more chronic and reflective of neurotic, psychotic or characterologic difficulties. For example, chronic general underlying anxiety or specific unconscious fears as of death, separation, passivity, or dependence may play a role in insomniac symptomatology. The specific features of the disturbances will vary from individual to individual.

Sporadic reactive insomnias due to transient psychological problems are usually best managed by the primary physician. They are characterized by some combination of shortened total sleep time, difficulty falling asleep, increased awakenings, early morning arousal, and decreases in REM and delta sleep. Support, guidance, and the short-term use of sleep medication are of great help. The importance of educating patients should not be underestimated. A physician's explanation that short-term sleep difficulties are normal concomitants of overstimulation, transient personal problems, or health concerns is often sufficient to relieve the insomnia or at least quell a patient's fears about it. Patients need to know that periods of relative sleep deprivation are a normal part of life that will not affect their physical or mental well being.

Conditioning is an important factor in the evolution of stress-induced insomnias into long-term sleep problems. A subject going through a period of intense psychological distress may spend long hours in bed, awake, tossing and turning, feeling anxious and uncomfortable. He or she may then become conditioned to associate the bed with arousal and discomfort rather than rest and comfort, and may begin to dread the arousal (and therefore the bed), making it still more unlikely that he will be able to relax and fall asleep.[8]

Patients with chronic psychophysiologic insomnia show some or all of the following sleep characteristics: shortened total sleep time, difficulty falling asleep, increased awakenings, early morning arousal, inconsistent sleep patterns, relatively elevated resting muscle tone and respiratory and pulse rates, and decreased REM and delta sleep time. Three factors contribute to the sleep disorder. First is such patients' generally aroused physiologic state, whch is present not only when they are awake but right through the hours of sleep. Second is their tendency to have poor sleep habits. Because of their difficulties getting adequate rest, these subjects develop a wide variety of behavior patterns and habits that are aimed toward effecting sufficient sleep but that in actuality disrupt sleep. For example, patients go to bed at irregular hours, take sleeping pills and alcohol, try to sleep late in the morning, or slip in some daytime naps. The third contributory factor is conditioning. As mentioned above, patients who have insomnia periods during which they experience anxiety and distress at bedtime may come to associate their bedrooms or beds with that uncomfortable state and may experience these feelings when simply approaching either bedroom or bed.

There are some basic treatment principles that can help patients in the midst of a brief period of insomnia (decreasing the chances that such an episode will become a more chronic problem) or patients with a persistent psychophysiologic insomnia. (See Table 14-2.)

One should instruct patients to avoid lying in bed, fretting, tossing and turning, and trying to sleep. Instead, if and when it becomes evident that they are not going to fall asleep, they should get up and out of bed and pursue some quiet activity like reading or listening to the radio. They should return to bed only when tired, relaxed, and ready to sleep. They must not try to make up for lost sleep by napping in the day, sleeping late in the morning, or trying to go to bed earlier that next night. Instead they should arise at the usual time and remain up until their usual bedtime, even if very tired during the day and even if they complain about the inability to perform properly during the day. That decrease in performance for a short period is more likely due to psychological distress than to sleep deprivation. It is worth repeating that periods of relative sleep deprivation are a normal part of one's life that will not affect physical or mental health, or even performance. Waiting until nighttime to return to bed will increase the likelihood that one will be able to fall asleep. Exercise during the day or during the early evening is often helpful in bringing about sleep. Whether one should exercise just prior to going to bed becomes a personal issue: some people feel comfortably exhausted and fall asleep quickly; others feel stimulated and find sleep still more difficult. Any of the well known sleep medications and minor tranquilizers are a helpful adjunct during these periods. They can help one reassociate bed with sleep and comfort rather than with helplessness and discomfort. Chronic use of medication should be avoided.

Education becomes particularly important in the management of insomnia in the elderly. Older people are often imbued with the idea that eight hours of good sound sleep is crucial to the maintenance of mental and physical health. They are not aware that sleep needs vary from individual to individual and that the normal aging process is associated with sleep changes. Even by age 30, stages 3 and 4 have begun to decrease and the number of awakenings, the total time awake, and the time it takes to fall asleep all have increased. By the seventh decade one has little delta sleep and may have several awakenings (making sleep seem fragmented), slightly diminished REM sleep time and often a general sense of a loss of the restfulness of sleep. The nighttime difficulties are compounded by the inadvertent or forgotten daytime napping which can further reduce the chances of a good nightime sleep. Before offering reassurances to the elderly, the physician must remember that depression with insomnia is a common disorder of the elderly. One must also remain alert to the possibility that the patient may be using alcohol or medications that fragment sleep. Once the contributing factors have been considered and either treated or ruled out, explanations and firm reassurances are usually very helpful.

With major mental illness, sleep fluctuates enormously. Acutely psychotic schizophrenic patients often show decreased sleep time, decreased REM sleep time, decreased delta sleep time, increased time to fall asleep, and increased number of awakenings. Chronic schizophrenics may have normal sleep or may show deficiencies of REM or delta sleep. Sleep disturbance is a common symptom of depression and in fact, so important a feature that whenever a physician is presented with a sleep disorder with no obvious precipitating cause, he should consider the possibility of a masked depression. Difficulty in falling asleep, early morning awakenings, fragmented sleep and at times excessive sleep are all symptoms of depression. Polygraphic studies of depressives often show an increased number of arousals and awakenings and decreased REM and delta sleep. Insomnia assoicated with depression, mania, and the schizophrenias usually responds to treatment of the primary disorder. As psychotherapy, antidepressants, lithium, or a neuroleptic begin to effect the appropriate changes, insomnia usually recedes. Should sleep difficulties persist beyond the period of acute illness one should consider whether the use or misuse of medication is playing some role in the persistence of the problem or whether there are other issues in the patient's life that have yet to be explored or defined. Hospital observation or an all-night polygraphic sleep study can often provide helpful clues for management. Management of sleep disorders that are symptoms of character disorders, phobias, or other ingrained difficulties probably will have to be turned over to a psychiatrist; such sleep difficulties should normally end with resolution of the underlying conflicts.

The Use of Medications as a Cause of Insomnia.

One of the most widespread but least suspected causes of insomnia is the use of medications that affect the central nervous system.[9] Barbiturates, benzodiazepines, glutethimide (Doriden), methaqualone (Quaalude), chloral hydrate, and similar sleep medications are all effective in inducing and maintaining sleep on a short term basis. However, by two weeks most hypnotics lose their effectiveness.[10] Patients often start increasing their dosage in an attempt to increase the effectiveness of their medications. Moreover, while these medications are effective in increasing total sleep time, they must not be thought of as agents that restore normal physiologic sleep. The barbiturates and barbiturate-like drugs (e.g., methaqualone (Quaalude), glutethimide (Doriden), ethchlorvynol (Placidyl), methyprylon (Noludar) are potent REM sleep suppressants that may also suppress delta sleep. The benzodiazepines have a lesser effect on REM sleep but suppress stages 3 and 4. In the presence of REM-suppressant medication, REM pressure accumulates. The result can be uncomfortable dreams and a feeling of restlessness and agitation in the middle of the night. Furthermore, unless the original cause of the insomnia is treated while medications are being used, the insomnia itself will break through in spite of the presence of the medication. The return of the original insomnia, combined with the distortion of sleep created by the medication, contributes to an increase in the sleep problems for which a cure was originally being sought. Meprobamate, chloral hydrate, and the antihistamines are other effective, though possibly less potent, hypnotics that do not have dramatic suppressant effects on REM or delta sleep.

Not only do sleep medications lose their effectiveness after being used for a relatively brief period of time but they contribute to a widespread syndrome termed *drug withdrawal insomnia*. Once patients have become accustomed to taking sleep medications, it becomes very difficult to withdraw them from the drug. Withdrawal of any of the REM suppressant drugs leads to a REM rebound that is associated with a feeling of agitation and often with vivid and frightening dreams. If patients try to stop their medication, they may have several nights of still more troubled sleep than they were having while on the drug or before they started it and may then, of course, reach for their medication again and more persistently. Patients must be informed that with withdrawal of sleep medication it could take weeks for their sleep to stabilize to comfortable and quiet rest. Sleep medication should be withdrawn slowly over an extended period of time. For example, barbiturates might be decreased by one dose a week. Even those medications that are not known to be REM suppressants may be associated with a drug withdrawal insomnia and should be decreased slowly over time to allow for the gradual return of normal sleep physiology.

Alcohol is commonly prescribed by physicians as a remedy for sleepless nights. While it may be true that for some patients, use of small doses of alcohol on an occasional and/or even regular basis may help induce sleep, in other patients the use of alcohol can be disruptive. Alcohol is a potent REM suppressant agent but also a short-acting drug. As such it may suppress a patient's first one or two REM sleep periods only to effect, on that same night, a REM rebound that is often a period of restless, agitated sleep. Chronic excessive alcohol use is associated with a deterioration of sleep architecture, decreased total sleep time, increased awakenings, decreased REM sleep, and possibly decreased delta sleep. On withdrawal of alcohol, a massive REM rebound may occur, with its accompanying restlessness, agitation, increased awakenings, and possibly nightmares.

The central nervous system stimulants—the amphetamines, methylphenidate, and caffeine—will predictably increase the time it takes subjects to fall asleep and increase awake time in the middle of the night. Furthermore, the amphetamines and methylphenidate (Ritalin) may decrease REM sleep and possibly stages 3 and 4.

The effect of narcotics on sleep becomes an important consideration for physicians treating hospitalized patients. Although the narcotics have been reported to have a stimulant and sleep-disruptive effect when tested in normal volunteers,[11] patients in pain experience a restful sleep when treated with a narcotic analgesic in the short term.[12] The effects of chronic narcotic use on the sleep of patients in pain is not known, but one should at least consider the possibility that the drugs are disruptive.

Sleep Apnea Syndrome

The sleep apnea syndromes are associated with both insomnia and hypersomnia. Because the majority of patients with these disorders present with excessive daytime sleepiness, the discussion is presented under the hypersomnias.

Nocturnal Myoclonus

A relatively rare disorder that has been associated both with insomnia and with excessive daytime sleepiness, nocturnal myoclonus consists of frequent, abrupt, regularly repetitive contractions of the legs that occur periodically throughout the night. The subject falls asleep but while asleep experiences these jerks, the result of which can be either frequent brief awakenings or brief arousals though not to full awakening. If the subject awakens completely, he or she is likely to complain of a disrupted sleep pattern—insomnia. If subjects are aroused by the jerking movement but not to full awakening, they report having slept all night yet feeling tired the next day, as if they actually had very little sleep. In truth, they did get little deep or uninterrupted sleep, as the jerking movements disrupted the sleep cycle. In both cases, the subject is not aware of the jerks and the physician must turn to the spouse for a history of jerking movements or excessive restlessness during the patient's sleep. The presence of morning leg cramps or pains can be helpful in making the diagnosis. All night polygraphic sleep studies with monitoring of leg movements can confirm the diagnosis. One should consider the possibility that the myoclonus may be associated with the ingestion of or withdrawal from a CNS-active drug. Although clonazepam (Clonopin) 0.5–2 mg at bedtime, diazepam (Valium), oxazepam (Serax), or lorazepam (Ativan) may be tried as treatment for this disorder, there is as yet no definitive cure.

Gastroesophageal Reflux

The presence of even a small amount of stomach acid in the lower esophagus due to gastroesophageal reflux can cause some patients to awaken or at least arouse to a lighter sleep. Helpful in making this diagnosis is the symptom of a burning discomfort in the lower chest during the night or in the morning. This cause of awakenings may be seen in patients who eat just prior to going to bed. They may awaken one or two hours later and may or may not have a sensation of burning. A change in eating habits is often successful in alleviating the nighttime arousal.

REM Interruption Insomnia

REM interruption insomnia is a term for repetitive awakenings out of REM sleep periods while nonREM periods are interruption free. The subject awakens approximately every 90 minutes in the night and may or may not remember a dream and may experience some associated distress. Some patients experience frightening episodes during which they are not sure whether they have been awake or asleep. This type of insomnia is usually associated with a history of psychological difficulties, a period of psychological stress, alcohol use or the presence of or acute withdrawal from medications that affect REM sleep time. Common, during withdrawal of REM-suppressant drugs, are arousals from frightening dreams.

Subjective Complaints of Insomnia Without the Presence of Objective Findings

There are some patients who complain of insomnia, who do not have any of the above listed disorders, and in whom all-night polygraphic sleep studies demonstrate no pathology. While hypochondriasis is an obvious possible diagnosis, one must be wary of forming that conclusion. A thorough psychiatric consultation is appropriate, keeping in mind that we do not yet know much about the functions of the different stages of sleep. It is quite possible that a subject whose sleep physiology looks perfectly normal by present standards may not experience the restorative aspects of sleep that cannot be measured. It is possible, too, that increased nonREM mentation or high levels of nocturnal physiological arousal contribute to a sense of not sleeping restfully and not feeling rested during the following day. For this diagnosis to be made the patient must have had all night sleep studies; therefore, a sleep laboratory would be involved in management. Generally, patients are reassured by the laboratory results that demonstrate normal sleep physiology and an explanation about the nature of their problem and the limits of knowledge about the restful, restorative aspects of sleep. They must be warned about forming bad sleep habits in an effort to cope with their problem. The principles of Table 14-2 should be followed.

Table 14-2.
Principles in Treatment of Chronic Psychophysiologic Insomnia After Consideration of Differential Diagnosis.

1. Reevaluate the patients anxiety/depression level and consider using tricylic antidepressants when suspicious of underlying or masked depression.
2. Reconsider the possible sleep-disruptive effects of medications or alcohol, particularly when taken to aid sleep.
3. Consider age. Educate the elderly about changing sleep patterns.
4. Once life-threatening illnesses such as sleep apneas or drug abuse are ruled out, patients should understand that decreases in daytime performance are more likely due to anxiety about sleeplessness than insomnia itself. People can usually do quite well in life getting less sleep than they would like.
5. Exercise and a rich daytime activity schedule will aid sleep.
6. Maintenance of a regular sleep schedule is helpful in achieving good sleep.
7. Eating just before bedtime may be disruptive to sleep.
8. If awake during the night, subjects should relax and avoid worrying about being sleepy the next day. If sleep does not return quickly they should try reading a good but unexciting book. If sleep still does not come they should not toss and turn and fret but get out of bed and pursue some hobby or work, until they feel ready to sleep. TV can be subtly stimulating for some subjects; when that is the case it should be avoided.
9. Avoidance of daytime napping, even though one feels very sleepy, is helpful in enhancing nighttime rest.
10. Short-term use of sleeping pills of any type can help patients begin to reassociate bed with comfort and rest rather than restlessness and discomfort.
11. Sedatives or respiratory depressants should be prescribed with caution for patients with loud snoring even though sleep apnea is not present.
12. Long-term use of hypnotics is usually inappropriate and is done more to give the physician the feeling he is doing something than to help the patient.
13. Some insomnias due to psychophysiologic arousal and some forms of idiopathic insomnia are simply not treatable with our present body of knowledge. As with many medical problems, patients must adjust and make do with a problem that will hurt them more if they worry about it than if they simply adjust to it. Physicians will be more comfortable taking such a stand if they have considered the appropriate differential diagnosis.
14. If in doubt, consult a sleep laboratory.

Disorders of the 24-Hour Sleep–Wake Cycle

Like all animals, humans are circadian creatures operating with "biological clocks" set in accord with cues and demands in the environment. While most individuals can rather easily alter the hours during which they sleep, their basic biological circadian rhythms cannot be shifted with such ease. For example, body temperature and the secretion pattern of a number of hormones may take an extended period to fully resume their usual relationship to the sleep-waking cycle when the latter is altered. Modern day technology has allowed man to function independently of the natural daylight–nighttime cycling and has allowed him to travel vast distances to points on the globe that may be out of phase with his own time schedule. Sleep-wake cycle disturbances are then very frequent in work situations involving variable time shifts and in subjects who travel across time zones ("jet lag"). In both situations, the individual is "supposed" to sleep at a time in the 24-hour day when his circadian rhythms are programmed for arousal and is "supposed" to be awake when his basic physiology is suited for sleep. Insomnia as well as daytime drowsiness results, and the loss of nocturnal sleep still further compromises an already disrupted situation.

Most humans average a sleep–wake cycle slightly in excess of 24 hours. Under normal circumstances the weight of environmental cues, particularly the solar day, forces an alignment of our inherent rhythms to the environmental clocks. There are some individuals, however, who seem to have an appreciably shorter or longer sleep–wake cycle than the normal or their biological clocks are not as responsive to environmental cues as is usual. The pressure of the shorter than 24-hour sleep–wake rhythm may cause the subject to experience the need to go to sleep earlier and wake up earlier than his or her environment demands. Subjects experiencing longer than 24-hour circadian rhythm may find themselves wishing to retire later and later and sleeping later and later in the morning.

Sleep–wake cycle disturbances can occur in individuals who do not keep to a regular sleep–wake schedule. Unemployment, retirement, periods of excessive work and physicial and psychological illness are just some of the situations in which subjects fail to maintain a regular sleep–wake schedule. If temporarily forced to live in accord with external rhythms, they may feel drowsy and not alert when awake and yet not be able to sleep at night. They may eventually lose their capacity to remain alert throughout a full wake cycle and to sleep regularly through a daily sleep period.

A highly motivated patient may correct these disorders by setting and strictly adhering to a schedule in accord with the solar day even though when first resetting rhythms he or she may feel tired and drawn at the time of arising. Eventually, the patient's biological clocks should reestablish themselves to be in accord with the standard day. Some individuals might find it initially impossible to get up at a set hour in the morning. These subjects may respond to a treatment program the general principle of which allows them to sleep later and later each day until they circle the clock and their desire to go to sleep is at the time of a standard bed time hour.[13] Once the subject reaches that part of the schedule he or she should force himself to maintain it by waking up at a set hour and going to bed at a set hour each night. Particularly important in increasing subjects' ability to go to sleep at night is a rigid schedule for morning awakening and a nap free work day.

DISORDERS OF EXCESSIVE SOMNOLENCE: HYPERSOMNOLENCE

Hypersomnolence, while of lower incidence in the general population than insomnia, is a common problem meriting medical attention. Patients complain of feeling tired, drowsy, or sleepy most of the time and fall asleep against their wills during the day. The polygraphic findings that typify the sleep of hypersomnolents vary with the nature of the primary disorder.

In the evaluation and treatment of hypersomnolence one might first consider whether or not the complaint exists despite seemingly normal nighttime sleep. Second, one might explore the idea that the problem results from disturbed nighttime sleep. Third, one might hypothesize the presence of a problem that is disruptive to both nighttime sleep and daytime alertness. Following a description of the patient's nocturnal patterns, a review of causes of hypersomnolence can be entertained. In order to provide a general organization for the evaluation of all sleep disorders, the order in which these causes will be discussed parallels the discussion of causes of insomnia. (See Table 14-1.)

Hypersomnolence Associated with Medical Illness

Hypersomnolence, like insomnia is a symptom seen in association with almost any medical, surgical, or neurological illness. Endocrine and metabolic disorders, hepatic failure, renal failure, chronic respiratory insufficiency, systemic infections, central nervous system infections, cerebrovascular disorders, head trauma, cancers located anywhere in the system, brain mass lesions or hemorrhages, and degenerative diseases are only a few of the numerous disease states in which excessive somnolence may be a symptom. Polygraphic studies may show normal, though excessive, sleep or in states of severe illness disruption of the characteristics defining the various sleep stages. As with insomnia, increases in somnolence may presage, accompany, or follow changes in medical status, and the symptom, therefore, should never be dismissed lightly. With resolution of the disease conditions, excessive somnolence usually subsides.

Psychological Causes of Hypersomnolence

Psychological factors and conflicts may result in the development of hypersomnolence in some individuals just as they may effect insomnia in others. The excessive sleepiness may be transient and situational as a means of dealing with an acute life change or stress or persist as a means of dealing with chronic unhappiness and tension. Some depressions, particularly those of bipolar affective illness, are more likely to present with hypersomnolence than insomnia. The symptoms may also be the only apparent sign of some difficult-to-detect personality disorders, often with deeply impounded rage or depression. The latter will require psychiatric referral for diagnosis and treatment.

The Use of Medications as a Cause of Hypersomnolence

The fact that misuse of medications or drugs with sedative–hypnotic effects can cause daytime hypersomnolence is obvious enough to merit little discussion except for the mention of three less apparent points.

Some patients, particularly the elderly, may develop daytime hypersomnolence while properly using therapeutic doses of medications and without recognizing the relationship of the sleepiness to the drug use. Patients should be educated about the possible prolonged soporific effects of medication taken the night or even the day before. Physicians should remain alert to the fact that some commonly used drugs, particularly the benzodiazepines (flurazepam, diazepam, and chlordiazepoxide) or their active metabolites, remain in the system for greater than 24 hours and may, therefore, accumulate day after day, resulting in the insidious onset of hypersomnolence. Chronic use of nighttime sedatives may disrupt more than help nighttime sleep and may contribute to unsuspecting subjects' daytime sleepiness.

Sleep Apnea Syndromes

The laboratory definition of the sleep apnea syndromes has been one of the major contributions of recent sleep research.[14] The syndromes are characterized by sleep-associated cessations of air flow lasting from 10 seconds to a minute or more and occurring from 30 to several hundred times during a night. The episodes can occur in any or all stages of sleep, and the patient is typically unaware of the respiratory compromise. Patients can experience cardiac arrhythmias during the apneic episodes as well as insidious and severe long-term cardiovascular effects, such as pulmonary and/or systemic hypertension. A decrease in air flow that is not a complete apnea is termed hypoventilation. With significant hypoventilation the presentation and sequelae are the same as with the sleep apneas.

Three types of apnea have been distinguished, and although these syndromes are being discussed under the heading of hypersomnias, the sleep symptom with which they present can be insomnia or hypersomnia, depending on the individual and the type of apnea. In central sleep apnea, the medullary respiratory center is periodically unsuccessful in triggering the respiratory musculature. Either just as the subject falls asleep or once he or she has been asleep for a variable period of time, the diaphragm and chest show decreases in respiratory movements and finally stop moving altogether. Breathing, hopefully, begins in response to the increasingly abnormal blood gases and usually is associated with a brief awakening. In obstructive sleep apnea, the walls of the upper airway, at the level of the pharynx, develop a hypotonia and collapse to obstruct air flow while abdominal and thoracic musculature continue with their respiratory efforts. In this syndrome the typical patient is a male adult with a complaint of excessive daytime sleepiness. The subject is not aware of his disrupted night time respirations and sleep patterns and feels only that despite having slept through the night, he is not well rested. He complains of being tired and somnolent the following day. The sleepiness is sometimes experienced as overwhelming, and patients with this syndrome may be misdiagnosed as narcoleptic. The daytime sleepiness is usually not as irresistible as it is in narcoleptics, and daytime naps may not bring any sense of refreshment. Morning headaches are a common accompaniment.

The diagnosis of apnea is made by observing the patient asleep; it can often be made by the patient's spouse. The sleeping patient with obstructive apnea exhibits loud sonorous snoring as he tries to move air past a closing upper airway. When the upper airway is completely occluded, breathing stops and there is a period of silence. Jerky, forceful breathing movements of the chest and diaphragm continue through the apneic period; finally with a loud snort, the obstruction is overcome and breathing and snoring begin again, until the next obstruction and the next silence. Polygraphic studies show the obstruction occurring as the patient falls asleep or after he has been asleep for a variable period of time. The period of apnea ends with an arousal from sleep to awakening or near awakening and in association with the awakening, the reestablishment of tone of the upper airway musculature and a loud snort as breathing begins once again. A well known subtype of obstructive sleep apnea is the Pickwickian syndrome, which is characterized by extreme obesity, hypersomnolence, cyanosis, periodic respiration, secondary polycythemia, right ventricular failure, hypoxemia, and hypercapnea. Physical abnormalities of the jaw and pharynx, neck, chest, and back may be associated with an obstructive sleep apnea, and sleep abnormalities should be specifically inquired about in the presence of micrognathia and mandibular malformation, kyphoscoliosis, adenoidal tonsillar hypertrophy, and goiter.

The third type of sleep apnea syndrome is the mixed type, in which both central and obstructive components are present. While the majority of patients with sleep apnea are male adults, the syndromes have been implicated in sudden infant death syndrome (especially the central type) and should be kept in mind in young children with hypersomnia, behavioral abnormalities, and very large tonsils (which could occlude the upper airway during sleep).

The symptom of excessive daytime sleepiness is not easily explained. Patients spend a good part of the night going from awake to stage 1 to stage 2 and then arousing from stage 2 as a result of the apnea. Possibly the continuous disruptions of sleep and the chronic sleep deprivation play a role. In addition, there may be persistent effects of the repetitive nighttime hypoxemia and hypercapnea. Possibly, too, these patients suffer from a disturbance in the basic mechanisms for maintaining sleep and wakefulness.

The diagnoses of insomnia or hypersomnolence with sleep apnea syndrome are being made more and more frequently as clinicians become educated about these disorders. Diagnosis is crucial since death by hypoxia is an ever present possibility. Weight loss and the correction of any structural abnormalities are often all that are needed for the treatment of the obstructive apnea. Some patients will obstruct only when supine; in such cases, any device that keeps them off their backs will prevent the apneas. A tennis ball in a sock pinned to the pajama top may suffice. Tracheostomy is definitive therapy. The tracheostomy is closed during the day and opened at bedtime, thereby by-passing the nocturnal upper airway obstruction. Once the tracheostomy is in place, the excessive daytime sleepiness usually disappears and normal blood gases are restored. In cases in which the upper airway obstruction is posing a major threat (e.g., when someone has many and/or prolonged obstructions or cardiac arrhythmias), the tracheostomy can be done first and then other measures implemented to correct malformations. Some patients lose weight more easily once the obstruction is relieved. The treatment of central apneas is more difficult. Medroxyprogesterone (Provera) 20 mg tid or qid may provide a beneficial respiratory stimulus. In fact, medroxyprogesterone may be beneficial in obstructive apneas as well because of the involvement of central mechanisms. A possible future definitive treatment of central apnea is the implacement of a diaphragmatic pacemaker that fires at night when respiratory rates fall below a certain level.[15]

Nocturnal Myoclonus

Nocturnal myoclonus is similar to the sleep apnea syndromes in that it, too, has been associated with both hypersomnolence and insomnia. It has been discussed under the insomnias.

Narcolepsy

Narcolepsy is a disorder mainly characterized by a persistent daytime sleepiness and recurrent brief "attacks" of uncontrollable sleep that intrude on one's waking hours. After the sleep "attack," which usually lasts 10–15 minutes, the patient may feel refreshed and alert. Before long, however, that alert feeling succumbs to the almost ever-present feelings of sleepiness and again, after a few hours, an irresistible urge to sleep will occur.

The disorder is usually manifested by sleep attacks plus one of several auxillary symptoms.[16] The sleep attacks and the associated symptoms of cataplexy, hypnagogic and hypnopompic hallucinations, and sleep paralysis are currently referred to as the narcoleptic tetrad. Any of the associated symptoms can occur alone, and as such they stand as an individual diagnostic entity. When sleep attacks occur alone, the diagnosis of narcolepsy becomes a more difficult one. In many cases, the auxillary phenomena will appear later in the history of the disease.

A narcoleptic will almost assuredly fall asleep when the lights are turned down in a room or when he or she is left in any situation conducive to sleep. In addition, there is usually a history of falling asleep at the most unlikely times such as when talking, working actively, or driving. Automobile accidents due to the patient's falling asleep at the wheel are a part of almost every narcoleptic's history. As many as 20 attacks a day are not uncommon, and although the periodicity of the "naps" may be totally unpredictable, it may at other times be quite regular. A history of hypersomnolence, sleep attacks, and any one of the associated symptoms is usually sufficient to make definitive the diagnosis of narcolepsy. It is intriguing that the nocturnal sleep of narcoleptics is usually restless and disturbed even when no associated symptoms occur.

Cataplexy refers to brief attacks of decreased muscle tone usually coincident to a burst of emotion such as laughter, surprise, sadness, or anger. Muscle-tone decreases range from a subjective feeling of weakness in one or more limbs to a near total paralysis that is sometimes accompanied by a fall, although consciousness is maintained. A decrease in muscle tone to the extent of a full body paralysis occurring in the transition from sleep to wakefulness or wakefulness to sleep is referred to as sleep paralysis. The paralysis can occur when a subject is first going to sleep for the night or upon awakening in the morning or in the middle of the night. Because the subject is awake when these attacks occur, they can be a frightening experience. The paralysis can usually be broken volitionally by the subject's forcing a movement or grunt. Hypnagogic or hypnopompic hallucinations are visual or auditory phenomena that occur in the transition between waking and sleep or sleep and awakening and, at times, simultaneously with sleep paralysis.

The age of onset of narcolepsy is usually between 15–55 years of age. The disorder then is present for life. The severity and the frequency of the attacks may remain stable or may increase with age, and remissions are rare and of relatively short duration. Although in as many as half of the cases reported a family history is present, the means of transmission is not clear. Usually the sleep attacks precede the appearance of the auxillary symptoms, but occasionally the reverse may be true. The cause of the disease is unknown. Physical and laboratory data are generally normal except in those rare cases that have had their onset following encephalitis, head trauma, or other medical, neurological, infectious, or toxic conditions. Although recently considerable advance has been made in our understanding of narcolepsy physiology, the diagnosis is still made mainly on the basis of the history. Polygraphic studies of sleep can be very helpful in confirming the diagnosis. Narcoleptic patients generally enter REM sleep immediately on falling asleep at night and on experiencing a daytime sleep attack. Often they will report a dream. A "multiple sleep latency test," which documents the patient's inclination to fall asleep at different times during the day, can also be helpful in establishing the diagnosis. The patient is given five opportunities to nap at 2 hour intervals over an 8.5 hour daytime period. Narcoleptics will usually fall asleep in less than 5 minutes and will often go directly into REM sleep.

The illness can be seen as a disorder in which the mechanisms for maintaining wakefulness are insufficient for suppressing sleep and particularly, REM sleep. The REM state may appear at unpredictable times, and certain characteristics of the REM state may become dissociated and appear unexpectedly. Thus, REM sleep might appear at sleep onset and the normal REM phenomena of muscle-tone inhibition and dreaming may break through or continue into wakefulness. Cataplexy and sleep paralysis may represent the low muscle tone of REM breaking into the waking state and hypnagogic hallucinations may represent the dream experience, again during waking time. In a similar fashion, sleep following a prolonged cataplectic attack will often begin with the stage REM, and a significant percentage of narcoleptics report a phenomenon often referred to as "waking dreams" in which REM mentation intrudes on normal waking mentation, compromising one's degree of attentiveness to the environment. The symptoms of narcolepsy can be so disruptive to normal life that it is not surprising that many narcoleptics have considerable emotional problems. Psychiatric evaluation and assistance is often invaluable as an adjunct to the pharmacological treatment of the disorder.

In subjects who do not show sleep onset REM periods over several polygraphic studies, who do not develop any of the associated symptoms, or who do not show a pathological inclination to fall asleep during the multiple sleep latency test, the likelihood of a psychological etiology of the symptoms is great. The sleep attacks in which nonREM sleep stages intrude into wakefulness might represent a form of narcolepsy, but for the present time, most sleep specialists will consider the diagnosis of narcolepsy only presumptive until at least one of the above criteria are met.

Treatment of narcolepsy is difficult and calls for continuous monitoring and adjusting of medication.[17] Amphetamines, methylphenidate (Ritalin) or pemoline (Cylert) are usually successful in suppressing the sleep attacks and increasing daytime alertness. Treatment should begin with the lowest dose needed to bring about the desired results. Patients can be expected to develop tolerance to these medications and, therefore, will require progressively larger doses. Periodically the drug will have to be stopped with the hope that one will be able to restart it at a lower, yet effective dose.

These medications have little or no effect on the associated symptoms, and the medications that reduce the frequency of the associated symptoms usually have no effect on the sleep attacks. The tricyclic antidepressants and the MAO inhibitors may each be effective in reducing the incidence of cataplexy, hypnagogic hallucinations, and sleep paralysis. Although their mechanism of action is unknown, both groups of drugs are potent REM suppressants. One would expect that their REM-suppressant qualities are related to their effect on the associated symptoms. Again, tolerance may occur and one should exercise some degree of caution when using the amphetamines methylphenidate (Ritalin) or pemoline (Cylert) in combination with any of these other medications.

Subjective Complaint Without Objective Findings

There are some patients who complain of a feeling of excessive daytime sleepiness without excessive daytime sleep; that is, they do not demonstrate an increased tendency or even ability to fall asleep during the day although they experience a vague but intense sleepiness and compromised alertness during the day that decreases their effectiveness in work and social settings. Physical and psychological evaluations fail to reveal the etiology of the complaints as do the normal appearing, all-night polygraphic sleep studies and daytime multiple sleep latency tests.

It is as if these patients' normal appearing sleep is in some crucial way nonrestorative or as if they have a subtle sleep–wake disorder with incomplete alert phases. Although one should be particularly careful in ruling out psychophysiologic hypersomnia and masked depressions, one must also be way of assuming that psychological factors must be the cause. Imipramine (Tofranil) or protriptyline (Vivactil) may be effective in doses lower than those used for antidepressant therapy, and occasional use of amphetamines, methylphenidate (Ritalin), or pemoline (Cylert), may provide symptomatic relief at particularly important times.

Disorders of the 24-Hour Sleep–Wake Cycle

See this title in the section on the insomnias.

Idiopathic Hypersomnia

Idiopathic hypersomnia refers to the symptom of excessive daytime sleepiness of unknown cause. Subjects with this symptom usually spend long nights asleep, 10 or 12 hours or more, and yet may feel tired and sleepy during the days, often requiring daytime naps. The hypersomniac feels his or her sleep to be deep and undisturbed and may even complain of an inability to wake up completely in the morning. Morning sleepiness and confusion can last up to several hours and because of its similarity to alcohol drunkenness, has been called "sleep drunkenness."

Like narcoleptics, these patients may complain of a persistent daytime drowsiness or sleepiness. They may, too, feel periodic increases in sleepiness at which time they feel the need to nap. This "sleep attack" is, however, much less compelling than that experienced by the narcoleptic. It can be resisted. Unlike narcoleptics, who sleep only a few minutes, hypersomniacs, when they nap, may stay asleep for hours. Polygraphic sleep studies reveal normal staging and patterning of sleep, and there is no association with any of the auxillary symptoms of narcolepsy. Our understanding of this disorder is too meager for any definitive statements about it to be made. It must be distinguished from the high end of the curve of normally long sleepers, and all other causes of hypersomnia must be ruled out. As our understanding of the causes of sleep symptomatology increases, idiopathic hypersomnia, like narcolepsy with no confirmatory signs, should become a vanishing entity. The diagnosis should now be made tentatively and the patient followed closely for other developments. Medications can be tried on a temporary basis. Amphetamines, methylphenidate (Ritalin), and even imipramine (Tofranil) or one of the other tricyclic compounds may be helpful. One should try to find the lowest effective dose. Counseling of family members may help them to develop a more flexible approach to the problem, and psychotherapy should be at least considered for the patient.

THE PARASOMNIAS

The parasomnias are sleep phenomena characterized by inconsistencies or dissociations of arousal; in these disorders, behavior usually associated with wakefulness appears during sleep.

Somnambulism, or Sleepwalking

Sleepwalkers may simply move around in bed, or they may walk around their rooms or house. On rare occasions, they may venture outside the house. Although subjects' eyes are open, they appear more to be staring blankly than seeing clearly. Behavior may be simple and stereotyped or it may encompass a full range of complex and purposeful activity. It is difficult to awaken sleepwalkers, and if they are aroused to consciousness they are usually confused. Episodes last up to several minutes, and subjects often return to bed themselves, or at least are easily led there. Amnesia for the episode is characteristic.

Somnambulism in childhood is not a rare disorder, and a normal and benign imbalance of neurologic maturational processes probably plays a role in its appearance. The activity does not mean that psychological difficulties are present in the child and most children will outgrow the symptoms. Such is not the case for an adult somnambulist. While occasional sleepwalking episodes may occur at times of serious psychological stress, persistent sleepwalking is often associated with more serious psychopathology. Organic causes such as epilepsy or the side-effects of drugs such as imipramine (Tofranil) must always be considered, and a thorough psychiatric evaluation is usually merited. Although motivational factors can often be deciphered for sleepwalking episodes both in children and adults, the hypothesis that sleepwalkers act out a dream has not been borne out. Polygraphic sleep studies have established that the somnambulistic episodes, rather than arising out of stage REM, when dreaming is common, arise out of stages 3 and 4, when dream mentation as we think of it is rare.[18] Nevertheless, the behavior suggests an intriguing interphase between the primitive psychological and the neurophysiological.

No effective treatment of the disorder has been established. Parents of child sleepwalkers should be assured that the symptoms do not necessarily represent psychopathology. One should inquire as to environmental stresses or medications that could be contributing to the appearance of the phenomena. Parents and child should usually be reassured that the patient will outgrow the disorder. Protecting the patient from harm is an important aspect of management. The subject, if possible, should sleep on the first floor, and potentially dangerous objects should be removed from the bedroom prior to bedtime. Windows and doors should be kept locked. If the somnambulism is attributable to a tricyclic antidepressant, reduction of the nighttime dosage should resolve the problem. Adults with persistent sleepwalking should be referred for a psychiatric consultation. The benzodiazepines, suppressants of stages 3 and 4, may be helpful in reducing the frequency of the episodes.

Night Terrors and Nightmares

Night terrors and nightmares are two clinically similar phenomena with nevertheless subtle differences that should be differentiated by the clinician.[19] A nightmare is a very frightening dream that arises out of REM sleep. The dreamer awakens, often with a startle, to full alertness, feels anxiety and dread, and has a quite thorough recall of the dream and its well developed plot. Night terrors, which include pavor nocturnus in children and incubus in adults, are sudden attacks of panic that usually occur out of stage 4 sleep. The phenomena are particularly dramatic, for from what appears to be a quiet and calm sleep, the subject suddenly bolts up, screaming in terror. Sympathetic nervous system activity is intense, and the subject sweats, his or her pupils dilate, pulse bounds, and respirations race. The subject is difficult to awaken to clear consciousness and can remain very agitated and in a cloudy mental state for as long as 20 to 30 minutes. Once alert, there is no recall of the phenomenon or dream content except for possibily a single terrifying image.

Night terrors can occur in both children and adults; even in infants as young as six months one can see crying and screaming episodes in the depths of sleep. Pavor nocturnus, like somnambulism, probably reflects a benign imbalance of central nervous system development that will spontaneously correct itself as the child matures. It is also possible that primitive psychological mechanisms play a role in etiology of the phenomenon and it is appropriate for the physician to look to personal or family stresses as possibly contributing to the occurrence of the terrors. If no such stresses are apparent, it is best to reassure parents of the benign nature of the symptom and encourage a "wait and see" attitude. It can be terrifying for parents to see their children in this agitated state; close contact between the physician and parents is often very helpful.

When night terrors occur in adults, significant psychological problems are more likely to be apparent, especially if the phenomenon is a persistent one. A psychiatric evaluation is indicated in most adults with night terrors, in children with a long standing history of the phenomenon, and in adults and children with a history of persistent nightmares. The benzodiazepines—for example, diazepam (Valium) 5–20 mg given at bedtime—may reduce the incidence of night terrors, probably by the mechanism of suppressing stage 4 sleep.

In somnambulism, night terrors and nocturnal enuresis, positive family histories are common and it is not uncommon for all three phenomena to be represented in the family. This occurence leads to hypotheses of disorders of arousal occurring in families, with the nature of the arousal disorder varying from person to person.[18]

Jactatio Capitis Nocturna

Jactatio capitis nocturna, sleep rocking or head banging, consists of rhythmic movements of the head or body prior to or during sleep. The phenomenon may begin about six months of age and will usually disappear in the middle childhood years. Less common is its persistence into adolescence and even adulthood. The rocking episodes can occur out of any stage of sleep. The etiology is not at all clear; organic and psychological etiologies have been suggested, and the phenomenon might well be a variant of disorders of arousal typified by somnambulism, enuresis, and night terrors. A family history of one of the parasomnias is common. No type of treatment has had consistent success; conditioning therapy and bedtime imipramine (Tofranil) (at up to standard antidepressant dose levels) have at times been helpful.

Nocturnal Bruxism

Nocturnal bruxism is teeth grinding during sleep. Patients are almost always unware of their symptom until their dentist tells them that their teeth are being ground down to smoothness or their spouses complain of a grinding noise in the middle of the night. The episodes occur periodically throughout the night and each burst may last 5–10 seconds. Polygraphic sleep studies show that the episodes arise out of stage 2 sleep. Psychological factors play a major etiologic role in this disorder, and psychotherapy is often helpful.

Sleep Paralysis

Sleep paralysis has already been discussed as part of the narcolepsy syndrome. It deserves mention on its own, however, because it is not an uncommon symptom in the general population, and its incidence is steadily increasing as physician's knowledge of and inquiry into sleep disorders increases. Subjects awaken in the middle of the night or in the morning and find themselves unable to move or talk. Although the episodes are benign, the subject, until he is educated as to the nature of this disorder, can be terrified when he awakens to find himself paralyzed. The paralysis can last from a few seconds to a minute and can usually be broken by a forced grunt or body movement or a touch from someone else. The phenomenon represents a dissociated aspect of REM sleep: the decreased muscle tone characteristic of that stage is persisting into the waking state. Psychological explanations have been proposed and psychotherapy might be helpful in alleviating the symptom; certainly education of the patient is crucial.

Hypnagogic and Hypnopompic Hallucinations

Hypnagogic and hypnopompic hallucinations, like sleep paralysis, are parts of the narcolepsy syndrome that deserve mention on their own because of their high incidence in the general population. As one is falling asleep (hypnagogic) or awakening (hypnopompic) patients may experience visual or auditory hallucinations. Usually the phenomena represent dream mentation intruding into the waking state. Less commonly a person under stress might briefly lose his sense of reality just as he is drifting off to sleep. Hypnagogic or hypnopompic hallucinations and sleep paralysis can occur together, the result of which is usually a frightening experience for the patient. Reassurance is the only treatment necessary after inquiry into other symptoms of narcolepsy.

THE RELATIONSHIP OF SLEEP TO OTHER DISORDERS

Although physicians often consider the effect their patient's illness may have on sleep, it is rare for them to consider that sleep, both normal and disturbed, can have profound effects on the nature and course of their patients' illness.

Medical–surgical problems in general disturb sleep. For example, postoperative patients in pain experience decreased REM and delta sleep and a fragmented sleep pattern, the duration of the disruption varying in some measure with the severity of the surgery. Severely ill patients may be chronically sleep deprived and particularly deprived of REM and delta sleep.[7] Whether such disturbances bear on ultimate outcome is uncertain but they should be considered in prescribing medications. Barbiturates and benzodiazepines, for example, will suppress REM sleep and stage 4 respectively, and both stages are already at lower than normal levels because of the patient's illness. At the same time, there are probably benefits to encouraging sleep over nocturnal restlessness and wakefulness. Attention to factors such as the conduciveness of the environment for sleep, daytime napping (which can contribute to night time insomnia), nurses' and doctors' routines that are without consideration for sleep, and medication that could be causing an arousal response may be more beneficial in alleviating in-hospital insomnia than sleep medication. Careful short-term, well-thought-out use of hypnotics can still be helpful. Before prescribing, one should remember, too, that respiratory irregularities can cause insomnia. If respiratory irregularities are suspected (see sleep apnea), respiratory suppressants are contraindicated, especially if other respiratory suppressants, such as the narcotics, are already being employed.

Normally blood pressure and cardiac and respiratory rates decrease with sleep onset, gradually reaching their lowest levels of the night around 4 a.m. The decline is not a steady one, however, because of the autonomic excitement that occurs with each REM period; in REM sleep blood pressure and cardiac and respiratory rates become variable and are generally higher than during nonREM periods. Energy utilization is greater in REM sleep.[20] In some patients, arrhythmias, nocturnal angina pectoris and ECG signs of ischemia occur more in REM than in nonREM sleep.[21] Even deep sleep may hold a potential danger to cardiac patients, as heart rate can decrease below a good perfusion rate. While the relationship between cardiac abnormalities and sleep stage needs to be further researched, it can be helpful for physicians to consider these issues when prescribing drugs that will affect sleep staging. For example, patients whose angina or arrhythmias occur one and a half hours after sleep onset or in the hours of the early morning may be having REM-associated occurences. No data are available for setting management guidelines in such cases but one should consider that barbiturates and narcotics are potent REM suppressors associated, too, with REM rebound upon their withdrawal. One has only one's clinical observations and judgment to use in balancing the possible benefits and hazards of REM-suppressant drugs. A very slow withdrawal of REM suppressants is essential.

Increased nocturnal gastric acid secretion and ulcer pain may also have a relationship to REM sleep, and the issues mentioned earlier apply here as well.[21]

A knowledge of sleep physiology may aid in the evaluation of severely ill patients. In comatose or stuporous patients the presence of sleep–wake cycling patterns in all-night or 24-hour polygraphic studies suggest the presence of a functional integrity that correlates well with recovery.[7,22,23] With serial studies, one may see improvement (or deterioration) in sleep patterns before any clinical changes become apparent.

Several neurological conditions are exacerbated during sleep: for example, carpal tunnel syndrome and nocturnal cramps of the foot or leg. Quinine hydrochloride (300 mg) and calcium lactate (600 mg) are helpful with the cramps. Tired arm syndrome, a condition seen in middle-aged women who over-work during the day, is characterized by aching or throbbing and numbness of the hand at night but not during the day. Rest is sufficient treatment.

Restless legs syndrome, a rather common problem for which no definitive treatment is available, consists of painful feelings of unrest and restlessness in the legs which arise upon the patient's going to bed or awakening in the night. Getting out of bed, walking, or continually changing positions are the only means of providing definite relief. Diazepam (Valium) or clonazepam (Clonopin) may be helpful. The problem is often seen in conjunction with nocturnal myoclonus.

Finally, the sleep–wake cycle may effect seizure activity. Some types of seizure discharges are activated during REM sleep and others during nonREM sleep. Inducing sleep is a well-established method for revealing seizure activity that may not be present in the awake period. Sleep deprivation will lower seizure threshold in epileptics and probably in normals as well.

Knowledge about sleep is no longer an interesting curiosity for doctors. An understanding of problems of sleep and the relationship of sleep to health and disease is an important part of any clinician's armamentarium.

REFERENCES

1. Rechtschaffen A, Kales A: A Manual of Standardized Terminology. Techniques and Scoring System for Sleep Stages of Human Subjects. U.S. Dept. of HEW, Public Health Service Publication No. 204, 1968
2. Aserinsky E, Kleitman N: Two types of occular motility occurring in sleep. J Appl Physiol 8:1–10, 1955
3. Wolman BB (ed): Handbook of Dreams: Research Theories and Applications. New York, Van Nostrand Reinhold Co., 1979
4. Feinberg I: Effects of age on human sleep patterns, in Kales A (ed): Sleep: Physiology and Pathology, A Symposium. Philadelphia, JB Lippincott, 1969
5. Hobson JA, McCarley RW: The brain as a dream state generator: An activation–synthesis hypothesis of the dream process. Am J Psychiatry 134:1335–1348, 1977

6. Kavey NB, Altschuler KZ: Sleep in Herniorrhaphy Patients. Am J Surg 138:682–687, 1979
7. Kavey NB, Altschuler KZ: Sleep patterns of surgical intensive care unit patients, in Chase MH, Kripke DF, Walter PL (eds): Sleep Research, Vol. 9. Los Angeles, University of California Brain Research Institute, 1980.
8. Hauri P: Insomnia and other sleep disorders, in Kagan F, Harwood T, Rickels K, Rudzik AD, Sorer H (eds): Hypnotics—Methods of Development and Evaluation. New York, Spectrum Publications, 1975, pp 11–28
9. Sleeping Pills, Insomnia and Medical Practice. Washington, D.C., National Academy of Sciences, Institute of Medicine, 1979
10. Kales A, Bixler EO, Tan T, Scharf MB, Kales JD: Chronic hypnotic drug use. Ineffectiveness, drug-withdrawal, insomnia and dependence. J Am M A 227:513–517, 1974
11. Kay DC, Eisentein RB, Jasinski DR: Morphine effects on human REM state waking state and nonREM sleep. Psychopharmacologia 14:404–416, 1969
12. Kavey NB, Altshuler KZ, Woodward AC: The effects of meperidine on sleep in the clinical situation, in Chase MH, Kripke DF, Walker PL (eds): Sleep Research, Vol. 9. Los Angeles, University of California, Brain Research Insitute, 1980
13. Weitzman E, Czeisler C, Coleman R, Dement W, Richardson G, Pollack C: Delayed sleep phase syndrome: A biological rhythm disorder, in Chase, MH, Kripke DF, Walker PL (eds): Sleep Research, Vol. 8. Los Angeles, University of California, Brain Research Institute, 1979, p 221
14. Guilleminault C, Tilkian A, Dement WC: The sleep apnea syndromes. Annu Rev Med 27:465–484, 1976
15. Farmer WC, Glenn WWL, Gee JBC: Alveolar hypoventilation syndrome studies of ventilatory control in patients selected for diaphragm pacing. Am J Med 64:39–49, 1978
16. Yoss RE, Daly DD: Criteria for diagnosis of the narcoleptic syndrome. Mayo Clin Proc 32:320–328, 1957
17. Dement WC, Carskadon MA, Guilleminault C, Zarcone VP: Narcolepsy: Diagnosis and treatment. Primary Care 3:609–623, 1976
18. Broughton RJ: Sleep disorders: Disorders of arousal? Science 159: 1070–1078, 1968
19. Fisher C, Kahn E, Edwards A, Davis D: A pyschophysiological study of nightmares and night terrors: The suppression of stage 4 night terrors with diazepam. Arch Gen Psychiatry 28:252–259, 1973
20. Brebbia DR, Altschuler KZ: Stage related patterns and nightly trends of energy exchange during sleep, in Kline NS, Laska E, (eds): Computers and Electronic Devices in Psychiatry. New York, Grune & Stratton, 1968, pp 319–335
21. Kales A, Kales JD: Sleep disorders. Recent findings in the diagnoses and treatment of disturbed sleep. N Eng J Med 290:487–499. 1974
22. Orr WC: The Sleep EEG in Neurological Diagnoses Am J EEG Technology 15: 169–178, 1976
23. Bergamasco B, Bergamini L, Doriguzzi T, Fabiani D: EEG sleep patterns as a prognostic criterion in post-traumatic coma. Electroencephalogr Clin Neurophysiol 25:374–377, 1968

Michael R. Milano, M.D.
Arthur R. Jacobs, M.D.

15

The Management of the Surgical Patient

The fact that the patient's need for a physician who is trusted, strong, and competent is most intense when he or she faces surgery has led to romanticization of the surgeon as a heroic figure. The surgeon's training, however, focuses on technical concerns. And the psychological demands of the surgeon's craft require that surgeons distance themselves emotionally from their patients during the operation itself. They may, therefore, have neither the time, training, nor inclination to support your patient psychologically through the period of diagnosis, operation, and convalescence. Consequently, the referring physician must often fill a void in psychological management.

The referring physician therefore plays an important role in all phases of the surgical process: diagnosis, referral, hospitalization, and recovery. This chapter will discuss each stage sequentially. The referring physician will have major responsibility for the sequelae of surgery, since psychological convalescence occurs long after surgical healing is completed and the surgeon's involvement has significantly diminished. The referring physician, however, is best equipped to deal with this responsibility since he or she begins with an established understanding of the patient and already has the latter's trust.

DIAGNOSIS AND REFERRAL

The most helpful interventions are those that occur *before* the surgical event itself. Preparation for surgery begins as the family practitioner evaluates the patient, takes a history, and begins to think of surgical referral. Two issues of general significance should guide the physician's approach to preparing the patient for surgery: whether the surgery is major or minor, and whether it will enhance or diminish the patient's quality of life. In addition, the physician must assess each patient, focusing on a number of specific topics, including patients' fears, their familiarity and past experience with surgical procedures and hospitalization, and the support available to them from family and friends.

Major or Minor Surgery

In general, major operations tax the patient's adaptive resources more deeply, and the referring family practitioner can prepare himself to provide more support for a patient undergoing an abdominoperineal resection than for someone anticipating a a cholecystectomy. However, vulnerable adults may have profound reactions even to minor surgery. For children, minor surgery is often fraught with fears of injury and separation from parents. In elderly patients, fears of physical deterioration, helplessness, or death may be reinforced by any anticipated surgery. An elderly patient with a mild organic brain syndrome may do well at home but become quite delirious or confused immediately postoperatively. Consequently, the seriousness of the anticipated surgery is only an inexact a priori guide to the patient's need for support.

Enhancement versus Diminishment

Much surgery is elective and leaves the patient less symptomatic and feeling better. Such procedures as elective hysterectomies for menorrhagia, cholecystectomies, and hernia repairs soon leave the patient feeling improved. This gain is a potent antidote to psychological distress, and fewer patients experiencing elective or curative surgery will be left with prolonged psychological disability. Psychological sequelae of depression and/or grief are more common when surgery results in a permanent deficit (e.g., amputation of a limb) or where it may uncover a fatal illness; the family practitioner faces new problems with these surgical patients.

Delay and Fears About the Diagnosis

A patient's reaction to the prospect of surgery begins when the symptom is first noted. The patient's response to that event can tell us a great deal about his or her future behavior. Some patients do not delay seeking medical advice because they are practical, scientifically oriented, and have a trusting, established relationship with their family practitioner.

Such patients usually cope with illness and surgery well. The anxious, hypochondriacal, or guilty patient who sees illness as punishment may or may not delay. But those patients who do put off seeking medical attention usually are using the mental mechanisms of avoidance and/or denial, and problems in the psychological adaptation to surgery are likely to follow.

Great tact and delicacy are required to explore the reasons for delay in seeking medical diagnosis or treatment. The anxious patient, guilty about his or her delay and fearing the worst, will be devastated by an accusatory, "Why did you wait so long?" The question, "Are you concerned that the surgery might discover a cancer?" may elicit anxiety and tears, but it paves the way for a more open and cooperative approach to referral and surgery. It provides an opportunity to deal with the patient's fears about the implications of surgery. Patients deny or delay because they fear "the worst." Usually a relatively positive outlook will be needed to keep the patient's anxiety from reaching panic levels. For example, a statement can be made about the effectiveness of modern cancer treatments, "Should that be the diagnosis." A failure to emphasize the hopeful aspects may drive the patient back to more avoidance and make cooperation with future treatment unlikely.

The patient's fears of the diagnosis should be discussed before the referral for surgery is made. Improper handling of the patient's fear of the diagnosis is probably the first and foremost cause of difficulty in surgical referrals and in many medical treatments. Failure to deal with it preoperatively can leave the physician with threatening information gained during surgery, but without any idea of how his or her patient can best handle such information.

Should the patient be told "the truth?" Information about how a patient will react to the discovery of a malignancy should be gained in the initial visit before referral. The patient with rectal bleeding and a suspicious rectal mass can be told, "You will probably need surgery to determine the cause of the bleeding. It could be a polyp or a diverticulum, and I guess you've even considered that it could be a cancer." It is safe to assume that all patients have considered the possibility of cancer. Using the term in a matter of fact way can be reassuring. This use of the word *cancer* is a trial balloon technique that allows you to evaluate your patient's emotional response to the potential diagnosis. Does he or she calmly ask for information? blanch but say nothing? burst into tears? The patient who responds with pessimistic anticipation can be reassured that you were merely reviewing all the possibilities as completely as possible and told that even if a cancer is found, modern treatment techniques are quite effective. This trial balloon technique can thus begin to provide you with the information you will need to help you determine what to tell your patient and at what time. A preoperative discussion of possible diagnoses also allows the family physician to deal with patients who mistakenly believe that they have cancer when they do not.

A 45-year-old Spanish-speaking male cried when visited by his family practitioner one week after surgery. Upon exploration of his feelings he stated that he interpreted a T tube and drain left in place after a cholecystectomy and common duct exploration as evidence that "something worse" was found. Of course, the "something worse" that he was responding to was his preoperative fear of cancer. Reassurance dispelled the anxiety he had been unable to communicate to his surgeon. Unsophisticated patients or those with cancer-phobia are prone to interpret drains, postoperative abcesses, and the like as evidence of cancer. This topic must be explored if the patient's fears are to be uncovered and dispelled.

Specific Fears of Surgery and Anesthesia

After the patient has been told of the need for surgical referral, common specific fears should be discussed.[1] These fears are usually related to individual personality traits or prior experiences with surgery and may be present regardless of the nature of the prospective surgery. Consequently, they can be explored prior to the patient's knowledge of specific details of the planned surgery and the patient's meeting with the surgeon. The first of these fears is that of surgery itself, the fear of "being cut." Patients with an especially intense fear of the surgical process frequently have a clear visual picture of the cutting, which is tinged with phobic anxiety. Nightmares about surgery, about "fingers being cut off," etc., are common even before any experiences with surgery. Such a patient may have had surgery in childhood.

Reassurance that these anxieties are normal often helps diminish them. The patient is better able to mobilize defenses for perceived dangers if such dangers are specifically discussed. Discussion leads to a more comfortable and actively cooperative patient and diminishes the likelihood of postoperative anxiety reactions. The following example describes the management of fears of surgery and the manner in which direct exploration modified the patient's acceptance of her illness.

A suburban housewife and diabetic in her mid 40s was admitted after a bunion that she had trimmed herself became severely infected. The possibility of amputation of her toe was discussed. As the surgeon left the room she began shaking, developed palpitations, dizziness, and a sense of impending doom—a full-scale anxiety attack. She demanded her clothing so she could go home. On inquiry about fear of being cut she stated, "I just can't stand the thought of their cutting the toe!" She continued that once the toe went, it would be the foot, the knee, then the whole leg would be whittled away. The question about "fears of being cut" led to the knowledge that the patient had a powerful visual image of surgery and falsely pessimistic anticipation of the outcome. Verbalization of these concerns, reassurance regarding her prognosis, and provision of a minor tranquilizer (benzodiazepine) allowed her to accept further treatment.

The second specific fear associated with surgery is that of anesthesia, which patients may describe as "being afraid of going to sleep" or "being afraid of being paralyzed." Some patients have very specific and understandable fears: for example, the patient with pulmonary disease may fear that anesthesia will trigger an asthmatic attack. However, for most patients the fear is based on what they *imagine* anesthesia to be. They may describe prior childhood experiences with anesthesia. They may have heard legends about being held down and overwhelmed. They may fear what they will do if they "lose control." Exploration of the specific fears can lead to specific reassurance. It is not necessary for the physician to be able to "do something" to remove such fears. For the patient the mere act of talking about such fears is the beginning of mastery. A preoperative visit from the anesthesiologist can also help change the experience from an anticipation of impersonal assault to one of friendly "going to sleep."

Previous Surgery

Before completing the referral process, the family practitioner should be able to answer several other key questions: (1) Has there been previous surgery? (2) What was the experience like? (3) Were there management problems with the surgeon or staff? (4) Were there postoperative psychological complications?

The patient's emotional response to surgery is usually determined by a stable set of psychological mechanisms. Consequently, the single best predictor of a benign postoperative emotional course is a history of having successfully negotiated a previous surgical experience. Previous encounters with postoperative complications may have left residual fears that must be discussed. Management problems are likely to occur again. It is easy to gather this data while doing the routine history of previous surgery.

A 35-year-old married woman was referred to a general surgeon for drainage of a pelvic abscess and excision of a perirectal fistula. Four years before she had had fulminant regional enteritis during her first pregnancy, necessitating a successful Caesarian section and a temporary ileostomy after bowel perforation and peritonitis. There had been numerous postoperative infections and the patient, a severely hypochondriacal woman, had needed psychiatric support and medication.

After seeming to accept referral for the currently planned minor surgery and seeing the surgeon, she returned to her family practitioner to report that all her prior fears of death had returned. Dreading the worst, she freely stated that she was too anxious to hear anything the surgeon had said to her. Only a second careful explanation by her family practitioner reassured her that this truly was a minor procedure with a low risk of complications. Her family practitioner offered to see her daily throughout her hospital course and offered her benzodiazepines to help blunt anxieties arising from her hypochondriacal fears about her body. She managed the later operation with little psychological or physical distress, and without medication.

Friends' or Relatives' Experience with the Same or Similar Surgery

Often the family practitioner will know from previous contact with the entire family whether the patient has relatives or friends who had the surgery he or she anticipates. This information is of special importance when the patient has lost a parent or sibling to a surgical illness during the patient's childhood. Frightening distortions, feelings of guilt, and fears of certain doom may persist, and the patient should be reassured that his or her case is different. Reassurance and stressing the increased effectiveness of new treatment techniques is essential. Since the fear stems from the patient's psychological identification with the victim as well as from realistic concerns, reassurances that the patient's case is not the same may help ameliorate the patient's anxiety but may not remove it. Continued support will be necessary, for the basic psychological identification with the victim will remain intact.

Previous Psychiatric History

Anxiety Symptoms

A history of anxiety symptoms per se is of less importance than anxiety focused specifically on anticipated damage to the patient's body. For example, the woman discussed earlier who needed surgery for an abscess and fistula had numerous fears about her body that antedated her first surgery. Fundamentally, she had "learned" her hypochondriasis from her mother. Where a patient's anxieties have always been focused on his or her body, considerable support and reassurance may be necessary. Minor tranquilizers and psychiatric consultation may be useful if the patient's distress is marked. Previous anxieties in other areas, like work or social acceptance, bear little relationship to the patient's psychological response to surgery.

Depressive Symptoms

The severely depressed patient may be a higher risk for death in the postoperative period.[2] In addition to exhibiting the physiological changes that accompany depression, such patients may be unwilling to cooperate in important postoperative tasks like coughing or may refuse to eat, threatening their metabolic nutritional status. Therefore, when surgery is elective, it should be deferred until a trial of psychotherapy and/or antidepressant medications alleviates the patient's depression. The chronically unhappy patient does not represent the same degree of risk for postoperative morbidity. (See Chapter 6 for help in the differential diagnosis of depression versus unhappiness).

Psychosis

For patients with a history of a previous psychotic break, there is no reason to assume that surgery itself will precipitate a psychosis. It is only when prior psychopathology has focused on body image, fears of physical damage, or unrealistic perceptions of the body, that preoperative psychiatric consultation is advised. For the acutely psychotic patient it is, of course, important to entertain the possibility of a medical cause of the psychosis. If possible, surgery should be delayed until the psychosis has been adequately treated. If there is little time for delay, a rapid antipsychotic regimen should be instituted. (See Chapter 7 for treatment details.)

Organic Mental Symptoms

The patient with a preexisting mild organic mental syndrome is prone to postoperative delirium (discussed later in this chapter). When such a patient is anxious or confused preoperatively, small doses of antipsychotic medication (for example, haloperidol 0.5 mg bid) should be instituted immediately. (See Chapter 7 regarding management of psychosis with organic brain syndrome.)

Pre-Operative Use of Psychiatric Medications

The family practitioner is frequently faced with the problem of referring patients on psychoactive medication for surgery. He may need to weigh the psychiatric consequences of discontinuing medication against the effects of such medication on other agents used for anesthesia. Phenothiazines can potentiate sleep time under anesthesia and narcotic effects post-operatively. The phenothiazines also produce relative alpha adrenergic blockade. Therefore, the use of an agent like epinephrine to treat hypotension would produce a paradoxical fall in pressure. However, phenylephrine (Neosynephrine) or Levarterenol (Levophed) can be safely used. The tricyclic antidepressants may potentiate the central depressant effect of some anesthetic agents; they do produce orthostatic hypotension and prolong cardiac conduction, and may potentiate the pressor effects of sympathomimetic amines. However, these effects can be dealt with by the anesthesiologist if he knows that the patient is taking such drugs.[3] There is, therefore, no need to cancel these antipsychotic or antidepressant agents prior to surgery, providing the anesthesiologist is made aware of their presence.

Monamine oxidase inhibitors, however, are known for their proclivity to produce hypertension in combination with sympathomimetics, and may also produce paroxysmal hypertension and/or coma in response to barbiturates or meperidine. MAO inhibitors should therefore be discontinued for 2 weeks prior to elective surgery. Lithium potentiates the action of muscle relaxants but need not be discontinued prior to surgery.

Support of Spouse or Family

The family practitioner may well know beforehand whether a supportive spouse and family are available. He is in a position to make crucial interventions based on this knowledge and on his or her previous relationship with both the patient and spouse. It is best to include the spouse in decisions about surgery from the time when a diagnosis has been tentatively established. This maximizes the availability of support systems for the patient.

From the very beginning some families may try to define the nature of the doctor–patient relationship according to the needs of the family rather than those of the patient. For example, the family that is involved and eager to help but uses denial as a prominent defense against fears of death can produce devastating consequences for the patient.

> The husband of a 48-year-old married woman convinced her surgeon of the need to keep the diagnosis from the patient. She had a necrotic metastatic lesion of her leg and after 2 weeks of hospitalization was panicked about the chemotherapy that had been recommended and instituted without any explanation. She would constantly ask nurses and house staff, "What's wrong with me?"
>
> The physician was finally able to help the husband understand how much his wife was suffering from not being told the truth. He was helped to understand that this policy had isolated her and had actually made it impossible for her to receive the emotional support of friends, family and doctors. The husband, therefore, agreed to allow his wife to be told the true nature of her problem. She responded quite well and was then better able to cope with her illness and the need for chemotherapy. It also allowed family and friends to be more supportive since they were no longer feeling the pressures of having to keep a secret.

In situations like the foregoing, the practitioner will have to provide considerable support to the spouse to help with *his or her* fears of surgery or cancer. It is these fears that have been projected onto the patient, who is then described as unable to accept the diagnosis. The spouse will not be able to help the patient without considerable help for himself or herself.

The tendency of physicians to be more frank in dealing with relatives than with patients bears closer scrutiny. There is no a priori reason to assume the relative is better able to deal with the more pessimistic news than the patient is. Moreover, the technique of hiding information from the patient rarely works, since the spouse cannot usually maintain the necessary facade. Consequently, the patient ultimately gets the message in a manner which suggests that it is news too terrible to share with him or her. It also implies that the patient cannot trust his or her physician. If the decision is made to withhold information from the patient it is usually best to treat the spouse the same way. No law requires us to do otherwise.

Under all circumstances it is important to continue to follow the lead of the patient rather than of the family. Eliciting patients' concerns about their diagnoses and recommended surgery preoperatively allows them to say, "Doctor, I don't want to know what's wrong. I only want you to take care of me." They may say this openly or they may indicate it covertly, by asking the physician to talk first with relatives. The patient may later change his or her mind and want to be more actively involved in treatment decisions.

OBTAINING INFORMED CONSENT

When the practitioner has informed the patient of the need for surgical consultation and has explored fears about the diagnosis, about being operated upon, and about anesthesia, he or she will have laid the groundwork for obtaining informed consent. This crucial detail is often relegated to the last minute, where both the physician and patient may feel pressured, therefore these earlier discussions will probably be more effective in truly informing the patient.

Securing informed consent need not require a detailed listing of every possible surgical complication. Most state laws require that the patient be given that information which is "reasonable" in helping him to accept the need for surgery. The majority of states define "reasonable" as that information which a "reasonable practitioner" in a similar community and of the same school of medical thought would have disclosed to his or her patient regarding the proposed treatment. The minority of states require the disclosure of that information which a "reasonable man" in the situation would deem significant in making a decision regarding treatment. In recent years, the "reasonable practitioner" statutes have been strengthened. The doctrine of "therapeutic privilege" also states that it is the physician's right and/or obligation to withhold information when he or she considers it to be in the best interests of the patient.[4] Indeed, "overinforming" the patient about every possible complication, or even obtaining consent on a form that details numerous possible complications, will not prevent lawsuits founded upon alleged lack of informed consent. However, the "list every possible complication" approach may stir up unnecessary anxiety and lead to avoidance of needed surgery. The patient needs to be provided with a reasonable amount of information, accompanied, where possible, with an attitude of realistic optimism. By systematically exploring the patient's capacity to cope with surgery, the practitioner sets in motion the process of coping. The later request for "informed consent" will be less likely to shock the patient.

The informed consent document is considered an important part of a surgeon's defense against malpractice suits. Obviously, most malpractice suits have at their core an untoward surgical result rather than a lack of information. The important variables are the manner in which the patient and the surgeon handle the adversity of postoperative complications. The patient who handles information comfortably and understands the need for surgery will remain cooperative when informed of complications and will cope with that adversity in the same way that he or she handled the need for surgery. "I always spend more time with patients who have postoperative complications," stated one surgeon, "and they are usually understanding of their setback and of me. In fact, they send me more referrals than patients who do well." Physicians who perceive their patients' need for support and who provide continued information are less likely to be sued than those who, out of fear or guilt, avoid their patients.

PREOPERATIVE PREPARATION

After the patient has been admitted to the hospital, the referring physician must make at least one preoperative visit. The procedure may need to be reexplained, for the highly anxious patient may retain little of the information given at the time of diagnosis. Indeed, the patient's capacity to retain information should be specifically monitored and is a useful gauge of his anxiety. Diagnostic procedures should be described and discussed and the patient should be given some idea of when they will be performed. Next, the patient should be informed of the time of his or her operation.

At this time the patient should be told about the sedative he or she will be given before leaving for the operating room, the method of anesthesia to be used, and the recovery room experience. Patients are often relieved to know that they will not be wide awake when wheeled into the operating room. For patients undergoing open heart procedures, emphasizing the supportive aspects of the surgical intensive care unit and recovery room and the presence of skilled nursing personnel may be expanded by a preoperative visit by a recovery room nurse. The more specifically reassurance is tailored to the source of the patient's anxiety, the better the result, e.g., patients with a history of respiratory disorders may be particularly anxious about anesthesia. As noted earlier, anxiety about anesthesia may also relate to deeper fears of separation, loss of control, or death and can almost always be dealt with by allowing for ventilation, followed by reassurance.

Patients in the immediate preoperative phase "worry"; that is, they have repetitive anxious thoughts about the immediate future. Janis has described the "work of worrying" as a necessary and helpful stage in preoperative preparation.[5] Such preparation helps the patient to face surgery with calm and preparedness. Patients whose questions are factual and pragmatic or scientific ("Will I have to eat small meals after my ulcer operation?") benefit most from being given specific information. They usually handle surgical stress well. Their worries tend to peak at the time of admission and immediately preoperatively, and they feel better soon after surgery. However, two disturbances of the process of worrying are commonly seen in surgical patients: anxious overquestioning and denial of need for support.

The Anxious Overquestioner

These patients are tense, feel helpless and overwhelmed, and express their neediness in an endless barrage of questions that often have little relevance to surgery. Plaintive and clinging, they follow each set of answers with more questions and fears, and focus on every possible complication. Patients' fears and concerns about dependency may be expressed about themselves, or they may be displaced onto others. Patients may appear personally unconcerned because they have displaced their fears of surgery and helplessness onto concerns for their children, spouses, parents, or businesses. Often the family practitioner is familiar with such patterns from prior medical treatment.

Anxious overquestioners cope with fear with requests for overprotection. Overprotection for them frequently is accepted as a basic mode of relatedness rather than as a disturbance. They frequently have had overprotected childhoods that they accept as normal. They overprotect spouses and children, and they do not see their innumerable anxious questions and pleas for reassurance as unreasonable.

Needless to say, such patients have the potential to stir resentment in medical and surgical staff. Their anxiety is contagious and unpleasant. The surgeon sees no positive "result" from each reassurance. Each question answered is followed by another, and the surgeon does not see the patient getting "better," that is, more independent and reassured. In fact, the patient has little immediate interest in becoming more independent. The nursing staff is plagued with requests for attention. Often the staff feel such frustration, irritation, and helplessness that they begin avoiding the patient.

Instead of allowing this course to unfold, the practitioner must begin to organize the patient's coping behavior early in the preoperative care. He or she may be the only person willing to deal with such a patient. Patients should be encouraged to worry about appropriate rather than inappropriate concerns. They should be encouraged to prepare a limited number of questions in advance of each visit. This emphasizes active coping and learning and puts limits on endless pleading questions. The emphasis is kept on active coping and patients are encouraged to do things for themselves throughout the hospitalization. They can be encouraged to practice coughing and deep breathing preoperatively. They may be told that they can expect a brief postoperative period of depression and that they should begin thinking of ways to cope with it. Minor tranquilizers may be useful and may decrease the need for analgesics.

> A very tense middle-aged housewife was seen prior to gall bladder surgery. She had been addicted to minor tranquilizers, necessitating detoxification several months before. She had many worries and fears about her surgery and, in addition, focused on worries about managing her family's impending move to a new home. She was told to leave this worry to her husband and children and to concern herself with preparing for surgery and the postoperative course. The procedure and postoperative pain were clearly discussed. She was told to practice coughing and to prepare for the possibility of a postoperative depression. She was seen daily and encouraged to prepare "two questions a day" for her surgeon. Small amounts of minor tranquilizers were permitted when she felt "very nervous." She remained tense but did well, was discharged on schedule, and at follow-up was living in her new home and preparing to resume full activities.

The family practitioner in this case stepped in to guide the patient's preoperative and postoperative course successfully. He was aware of the potential conflict between a surgical staff who wanted the patient to be independent and a patient who coped in a different fashion. He did not try to stop the overworrying entirely, but instead helped the patient to focus on coping rather than on helplessness.

The Anti-worrier

At the other extreme are the patients who appear to experience no anxiety. They may jocularly greet their doctor and ask them about their golf games or engage them with irrelevant questions. They may be preoccupied with business affairs or talk about other areas of their lives over which they feel in greater control. Male patients of this type commonly make sexual innuendos in conversation with staff nurses, and the family practitioner will often be familiar with patterns of noncompliance with previous medical recommendations. The patient who professes such unconcern preoperatively may in the immediate postoperative period display great helplessness and/or falsely accuse his or her physicians and nurses of poor care and faulty preoperative preparation. This change usually occurs with the emergence of the feared "weakness" produced by the surgical procedure. The patient seeks to compensate by trying to gain control of the medical staff. The criticism is one way of achieving this.

Preoperatively, these patients should be given permission to worry. "Everyone experiences some worries about surgery" offers the patient an opportunity to begin self-preparation. A study of cardiac surgery patients showed that patients who were interviewed preoperatively suffered a lowered incidence of postoperative delirium than those not interviewed.[6] Notable, however, is the proclivity of the anti-worrier to deny his need for support or preparation. Most commonly, the best attempts at preparation do not forestall the patient's postoperative distress nor do they spare the physician or nurses from unjust criticism.

> A 50-year-old truck driver was hospitalized with rectal bleeding. He was informed of the need for an abdominoperineal resection and apprised of the possible consequences. At no point did he express fear about cancer, the surgery, or colostomy to either the family practitioner or the surgeon. He spoke only of his recent sexual adventures, his power in the trucking business and his close ties to the underworld. When surgery was mentioned he brushed it off with "Doc, I know you're a wizard. I'm not worried about a thing." Postoperatively, he became extremely anxious, cried frequently and criticized his doctors and nurses for not telling him how much pain there would be. For weeks he refused to care for his colostomy. Throughout the hospital course he resolutely denied any concern about the surgery terminating his sexual potency. Only after several stormy weeks; when physical recovery was near completion, did his distress diminish.

Dealing with such patients preoperatively and postoperatively requires a large measure of good grace on the part of the family practitioner.

The best preparation frequently accomplishes little in altering the patient's perception of surgery or his or her response to it. Postoperatively, gratitude is rare but criticism, demands, and scorn are in abundance. At the very least, comprehension of this coping pattern helps the family practitioner (and the surgeon) avoid "taking it personally."

POSTOPERATIVE MANAGEMENT

For uncomplicated patients who are coping adequately, the most neglected time of need may be the immediate postoperative period. Adequate preparation for this time is essential. Patients should be told specifically about the type of pain they will experience and should be assured that pain medication will be available. They should be told of the need to cough and breathe deeply postoperatively after general anesthesia and of the need to ambulate with help as soon as practical. Patients who were given specific instructions regarding what kind of pain to expect and what they could do to relieve it (e.g., how to get about in bed) required significantly less pain medication and were discharged several days earlier than those who were not.[7] The more carefully postoperative instructions are built about patients' active participation in the recovery process, the more their psychological and physical recovery will be facilitated.

The family practitioner who scrubs on operations may be able to visit his or her patient in the recovery room. Such a visit may be quite important. Many patients, especially women who have had one-stage mastectomies, describe the shock of learning of their diagnosis by self-examination in the recovery room. Patients who have been semiconscious during surgery may be irritable, anxious, and show signs of recent psychic trauma. Manzer et al. state that those posthysterectomy patients who showed childlike, demanding, and uncooperative behavior in the recovery room went on to a poor psychological acceptance of their surgery.[8] A brief visit in the recovery room may be highly supportive. Keep in mind that apparently stuporous patients in the recovery room (and even in the operating room) have been able to recall much of what has been said around them.[9]

Undermedication for pain is a common error. The physician's fears of addicting his or her patient can play too great a role in management. (This subject is discussed in more detail in Chapter 16 on the management of pain.)

The patient who has undergone surgery and is awaiting the results of a biopsy is under great stress. These patients observe other patients with successful surgery leave, while they grapple with the fear of cancer. Sometimes three to five days or longer may elapse before a definitive tissue diagnosis and node count is available. For the doctor not much is happening, but patients regularly report this as a time of peak psychological stress. Brief visits to the patient should continue through this period to prevent the development of feelings of abandonment or despair and to prepare the patient for the probable outcome and the next stages in treatment.

Continuity of care is essential during the postoperative period, and here the primary practitioner can play a crucial role. Of course, there are occasions when vacations or brief trips remove the physician from contact with the patient. The patient should be prepared for this several days beforehand and personally introduced to the covering physician. More commonly, the patient's sense of abandonment may come from the natural letdown in attention in the convalescent stage of successful surgery. Unique circumstances may heighten this feeling of abandonment. The classic example is the kidney donor who, preoperatively, is the center of his family's and physician's attention. Postoperatively he or she is relatively neglected as attention shifts to the organ recipient and focuses on whether the transplant will survive. Donor patients often feel forgotten, and they may become embittered and regret having made the sacrifice.[10] A few brief postoperative visits and direct discussion of the issue can prevent this.

It is in the postoperative period that the physician also is faced with decisions about "telling the truth" to a patient with metastatic cancer or some other illness with a bad prognosis. Such a decision is not the sole prerogative of the surgeon, and most commonly family practitioners will be in the best position to decide how to deal with their patients. They will know how their patients have responded to past illness and to past misfortunes. They will have raised the possibility of cancer in their prereferral discussions. They will know the family of their patients. In short, their patients will have had prior opportunity to inform these practitioners about how to handle a discussion of such an illness. This information should be shared with the surgeon to facilitate the patient's management. This issue is discussed in greater detail in Chapter 17, on the Management of the cancer patient.

Despite the best psychological attention, some patients will show significant psychological disability after surgery. Titchener, et al. found that 15 percent of 200 surgical patients worsened psychologically despite successful surgery.[11] Two clinical phenomena appear to be predictive of long-term psychological difficulties. First, when the physician notes the appearance of new anxiety postoperatively, coupled with a forced change in the patient's style of coping, difficulty may be anticipated. The case example of the truck driver with a colostomy typifies the switch from a jocular, devil-may-care attitude to a fearful, helpless, but intensely critical mode of coping. This patient was able to resume his prior psychological coping patterns when he had recovered physically. Psychiatric intervention would have been necessary had his coping defenses remained shattered after he recovered physically. Fortunately, this man was able to resume an action-oriented, masculine role as a truck driver and this compensated for his loss of sexual potency. Had his surgical illness required that he assume a desk job, then psychological rehabilitation might have required construction of an entirely new system of self-esteem.

The second phenomenon predictive of long-term psychiatric consequences is the patient's experiencing surgery as a punishment. Postoperative guilt is a strong feature of such a patient's course. Such patients ask, "Why me? What did I do?" They worry about rejection by spouses and children and see their future grimly. They constantly expect the worst. Linking such negative anticipations to repressed guilt may require psychodynamic exploration which may be difficult for the family physician unless he is aware of the link between guilt and the expectation of punishment. For these patients pain and suffering are evidence of prior wrongdoing. Where such guilt-laden ideas dominate the patient's response to surgery, referral for psychiatric help can be useful in helping the patient deal with the psychological aftermath of the surgery.

> A 50-year-old woman responded to a mastectomy with profound and immediate unhappiness. In the days after surgery she ruminated about why this had happened to her and anticipated death from cancer despite reassurance that cure was aloost certain. She confided in her family physician that she still felt doomed and depressed. Further discussion of her problems revealed that her mother had had breast cancer and had recently been placed in a nursing home for a severe chronic dementia. The patient had always cared for her mother, and had felt extremely guilty about not being able to continue to care for her. They had always been the "perfect" mother and daughter. She strongly denied resentment toward her mother, though these feelings were apparent to her doctors. In retrospect she could see that her guilt and some depression had been present even before the discovery of cancer. The patient herself wanted psychiatric referral. Brief therapy and antidepressants markedly altered her adaptation to surgery and within months her usual optimism and vigor had returned.

POSTOPERATIVE DEPRESSION

Frequently, a psychiatric consultant will be asked to see a "depressed" or crying postoperative patient. The postoperative patient who cries deserves careful diagnostic attention. However, true endogenous depression or schizophrenia are rare postoperatively.[12] Let us look at three possibilities that the physician must consider in evaluating patients who cry in the immediate postoperative period.

First, patients may be temporarily overwhelmed by grief concerning their diagnosis or anxious about their eventual recovery. Such patients freely discuss the intensity of their psychological distress and correlate it with concerns about their medical condition. Most commonly, these patients will have coped with life well and will have a successful prior adaptation. They have handled past illness satisfactorily and just want to be well and to return to their prior lives. Issues of guilt or blame will be minimal, and their concerns will be oriented toward the future rather than the past. Patients need to talk about these concerns. Support and reassurance are readily accepted. Questions about the tearfulness should be followed by hopeful reassurance about the potential for treatment and a return to normal life activities. Do not make the mistake of ordering an antidepressant when the patient really simply needs to talk over his or her concerns.

Second, patients may be responding to anxiety or guilt that they were unable to express preoperatively. These patients are less able to relate their distress directly to their ongoing surgical illness. Patients may be anxious about having to change their life style and may be experiencing collapse of their customary coping mechanism. Guilty preoccupations may be emerging and an unrealistically pessimistic view of the future may underlie their tears. Such patients should be followed closely. They may develop the symptoms of major depressive disorder and require antidepressant treatment. However, more complex problems which antedated the surgery may be emerging. Psychiatric consultation may be required to develop a treatment plan.

Third, patients may be suffering from an acute delirium in which crying is a manifestation of the emotional lability characteristic of an organic brain syndrome. Postoperative delirium frequently manifests itself in tearfulness that may be spontaneous or may be expressed in loud, persistent shouts about pain. In both cases the patient's confusion is the real problem. The patient's fear is a response to his or her inability to comprehend the situation. If the difficulty is misdiagnosed, the physician may choose inappropriate therapies. Antidepressant medication may exacerbate the patient's delirium, and long, detailed explanations of the patient's condition may further increase his confusion.

PSYCHOLOGICAL APPROACHES TO SPECIFIC TYPES OF SURGERY

Mastectomy

At the time of the initial visit to her family practitioner, the woman with a breast lump is obviously highly anxious. In the diagnostic session the groundwork is laid for assessing and mobilizing the patient's adaptive strengths as well as planning the future surgical course. In gathering the history of discovery of the lump, the following questions should be asked: When was the lump first noticed and by whom? Was there a delay? Are there specific fears and anxieties? What are they? Was the patient fearful that cancer would be discovered?

The experienced practitioner can usually make a good estimate of the likelihood of malignancy based on the history and physical examination. The possibility of cancer should therefore be stated to the patient and her response observed. The patient should be encouraged to ask questions either immediately or during her first appointment with the surgeon.

Some women will immediately ask about the type of surgical procedure they may need. The family practitioner and the surgeon can both provide a full explanation of the alternatives. A consistent and informative approach will usually gain the patient's trust. Optimism is important. The patient should not fear that a diagnosis of cancer is an automatic death sentence. Eliciting specific fears of the surgery or anesthesia will help prevent flight or denial. Some women will need time to allay their fears and uncertainties and may seek a second opinion.

It is essential to involve the spouse early in the process leading to surgery.[13] Women who are insecure regarding their sexuality may project their concerns onto their spouses and erroneously anticipate that they will reject them. Spouses should be alerted to this concern and encouraged to be reassuring from the start. Unpartnered women or women with rocky marital or sexual relationships may feel especially threatened by this illness and the loss of a breast. Women with young children are most poignantly concerned with the fear of death and with concerns about their children. The family practitioner who is aware of these needs and able to listen to his patients' differing concerns will help them to continue to cope with life by reassuring them and encouraging them to plan for the future. The usual patient's primary concern will be with cure and longevity and only secondarily with her appearance.

The women most typically at risk for the psychological consequences of diminished self-esteem are not necessarily the young or the unpartnered, but rather those whose sexual pride and feelings of attractiveness are closely and specifically tied to their breasts.[14] The woman who is proud of large breasts or ashamed of small breasts is more affected by the thought of losing a breast than the woman whose pride focuses on her children, her job, her face, or other unaffected attributes. Sensitivity to this issue and specific attention to these consequences of mastectomy may be a critical issue in the patient's acceptance of surgery.

A 33-year-old unmarried woman had delayed surgery for about four months. She was seen after refusing a radical mastectomy. In the interview, she revealed that all the women in her family were "well-endowed." During adolescence she had always been relatively flatchested and was teased by her family. With each pregnancy her breast size had increased and she had begun to feel she was beginning to match her sisters both physically and emotionally. To her dismay, the doctor was telling her she would have to give up her breast. To this woman, it meant the loss of her hard-won struggle for status in the family system. Eliciting and discussing these fears allowed her to put some of these issues in better perspective. The process of bringing such concerns to consciousness and discussing them objectively can often diminish their power. This patient was able to agree to have a subtotal mastectomy. Patients of this kind may be interested in breast reconstruction and can be informed of this possibility. It can make the prospect of mastectomy more tolerable. Ultimately only a small percentage of patients will have the procedure done.

It is not uncommon today for informed patients to have specific requests for staged surgery, for partial mastectomy, or for treatment other than mastectomy. These requests are not necessarily an index of distrust or noncompliance. The lay press is filled with articles about breast cancer, and patients often shop for opinions that meet their own emotional needs. In addition, there are valid differences of opinion about the best surgical options for specific breast cancers. Considerable flexibility and openness will be required to help your patient accept the best treatment plan. Adequate knowledge of the personal factors noted may be crucial.

After surgery, most patients worry intensely until the pathology report returns and their therapeutic course can be fully outlined. Here a few daily words of support are especially helpful. Otherwise, the patient feels abandoned at her time of greatest tension and uncertainty. Patients are more likely to turn to their family practitioner than to the surgeon during this time.

Shame is most evident in reluctance or refusal to view the scar or wound. The doctor should be alert to this reaction and deal with it directly. At some point, he may have to assist the patient in viewing the wound. Helping the patient to talk about her feelings beforehand will actually diminish their intensity. Shame may be pathological when the patient is unable to let herself and/or her husband see the wound months after surgery. The patient should be provided with information about prostheses and cosmetic surgery and told about the several existing self-help groups. Some groups, such as the American Cancer Society's Reach for Recovery, offer assistance to the postmastectomy woman only immediately after the surgery—generally while she is still in the hospital. Others, such as the New York metropolitan area's SHARE (Self Help Action and Rap Experience for Post Mastectomy Women), provide ongoing "rap" sessions that women can attend for weeks and months. An early active approach by the physician to these issues pays large dividends, for intense shame or guilt may prevent some women from asking appropriate questions and may lead to non-compliance with further treatment.

Even without adjuvant chemotherapy, the period of adjustment after mastectomy may last for up to a year. The most commonly described delayed postoperative psychological complications are sexual dysfunction and depression.[15] Since these are usually of late onset (6 months to 2 years after surgery), the family practitioner may be the physician in the best position to identify these problems. The pertinent information may come from the patient's spouse.

Sexual problems may arise from anxiety and concern in either the patient or her husband. Abandoning an active sexual life may stem from the general lethargy and loss of interest in life seen in depression. Appropriate treatment of the depression, as outlined in Chapter 6, should bring a return of sexual interest and activity. More commonly the patient simply does not adjust to the change in body image and the sense of diminished attractiveness. Jamison et al. describe both the mastectomy patient and the spouse as experiencing equivalent distress and report that rarely are spouses able to communicate with each other preoperatively.[16] Frequently, the patient, seeing herself as damaged, displaces her feelings onto her husband and feels or states, "He couldn't find me attractive anymore." Such couples don't discuss the problem and quietly allow their sex life to slip away. Including the spouse in early discussion about the need for surgery and encouraging communication counteracts these trends before they become ingrained. The question, "Do you think the operation will affect your marital life or sex life?" can be asked before the patient goes home. The expectation of rejection can then be dealt with openly with both husband and wife. A frank supportive talk with the spouse regarding his concerns about future sexual relations can also be very helpful. He can be told what his wife's chest will look like so that it does not come as a shock. He must be alerted to her special sensitivity to his reaction.

> A 58-year-old postmenopausal woman was seen on the fourth postoperative day after her second radical mastectomy. Anxiety and nightmares were a reflection of her previous hypochondriasis and feelings of guilt. They had been present after the first operation 5 years before. Ventilation and appropriate medication were helpful, but after return home the patient and her husband failed to resume their prior active sex life. The patient had been a buxom woman who viewed this as her major sexual asset. Both she and her husband described the importance of breasts in their sexual activity. They had had a restricted and highly conventional sexual life in other areas of foreplay and sexual interaction. They first experienced a period of grief for their lost sexual routine. With encouragement and advice from their physician, they were able to embark on new varieties of sexual experience and developed a new sense of pride in being experimental and open minded. They viewed this as compensation for their loss of the patient's breasts.

Therefore, for the family practitioner, the most important management time may be the months after surgery. But he can help his patient only if he inquires directly about her psychological and social progress. Has she resumed her work and her social and sexual life in a manner appropriate to her medical state? One year after mastectomy 80 percent of women do as well as before (assuming a probable cure).[17] If problems persist, then marital consultation, medication, and/or psychiatric referral should be considered.

Colostomy

The family practitioner with a patient facing a permanent ileostomy or colostomy will, of course, be aware of many of the same phenomena encountered in mastectomy patients. The patient loses a major organ, the rectum, and must confront the daily visual experience of a permanent ostomy. The patient must learn the skills of ostomy care and cope with both the illness and his or her feelings about his illness. Feelings of shame and humiliation about odor, spillage, appearance, and the like are commonplace. Fortunately, advances in appliances and surgical technique have lessened these problems, and postoperative instructions by ostomy nurses, the surgeon and/or the family practitioner can usually make the adaptive process successful. Unless there are serious surgical or psychological consequences, the technical aspects of ostomy care are usually trouble free. However, patients must be educated about these facts of ostomy care. If possible, the patient can be introduced to someone like themselves who has made a successful adjustment and can answer specific questions. A local ostomy club can provide volunteers.

The family practitioner should be aware, however, that the consequence of a permanent ostomy must be seen in the light of the patient's underlying illness. Patients with a permanent ileostomy after colectomy for ulcerative colitis are usually young people. Postoperatively their overall health is usually much improved, and this is a major positive factor in rehabilitation. They are better able to cope with the ostomy since surgery has given them relief from previously disabling illness. Delayed depressive reactions are rare, and an enhanced quality of life should be the norm.[18] The other large group of permanent colostomy patients are usually males undergoing abdominoperineal resections for rectal cancer. Here both the patient and family must cope with the issue of cancer and with advancing age. Although colostomy care is easier than ileostomy care, these patients do not experience the enhanced postoperative health of the colitis patient. Organic impotence also frequently follows dissection of the sacral plexus.[19] These factors complicate the postoperative adaptation of these patients. Depression, discouragement, and feelings of worthlessness are therefore frequently encountered.[20] Again, only the family practitioner may be available to pick up such symptoms postoperatively and to explore the problem with patient and spouse.

The patient prone to feelings of shame will most often anticipate rejection and social unacceptability as soon as the prospect of an ostomy is broached. The family practitioner can emphasize to such patients that improved ostomy techniques have made spillage, odor, and so on controllable problems. Postoperatively the patient must be given intensive practical guidance. Where this fails to reassure the patient, the sources of the feeling of shame can be directly explored in greater detail. Patients can be helped to review early life experiences which may have created this hypersensitivity. Psychiatric consultation may prove helpful.

> An 81-year-old woman adamantly refused to view her postoperative transverse colostomy and to begin self-care. She knew that she was cured of cancer, but was "too ashamed" of what she would look like. A few questions about other sources of shame revealed that she had been an adolescent bedwetter and had been humiliated by her siblings. The feeling of shame had lasted long after the bedwetting and teasing stopped, and she had never been willing to look at herself "down there." After discussing this, she was willing to be seen by her ostomy nurse and became proud of her eventual mastery of the ostomy.

It is important to recognize that openness in talking about shame is in itself an antidote to the inner message, "Keep it hidden. If they know, they'll reject you." Merely talking with another breaks the cycle of hiding the problem and feelings. In the above example, once the problem of shame was identified, the physician took a history of the specific feeling of shame. When the patient revealed the deeper historical roots of this feeling, the patient felt truly "understood" and was able to move forward. When the despair is found to be related to depression, rather than simple shame, treating the depression usually provides relief.

The patient with an abdominoperineal resection presents a number of special difficulties. Phantom rectal sensations may be puzzling and frightening. The patient should therefore be alerted to their possible occurrence and reassured that this is a normal postoperative phenomenon that will gradually disappear. The patient may experience profound shame, rage, or diminished self-esteem about his postoperative impotence. Therefore, it is important to discuss with the patient and spouse the possible use of manual and oral techniques of sexual stimulation and/or of penile prosthetic implants that simulate erection. The physician must take the initiative in discussing these issues. The patient will usually be grateful for the opportunity to express his feelings, and you will have a chance to make constructive suggestions. Chapter 9 discusses the management of such sexual problems in greater detail.

It is important to note that even the patient with a temporary colostomy may be seriously concerned about appliance care and may be obsessed about "being different" while the appliance is in use. The patient may not believe that the ostomy is temporary, and the basis for such mistrust must be explored. Careful education of the patient and attention to the cause of distress can almost always tide the patient over until reanastamosis is accomplished.

Hysterectomy

The management of the hysterectomy patient is discussed in detail in Chapter 4.[21, 22]

Amputation

Frequently the family practitioner is faced with an elderly patient undergoing amputation for vascular disease. There will have been a prior history of treatment for chronic peripheral vascular disease, with antecedent pain and loss of function of the limb. The elderly patient may not understand the procedure, and chronic memory disturbance may impede preparation for surgery. While amputation may relieve pain or be lifesaving, many patients respond with a profound sense of hopelessness and/or depression.[23] Prior chronic medical problems and unemployment seem to predict a poor medical and surgical course, with limited recovery. Such patients may have difficulty pursuing rehabilitation and may initially refuse surgery. Their sense of hopelessness should be countered by active rehabilitative efforts and, where true depression is present, the use of antidepressant drugs (see Chapter 6).

Over months or years of conservative treatment, many patients with vascular disease will have adjusted to the possibility of losing the limb. Indeed, relief of pain may leave the patient feeling better after amputation. Under these circumstances, intense responses of grief and loss are attentuated. A special note should be made of phantom pain. Phantom sensations are ubiquitous after limb amputation, and phantom sensations of breast and rectum may also be present after mastectomy or abdominoperineal resection. Patients should be asked about their presence since they are relieved to know these are normal. Persistent painful limb phantoms are uncommon, however, and are most often seen when a very painfully diseased extremity is amputated.[24] Frequently, it occurs when the patient is clinically depressed. Antidepressant medication may then be efficacious for both pain and depression (see Chapter 6). Unresolved grief reactions in highly perfectionistic patients who strongly prize their independence may also lead to the appearance of chronic phantom pain. Here psychotherapy should be considered. Some patients with persistent phantom pain have been closely identified with an amputee in early life. Others openly mourn the lost limb and will want to know how it was disposed of to complete the mourning process.[25]

A 68-year-old married woman experienced a series of amputations for vascular disease. Postoperatively, she complained of severe stump pain and was progressively less able to pursue rehabilitative measures. She had devoted several years to caring for a diabetic older sister (also a patient of the family practitioner) who had died several years before following an amputation. When questioned about missing her sister, the patient grimaced and immediately experienced acute spasms of leg pain. She saw little hope for herself. This woman was given small doses of antidepressants for several weeks and was actively encouraged to express her grief for her sister and for her own leg. Her pessimistic identification with her sister was challenged. Over a span of 2 weeks, she began to describe herself as "back to normal" and actively began to use her prosthesis.

Less frequently, the family practitioner will have to deal with patients whose amputations are due to trauma or cancer surgery. This group of patients is usually younger and they are losing a functioning, pain-free extremity. The trauma patient may also have a superimposed transient traumatic neurosis in the early postoperative days. Thus, the patient with an acute traumatic neurosis will be experiencing all of the problems of coping with surgery and, in addition, will be reliving the traumatic experience in nightmares and in repetitive daytime remembrances. This patient will be easily startled and overtly anxious. Ventilation is essential, and the patient should be reassured that these psychological symptoms are unavoidable and will decrease gradually over time. Benzodiazepines and hypnotics may be prescribed if anxiety is intense. (See Chapter 5 on the management of anxiety.)

Plastic Surgery

More patients request elective cosmetic surgery each year. The process often begins with a discussion with the family practitioner. Olley has delineated the necessary screening interview and the themes to be covered when evaluating a patient for elective plastic surgery:[26] (1) What is the nature of the cosmetic defect and what are the patient's feelings about it? (2) Why has the patient decided to seek surgery at this time? and (3) What type of anatomical change is desired by the patient?

Contraindications to surgery are as follows:

- The procedure is being requested mainly because of pressure by others and is not desired by the patient. Adolescents may be pressured by parents, and the physician must assess the motivation of the adolescent himself or herself. Similarly, an adolescent may have unrealistic expectations of what surgery can accomplish and may gain his or her parents' consent against their own best judgement.
- The patient can describe the "deformity" only in vague, nonspecific terms. Most patients desiring cosmetic reconstruction have been

aware of the deformity for a long time and can describe it in exquisite detail.

- Other, more severe physical abnormalities are being ignored by the patient.
- The patient has had previous cosmetic surgery with apparent success but has continued to be dissatisfied. Perfectionistic patients may focus their concerns on their bodies and may want to change everything. Such quests end in failure for the patient.
- The patient has magical expectations about how others will change their attitudes toward the patient after surgery. For example, it is reasonable to expect that an improved nasal contour will allow the patient to experience lessened self-consciousness. However, the expectation of a new life or an entirely different self is unreasonable and the expectation of such results predicts trouble.
- The deformity has unrealistically served as an excuse for personal failures.
- The deformity is part of a psychotic thought process.

The benefits available through cosmetic surgery are increasingly clear, and the issues listed above offer only the briefest guide to assessing patients. In the main, plastic surgery patients are pleased with their enhanced appearance.[27] Fears of symptom substitution are usually unfounded, and psychoses are not precipitated by removing an external deformity. A good screening interview by the family practitioner before referral to a plastic surgeon will eliminate those grossly unsuited for surgery or those who require psychiatric evaluation and treatment before surgery.

SUMMARY

Although the surgeon does the patient's surgery, the patient's psychological problems are often best dealt with by careful preparation and evaluation by his or her personal physician, who then maintains a vigilant eye for delayed psychological complications. These efforts can make the difference between true surgical success or failure.

REFERENCES

1. Deutsch H: Some psychoanalytic observations in surgery. Psychosom Med 4:105, 1942
2. Kennedy J, Bakst J: The psychological parameter in cardiac surgery. Bull NY Acad Med 42:811, 1966
3. Kosanin R: Anesthetic considerations in patients on chronic tricyclic antidepressant therapy. Anesthesiology Review 8:38–41, 1981

4. Barber B: Informed Consent in Medical Therapy and Research. New Brunswick, NJ, Rutgers University Press, 1980
5. Janis IL: Psychological Stress: Psychoanalytic and Behavioral Studies of Surgical Patients. New York, John Wiley & Sons, 1959
6. Kornfeld DS, Heller SS, Frank KA, et al: Personality and psychological factors in post-cardiotomy delirium. Arch Gen Psychiatry 31:249–253, 1974
7. Egbert LD, Battit GE, Welch GE: Reduction of postoperative pain by encouragement and instruction of patients. N Engl J Med 270:825, 1964
8. Menzer D, Morris T, Gates P, Sabbath J, Robey H, Plant T, Sturgis SH: Patterns of emotional recovery from hysterectomy. Psychosom Med 19:379, 1951
9. Levison BW: States of awareness during general anesthesia. Br J Anaesth 37:544, 1965
10. Kemph JP, Bermann EA, Coppolillo HR: Kidney transplant and shifts in family dynamics. Am J Psychiatry 125:1485, 1969
11. Titchener JL, Zwerling I, Gottschalk LA, Levine M, Silver H, Cowett A, Cohen S, Culbertson W: Consequences of surgical illness and treatment. Arch Neurol Psychiatry 77:623, 1957
12. Cobb S, McDermott NJ: Postoperative psychosis. Med Clin North Am 22:569, 1938
13. Ervin CW: Psychologic adjustment to mastectomy. Med Aspects Human Sex 42, February 1973
14. Renneker R, Cutler M: Psychological problems of adjustment to cancer of the breast. JAMA 148:833, 1952
15. Maguire P: The psychological social sequelae of mastectomy, in Howells JG (ed): Modern Perspectives in the Psychiatric Aspects of Surgery. New York, Brunner/Mazel, 1976, p. 390
16. Jamison KR, Wallach DK, Pasnau RO: Psychosocial aspects of mastectomy. II. The man's perspective. Am J Psychiatry 135:543, 1978
17. Jamison KR, Wallach DK, Pasnau RO: Psychosocial aspects of mastectomy. I. The woman's perspective. Am J Psychiatry 135:432, 1978a
18. Druss RG, O'Connor JF, Stern LO: Psychologic response to colectomy. I. Adjustment to a permanent colostomy. Arch Gen Psychiatry 20:419, 1969
19. Stahlgren LH, Ferguson LK, Influence on sexual function of abdominoperineal resection for ulcerative colitis. N Engl J Med 259:873, 1958
20. Sutherland AM, Orbach CE, Dyk RB, Bard M: The psychological impact of cancer and cancer surgery. I. Adaptation to Dry Colostomy: Preliminary Report and Summary of Findings. Cancer 5:857, 1952
21. Roeske NA: The emotional response to hysterectomy. Psychiatric Opin 15:11, 1978
22. Lindenmann E: Observations on psychiatric sequelae to surgical operations in women. Am J Psychiatry, 98:132, 1941
23. Caplan LM, Hackett TP: Prelude to death: Emotional effects of lower-limb amputation in the aged. N Engl J Med 269:1166, 1963
24. Parkes CM: Factors determining the persistence of phantom pain in the amputee. J Psychom Res 17:97, 1973
25. Kolb I: Psychology of the amputee: Phantom phenomena, body image and pain. Coll Papers, Mayo Clin 44:586, 1952
26. Olley P: Psychiatric aspects of cosmetic surgery, In Howells JG (ed): Modern Perspectives in the Psychiatric Aspects of Surgery. New York, Brunner/Mazel, 1976, p 491
27. Edgerton MT, Jacobson WE, Meyer E: Surgical psychiatric study of patients seeking plastic (cosmetic surgery): Ninety-eight consecutive patients with minimal deformity. Br J Plast Surg 13:136, 1960

Donald S. Kornfeld, M.D.

16

The Management of Pain

> To exert an influence on pain, it is more useful to know the minds of men than their physiology. [Charles Aring[1]]

Since pain is a subjective experience, it seems appropriate that a psychiatrist advise regarding its management. Too often when requested to evaluate a patient with pain the psychiatrist is asked to distinguish between "real pain" and "psychogenic pain." This is a meaningless differentiation, since all pain is subjectively experienced. However, the question does speak to an important consideration: How should the pain best be treated? Can some type of treatment directed at the patient's emotions aid in pain relief? But to ask the question, "Is the pain real?" has implications for both the physician and patient that can guarantee therapeutic failure. The question implies that "psychogenic pain" is imaginary and therefore not a legitimate complaint. The question may even suggest a conscious attempt to deceive or malinger. These overtones will doom any therapeutic efforts. Should the treating physician refer the patient for a psychiatric evaluation on that basis, his or her efforts will fail. The patient has been placed in the untenable position of having to prove that nothing the psychiatrist can do will work, for if the latter is successful, the patient has been demonstrated to have an unreal "psychogenic pain." Therefore, referrals of this kind are usually self-defeating.

Most patients with chronic pain are not referred to a psychiatrist and rightly so. The primary care physician should be able to manage these patients. The understanding of certain basic principles can make the job easier.

First, if we are to successfully treat the patient with pain, we must distinguish *pain* from the *complaint of pain*. Pain, as a totally subjective experience, is unique for each individual. The complaint of pain, however, includes the patient's subjective experience, his or her emotional responses to and reporting of it and, finally, our response to the patient's complaint. This subjective sensation experienced by patients can therefore produce a variety of emotional reactions in those about them: sympathy, fear, rage, and combinations of these. As physicians we must concern ourselves with both sides of this equation, since our own subjective reactions to the complaint of pain can influence our decisions regarding its management.

Pain is part of a system designed to protect the body from injury and, therefore, its presence presumably signifies trouble and stirs up anxiety. However, pain and the complaint of pain also become useful in the development of our relation with others. For example, an infant's cry of pain, hopefully, gets a comforting response from its parents. In this way, pain and its relief can be associated with the receipt of love and affection. Unfortunately, there are some family situations where a loving response can be elicited from parents or other supporting figures only when the individual seems to be in physical pain. The consequences of this pattern for future behavior are apparent.

The word *pain* is derived from Latin and Greek roots meaning "punishment," and the ways in which pain and punishment are linked in early life can affect the adult's response to pain. For example, painful punishment is used by some parents who then remorsefully provide the child with love and considerable closeness. For children treated that way, the expression of pain is seen as the only way of eliciting affectionate and loving responses from the people around them. For others, pain can provide punishment and relieve guilt for thoughts or actions that have elicited guilt.

What about the physician's response to the patient with pain? The complaint of pain usually evokes sympathy and the desire to help. Our training as physicians provides us with the tools to do this quite effectively. Too often, though, the treatment of the patient with pain becomes a source of conflict for the treating physician. He or she worries about overmedicating patients who have "real pain," out of a fear of addicting them. The physician struggles with a decision to recommend surgery for a patient who does not respond to more conservative treatments. The physician finds himself getting angry with the patient whose pain persists despite all forms of treatment. These patients can be the most difficult we are asked to treat because they create conflict within us. Out of frustration, they can make us feel helpless, guilty, and angry.

We must appreciate that a physician's reaction to pain is just as colored by early experiences as is a patient's reaction. The physician who was raised to be a stoic may respond less sympathetically to the "weak" patient who openly complains than to the "strong" patient who suffers in silence. On the other hand, the physician raised in a setting in which it took a dramatic display to get attention may easily underestimate the degree of true suffering being experienced by a stoical patient.

THE PLACEBO RESPONSE

The effect of emotions on the perception of pain is well known to all of us. Who has not observed the tearful child with the bruised knee who appears to get prompt relief when his or her mother "kisses it to make it well." This is probably the earliest use of the placebo response. What about the wounded soldier, or the injured athlete who appears to feel no pain until the battle or game is over? Were there no painful stimuli in the central nervous system? Apparently some central mechanism modifies the perception of these signals. Some recent work suggests that the endorphin system of internally secreted morphine-like substances may play a role in these responses.[2]

Despite these observations, a patient's favorable response to a placebo is sometimes used as evidence that his or her pain is not "real." Knowledge of Beecher's work with placebos should dispel this notion. Among a group of postoperative patients, 40 percent responded with pain relief to a placebo injection.[3] Unfortunately, placebo injections are still used to determine if pain is "real." Obviously, a positive response merely establishes that the patient is a placebo responder, a designation that applies to approximately one-third of our population. No specific psychological characteristics have been determined to predict placebo responsivity.[4]

Conversely, emotions can also intensify the perception of pain. The continuum of pain severity has three significant points. The *discriminatory* point at which any sensation is felt, the *emotional* point at which the sensation is identified as "pain," and the *motivational* point at which the pain is considered to be "intolerable. Anxiety and antianxiety agents can affect the emotional–motivational components while the sensory discriminatory component is unaffected.[5] Beecher has suggested that the basic need in many clinical pain situations is sedation rather than analgesia.[6] The application of these observations will be discussed later.

THE MANAGEMENT OF "REAL" PAIN

Acute Pain

The treatment of postoperative pain or pain related to cancer is often considered to be fairly straightforward. Not so. Our emotional conflicts can obstruct the provision of good care. We tend to overestimate our patients' potential for addiction and to underestimate the analgesic power of the physician–patient relationship.

Egbert et al. have demonstrated that adequate preoperative patient preparation with regular postoperative follow-up can significantly reduce the need for narcotics and shorten hospital stay.[7] In this study, the anesthesiologist, prior to abdominal surgery, told patients what type of pain to expect and how to reduce it by specific techniques for breathing and moving about in bed. The patients were then followed daily postoperatively and these instructions were reinforced. The treated patients used half as much narcotics and left the hospital two days earlier than untreated patients. In addition to the value of the specific advice, this approach introduced another device for lowering anxiety: it gave the patient a greater sense of participation in his or her own care.

The excessive concern of physicians regarding the possibility of addicting their patients to narcotics is often related to their confusing physical dependence with true addiction. The former is quite commonly produced in hospital patients, but the latter quite rarely. Addiction is a behavior pattern of compulsive drug use characterized by overwhelming involvement with the use of a drug and with the securing of a supply, as well as a tendency to relapse after withdrawal.[8] The development of addiction is very rare in medical patients with no history of addiction. Patients are as concerned as we are about addiction. Unless a patient has very specific emotional needs that coincide with this illness experience, addiction is highly unlikely to occur. The physical dependence that can occur is easily managed by gradually tapering the narcotic dose.

Excessive concern regarding addiction was well demonstrated in a study by Marks and Sachar, who found that a high percentage of house officers tended to overestimate their patients' potential for addiction and, as a consequence, undermedicated them. For example, 75 percent of the doses of meperidine (Demerol), usually 50–75 mg q 9 hr prn, prescribed for a variety of serious medical and surgical problems, were found to be inadequate for severe pain. Pharmacological studies show that 75–150 mg q 3 hr are necessary, depending on the patient's weight and previous tolerance for the drug. Ironically, undermedication may actually increase the potential for addiction by forcing the patient to remain in pain for a prolonged period of time, thus increasing the craving for every analgesic dose.

The patient with underlying emotional problems is just as likely (if not more so) to become addicted to a course of low doses designed to prevent the occurrence of addiction. A patient whose pain is inadequately treated will certainly never believe that his or her physician cares about him. This will defeat any opportunity for dealing with underlying emotional problems and prevent the physician from using himself therapeutically. On the other hand, if a relationship of confidence is established it can do much to relieve both the pain and the anxiety. That constructive atmosphere can then do a great deal to reduce the need for narcotics.

Concern regarding addiction often plays a special role in the management of the patient with sickle cell anemia, which therefore serves as an excellent example. The patient presents with few or no physical findings. The only treatment is usually narcotics for analgesia. The physician becomes overly concerned about addiction and undermedicates the patient. This is easy to do since many of these patients have developed a tolerance for these drugs. The undertreatment produces an angry patient whose demands for pain relief only escalate, producing more anxiety and then anger in the treating physician. Too often, the physician then scolds the patient and includes a lecture on the evils of narcotics. (You know how much good that does!)

In my experience such patients are best managed if their pain is treated adequately at the outset. The initial narcotic doses should be large enough to provide pain relief and create a sense of trust in the physician. At the time of a crisis patients cannot deny the existence of their illness and its consequences. Anxiety is therefore often an important component of the illness and requires treatment. The phenothiazines can be helpful in this regard. They may be added to potentiate the narcotic effect and reduce the patient's anxiety (e.g., chlorpromazine, 25 mg IM, tid or qid). The short course of narcotics required to treat the usual sickle cell crisis is not likely to addict the patient. The patient who does become physically dependent may be withdrawn quite easily when the crisis ends. Of course, emotional factors can play a role in the triggering of the sickle cell crisis and in the patient's pain behavior. However, these issues cannot be dealt with while the patient remains in pain and they will never even be discussed with a physician who is perceived as unsympathetic to the patient's suffering.

Table 16-1 contains information that can be helpful in selecting an appropriate narcotic, dosage regimen, and route of administration. Narcotics do not eliminate the perception of pain; instead they affect patients' affective response to pain. At equivalent doses they are comparable in efficacy. However, note the differences in potency and duration of action. For example, meperidine (Demerol) is quite short acting and should be ordered at least once every 3 hours, whereas methadone can be ordered once every 8–12 hours. Methadone, codeine, oxycodone (in Percodan) and levorphanol (Levodromoran) are all superior to morphine when given orally.

Note that pentazocine (Talwin) has narcotic antagonist activity; this drug, therefore, should never be given in association with a narcotic since

Table 16–1
Narcotic Analgesics

Generic Name	Trade Name	Dose (mg) Subcutaneous	Dose (mg) Oral	Duration (hr)	Distinguishing Features
Morphine		10	60	4–5	
Hydromorphone hydrochloride	Dilaudid Hydrochloride	1.5*	7.5*	4–5	
Codeine		120*	200*	4–6	
Oxycodone	(in Percodan)	15*	30*	4–5	
Levorphanol tartrate	Levo-Dromoran	2*	4*	4–5	
Methadone hydrochloride	Dolophine Hydrochloride	10*	20*	8–12	Less euphoria
Meperidine hydrochloride	Demerol Hydrochloride	75*	300*	2–4	Little constipation or biliary spasm
Anileridine hydrochloride	Leritine Tablets	30*	50*	2–3	Little constipation or biliary spasm
Pentazocine hydrochloride	Talwin Hydrochloride	60*	180*	2–4	Mixed narcotic agonist–antagonist

Source: Shimm DS, Logue GL, Maltbie AA, Dugan S: Medical management of chronic cancer pain. JAMA 241:2408–2412, 1979.
* Dose produces same analgesic effect as morphine, 10 mg subcutaneously.

it will counteract its effectiveness. It can also precipitate withdrawal symptoms if a patient is abruptly switched to it from a narcotic.

In treating patients with severe pain do not overlook the potential benefit of aspirin and acetaminophen. These drugs exert their analgesic properties peripherally and in that way differ from the central action of the narcotics. They can, therefore, offer a supplemental form of pain relief via a different mechanism of action. Of course their effect on the gastrointestinal tract, blood clotting, and bone marrow must also be kept in mind.

Try to be aware of the effects of anxiety on pain. As Beecher has pointed out, reducing anxiety can affect the need for narcotics. The prescription of diazepam for patients in a coronary care unit reduced the need to prescribe narcotics there.[10] Although the phenothiazines can potentiate narcotic action centrally, their effect on pain is probably also related to their ability to lower anxiety.

Chronic Severe Pain

Dr. Cicely Saunders, the English physician who founded St. Christopher's Hospice, has taught us a great deal regarding the management of chronic severe pain in cancer patients.[11] She points out the need to help each patient distinguish pain from fear and depression. In this way the appropriate drug can be prescribed for each of these painful affects, and narcotics need not be used as a universal treatment. On the other hand, Saunders and her associates have little concern about the patient's becoming dependent on addicting substances. They have not found the development of tolerance to be a problem.[12] For patients in constant pain, narcotic drugs are prescribed around the clock and not as needed (of course, the patient is allowed to refuse a dose). Additional doses are also made available as needed. The patient is allowed to have an additional less potent analgesic at the bedside to be taken orally. Such a treatment plan reduces the usual anxiety that patients experience anticipating the return of the pain or the need to suffer should the time interval between doses be too long. Phenothiazines such as chlorpromazine can also be used to reduce anxiety and potentiate the narcotic effect. Their antiemetic effect also can be helpful. A dose of 25 mg po of chlorpromazine may be adequate without oversedating the patient. Care should be taken not to overdose the patient and produce daytime somnolence. Dextroamphetamine, 5 mg, once or twice a day, can potentiate the narcotic effect and neutralize the prescribed narcotics' sedating effects.[13] It should be possible to find a combination of drugs and a dose schedule that will provide pain relief and still allow the patient to be alert. The sedative effect of the phenothiazines can be utilized by giving a larger dose of chlorpromazine at bedtime. Haloperidol 10 mg hs, also has been reported to potentiate analgesic effects when used in this way.[14]

PSYCHOLOGICAL COMPONENTS IN THE ETIOLOGY OF PAIN

Emotional factors can play a more direct role in the production of pain. The problem in the management of such types of pain is that too often the physician is so concerned that he might miss something organic that he devotes all his time and energy (and the patient's money) to ordering more and more elaborate tests. When these are found to be negative the patient is left with reassurance that "Nothing is wrong," and his or her pain. Why is it that some physicians are so concerned that they might miss something like a brain tumor—a very rare disease with a guarded prognosis, even with treatment—yet are not particularly concerned that they will miss an emotional problem—a very common disorder that, with treatment, has a good prognosis?[15]

The diagnosis of "functional" pain or of "psychogenic" overlay should not be a diagnosis of exclusion. The search for positive diagnostic elements can establish a basis for treatment.

The psychophysiologically produced pain is perhaps the easiest for physicians to understand. For example, it seems clear enough that tension headaches are related to spasm of muscles in and around the head. The treatment also seems obvious: the use of a mild analgesic like aspirin plus a minor tranquilizer such as diazepam (Valium) or oxazepam (Serax); (see also Chapter 5 regarding the use of these drugs). Relaxation exercises or biofeedback also are quite effective. The former requires no special equipment, is essentially without side effects, and can be easily taught to the average patient (see Chapter 5). However, the underlying issues that produce the tension should also be dealt with to assure relief of symptoms and to prevent recurrence.

Most patients are eager to talk to their physicians regarding their problems. Physicians must provide them with the opportunity to do so. This means setting aside the time and being willing to ask a few leading questions. For example you may say, "These kinds of headaches are usually related to tension or worries. What's been troubling you?" It may be helpful to ask the patient who cannot consciously make these connections to keep a diary, recording specifically what is going on at those times when the pain occurs. Where you already have an adequate history (the preferable method), you can say, "I know that your husband's mother has recently had to move in with you. That can provide a great deal of tension in a family. Tell me what it's been like." In some situations ventilation alone is effective. Chapters 3 and 8 deal further with other office psychotherapy techniques that can be utilized to deal with such problems.

Psychogenic Overlay

What about patients with a "psychogenic overlay" to their symptoms; for example, the patient with a low back pain that fails to respond to treatment? Here we often are dealing with a patient who has found that a symptom provides some relief from an intolerable situation; for instance, the overburdened homemaker or the employee in conflict with his or her supervisor. The emotional factors are unconscious and can affect the patient by lowering the threshold for pain, interfering with the ability to ignore the pain, or actually increasing the symptomatology by intensifying muscle spasm.

In exploring such issues, you must be careful not to imply that a physical pain does not exist. Most patients can accept the notion that tension or worries are making their physical problem worse. They are often eager to discuss these personal matters so long as we do not suggest that the basic medical problem is not legitimate. It is, therefore, essential that all the physical treatments continue while an effort is being made to relieve the sources of emotional pressure.

> A 40-year-old mother of five was troubled by persistent sciatica. The usual conservative measures failed to relieve the symptoms. Her daily activities were becoming increasingly limited. She was referred to an orthopedist who found no indications for surgery. In reviewing her life situation he learned that her husband, a successful executive, had been drinking excessively for years.
>
> The patient was eager to talk. She had been a long-suffering wife, who assumed she had to fill in wherever her husband was unable to function. She could not admit to herself or to others the anger and resentment she felt toward her husband. She felt obliged to be, as she later put it, "superwife" and "supermother." The only acceptable excuse for not doing everything was a physical illness. Her sciatica was quite real; however, her use of it was determined by her emotional state.
>
> The birth of this woman's last child, less than two years before, had probably been the last straw in the face of the husband's continued drinking. There was a growing awareness that she could no longer deceive herself regarding the severity of his alcoholism. He had promised to stop drinking and failed just once too often. Her reaction to the sciatic pain was a plea for help expressed in the only way she could find acceptable.
>
> The patient's sessions with her physician provided her with an opportunity to ventilate her feelings to an authority figure from whom she could

derive approval and support. The physician also helped her to realize that she need not be physically ill to justify a reduction in her whirlwind schedule. In the meanwhile, the husband was encouraged to seek hospital treatment for his alcoholism.

The patient was also started on a regular physical therapy program for which she previously "had no time." There was gradual improvement in the low back pain and considerable improvement in the patient's mood, as she began to feel more in control of her own life.

Conversion Reaction

A conversion reaction is a physical symptom that involves the musculoskeletal system or organs of special sense that is caused by unconscious conflict. Pain may represent such a conversion symptom. In many instances the symptom may have begun with an illness that provided the patient with a crystal around which the system became elaborated. The diagnosis should not be based merely on the absence of positive physical findings. Instead it should be based on positive answers to the following questions:

1. Based on this individual's personality structure, would one assume that he or she would use a physical symptom—in this case, pain—as a means of dealing with some emotional conflict?
2. Is something occurring in the individual's present life that would account for conflict and thus, create a need for a physical symptom?
3. Does the symptom—in this case, pain—appear to resolve the conflict with which the patient is struggling unconsciously?

An individual with a conversion reaction does not have to have a hysterical personality.[16] In the typical series of patients with conversion reaction, no more than 50 percent may fit the hysterical personality type. A combination of obsessive and hysterical traits is common. There are some general principles one can follow in trying to answer the first question, referring to personality types. Individuals, who in the past have manifested overt psychiatric symptomatology at the time of stress, are most likely to continue with that pattern. Depression, anxiety, or a psychotic break are more likely to return under stress than a physical symptom if that has been the patient's manner of dealing with stress in the past. However, for an individual in whom past stress has not produced overt emotional manifestations, one can assume that a physical symptom may be the only acceptable way of dealing with conflict.

Engel, going one step beyond these general principles, has characterized a type of person who believes he will repeatedly suffer from one painful disability or another.[17] These pain-prone people are chronically depressed, pessimistic, gloomy, guilty, and self-deprecating individuals who always appear to have been defeated in life and yet who do not seem to learn from their experiences. Unconsciously many of them cannot tolerate success and must pay a price of some kind because of the guilt associated with it. In their family backgrounds, there is much aggression, suffering, and pain, very often with harsh, punitive parents. Violence and aggression, or threats of it are used as a means of control. In the past there may be a history of a painful experience that is recalled to consciousness at such times as the individual needs it for emotional reasons. This personality type does exist, but this is not the only type of individual who uses pain to deal with unconscious conflict.

Having considered the patient's personality, the clinician should then ask, "Why now?" It is very unlikely that by asking the individual, "Is anything upsetting you?" you will get a very helpful response, since many of these patients have developed their physical symptoms as a means of repressing their painful emotions. The most effective way of determining a positive answer to the question of "Why now?" is to take what is referred to as a parallel history: that is, to elicit the history of the pain in the usual medical manner and then return and take a history of the patient's life events and situations. When you superimpose one history upon the other it may become clear why the individual has felt the need to develop a particular symptom at that particular time. A family member may provide a fuller history of emotionally stressful factors than the patient. Has the patient experienced a recent failure, with unexpressed guilt or rage? Has the patient achieved a recent success for which his or her unconscious demands punishment? Has the patient suffered a real, threatened, or fantasied loss that has evoked a mourning response? Is this the anniversary of such a loss?

Finally, does the symptom resolve a conflict for this patient? A positive answer to this question helps confirm the diagnosis. The patient with sciatica described earlier is a good example.

In one study these three criteria were found to be the most reliable in making the diagnosis of conversion reaction.[18] Traditionally, it was felt important that a conversion be found to have special symbolic significance. This was not found to be a useful criterion. Such symbolism usually reflects more the creative imagination of the examining physician. Similarly, *la belle indifference,* an apparent indifference to one's plight, classically attributed to these patients was not consistently present.

Establishing a positive diagnosis of conversion reaction does not mean that the issue can be resolved by a brilliant interpretation. Very often the patient has too much of his or her self-esteem wrapped up in the physical symptom and to confront him directly may, in some instances, be counterproductive. We must allow the patient a facesaving way out of the situation by providing simultaneous physical treatment.

The patient should sense your expectation that the pain will respond to such treatment. The patient must then be given an opportunity to discuss the areas of conflict that have emerged in your earlier history taking. Where indicated, special help should be provided: for example, where marital conflict exists you will have to meet with the spouse. Advice regarding marriage counseling may follow. If there are problems with a child, a referral for appropriate help can be arranged. All the while, the physical therapy goes on. The emotional problems should be treated as complications of the illness, not as its cause. The approach is similar to that outlined for the patient with psychogenic overlay.

Generally, these patients do well; even those patients who are unable to verbalize their difficulties may still benefit from your supportive manner and the respite from their problems that a brief hospitalization provides. Their pain is a cry for help, and your response speaks to that need. They are not indifferent to their difficulty. Many of them are anxious and depressed about their situation and are eager to be relieved of it. The patient receiving both physical treatment and "talking" treatment can attribute the relief of his pain to the physical therapy. In the meantime, the patient has become better able to deal with the problems with which he or she has been struggling. This support is best given by the primary physician. If referral for psychotherapy is absolutely necessary, the primary physician should continue physical treatment. It is when the primary physician completely abandons the patient, suggesting that the pain is "all in your head," that the patient becomes resentful and more resistant to all forms of treatment.

DEPRESSION AND PAIN

What role does depression play in the management of pain? Can we assume that depression is a necessary concomitant of chronic pain or does depression set the stage for chronic pain? Regardless of which came first, if a patient is truly clinically depressed, then the appropriate treatment of that depression will help. When depression precedes the pain or appears simultaneously with it, the pain is more likely to be completely relieved after successful treatment of the depression. When depression follows the onset of pain, successful treatment of depression can provide increased tolerance of pain.[19]

Tricyclic antidepressants, electroshock treatment (EST),[20] and monamine oxidase inhibitors,[21] have all been reported to be effective in the treatment of chronic pain disorders. The tricyclics, sometimes used in combination with a phenothiazine or haloperidol, have been successfully used in the treatment of pain associated with post-herpetic neuralgia,[22] diabetic neuropathy,[23] rheumatoid arthritis,[24] thalamic syndrome, phantom limb, and causalgia.[25] (Phantom pain is discussed in more detail in Chapter 15).

The patients in the studies cited did not all meet the criteria for clinical depression, although some depressive components were usually present. What is clear is that with adequate doses of an anti-depressant, given long enough, a significant number of patients did respond. For some time it was thought that this response represented the successful treatment of a depressive equivalent—pain. However, Taub points out that in his series pain relief antedated the lifting of mood and not vice versa.[22] There are also animal data which suggest that the tricyclics may have direct analgesic properties.[26] Other work suggests that morphine and the tricyclics have common parallel actions within the brain.[27]. It therefore seems likely that pain and mood are influenced by closely related centers within the nervous system.

A 59-year-old businessman experienced the gradual onset of lancinating pain around the right thorax. X-ray examination revealed calcific spurs at T8 and T9. The patient was treated with salicylates, biofeedback, acupuncture, self-hypnosis and nerve blocks. No treatment provided more than temporary relief. Over the course of 18 months, his pain worsened and he was maintained on codeine 400–600 mg/day, which was also becoming ineffective. Dorsal rhizotomy was being considered. He was sent for psychiatric consultation.

The patient reported that because of the pain he was finding it quite difficult to continue at work, where he had considerable responsibility in a family business. He was anorectic and had lost approximately 15 pounds. He had no interest in formerly pleasurable activities. His sleep was interrupted, and he awakened early each morning with pain.

The patient also revealed that about two years ago, at his brother's urging and against his own better judgment, they had purchased a new and larger business. As the patient had feared, there were many problems which he felt were insoluble because he could not obtain competent help. He had always tended to defer to his more aggressive brother and now felt his pain made it even more difficult to deal with him. The patient felt himself caught in a downward spiral, with his pain the basic cause of his difficulty.

He was started on amitryptyline 25 mg bid and 50 mg hs. This more sedating tricyclic was chosen so that it could be given at bedtime to help with the patient's insomnia. His sleep did begin to improve within a week.

The dose was gradually increased at 25-mg/day increments each week, to a total dose of 150 mg. Gradual improvement began at 4 weeks, with almost complete pain relief 8 weeks after start of treatment. Codeine was gradually reduced until the patient required only an occasional sallcylate. With the improvement in his mood, the patient began to deal more effectively with his business problems, and his interest in his social life, golf, and other activities also returned. He was maintained on amitryptyline 150 mg/day for 8 months, 100 mg for 6 months and then 75 mg, which has been his maintenance dose for the last year.

The tricyclics are slow acting, and the therapeutic dose can vary widely among individuals. Therefore, you must allow enough time (4–6 weeks) and give adequate doses (up to 300 mg/day) to insure a response. A more detailed discussion of the use of tricyclics can be found in Chapter 6. Some reports indicate that the combination of a tricyclic with a phenothiazine may be more effective than the tricyclic alone.[22,25] The sedating tricyclic amitryptyline can be given at bedtime to promote sleep (50–75 mg), while a less sedating phenothiazine or haloperidol is used during the day. For example, typical regimen would be amitryptyline 50–75 mg hs with trifluperazine (Stelazine) 1 mg tid or haloperidol (Haldol) 0.5 mg bid. Sleep improvement should occur early, with pain response developing after a 2–4-week interval. Most patients report their pain persists but is easier to bear, and an occasional patient will report complete relief.

PAIN ASSOCIATED WITH COMPENSABLE INJURY

In an important series of papers, Hirschfeld and Behan have described what they refer to as the *accident process*.[28–30] These investigators' data suggest that the patient with prolonged disability following a compensable accident may be using the accident and its apparent consequences to resolve a problem that began prior to the accident itself: for example, the worker, in conflict between his desire to be free of his dead-end job and his need to work to support his family and maintain self-esteem; the overburdened wife and mother working outside the home, in conflict between her desire to be rid of this double burden and her family's need for additional money. These anxious, depressed, conflicted individuals can precipitate an accident through an act of carelessness. Such "accident proneness" is not a lifelong characteristic, but rather a temporary trait to which we are all susceptible under specific circumstances. It is not necessary that one unconsciously wishes to be injured but rather that one is preoccupied with personal concerns or experiencing psychomotor retardation associated with depression. It is not surprising that such individuals will then cling to the painful disabilities that appear to resolve their conflicts.

Unfortunately, our workmen's compensation laws, which pay workers primarily for their lost capacity to earn a living rather than for their injuries per se, reinforce the problem. The early award of a lump sum for injury might help in some situations to reduce prolonged disability. Otherwise our efforts to relieve our patients' pain so that they can return to work may be in conflict with their own unexpressed needs.

How to treat such patients? Hirschfeld and Behan say, "In accidental injuries the physician is not just the therapist, he is the therapy." It is essential to take a detailed history of the events surrounding the accident and then to get to know as much as possible regarding the patient's life circumstances prior to the accident. It is this latter knowledge that may provide the information needed to construct a total treatment package, one directed at both the injury and the patient's underlying distress. For example, a depression may require treatment; marriage counseling may be needed; an industrial worker may need advice regarding how to make a job change. All the while, physical therapies continue. It is essential that the patient's family physician direct the treatment effort. While specialists can offer specific expertise, they do not have the relationship with the patient needed to treat his or her total needs.

Dr. Wilbert Fordyce of the Pain Clinic at the University of Washington recommends an approach that he believes can reduce the likelihood of chronic disability in cases of injury.[31] He believes the doctor should communicate clearly that he expects complete recovery by a specific date. Initially the physician decides what is a realistic time to allow for healing of the acute injury (perhaps he can then add a few days just to be safe). The patient is told he must restrict his activities until that time. Bed rest is ordered, if indicated, for a specific number of days. The patient is given an analgesic and told to take it regularly, not just as needed. He is then given a specific graduated plan for return to activity. Analgesics are withdrawn gradually, again on a specific schedule. Fordyce points out that disability is sometimes prolonged because patients feel pain with movement and fear they will damage themselves if they continue activity. They must be reassured that activity is not harmful after the acute phase of an injury even if pain occurs, and that their activity level will probably be able to increase faster than their pain level will decrease.

When such a regimen fails, it should suggest that emotional variables are at work. This is a critical period. If such a treatment failure leads only to further efforts with different forms of physical treatments, the prognosis is for prolonged disability. Instead the detailed life history, taken during the period of physical treatment, should serve as the basis for additional psychiatric intervention by the primary physician. Of course, this approach will require longer office visits, but it will probably save time and money when one considers the total effort that is usually expended for the entire period of a prolonged disabling injury.

ACUPUNCTURE IN PAIN CONTROL

How valuable can this ancient technique be in pain management? The dramatic reports of its use for surgery do not reflect standard practice in China, where it is probably used successfully in less than 10 percent of surgical procedures. Acupuncture is more commonly used for the treatment of chronic pain, and a much higher rate of success has been reported with this use, in both the Chinese and the Western literature.[32]

Acupuncture is based on the traditional Chinese concept that life forces travel through meridians that transverse our bodies. The manipulation of acupuncture points on these meridians is supposed to restore homeostasis to the system. Currently, there are two main theories as to why acupuncture is successful in pain relief. The first is based on the gate theory of Melzack & Wall.[33] These researchers postulate that within the nervous system the well-myelinated C fibers carry slower, more chronic pain signals. These signals are transmitted through the substantia gelatinosa of the spinal cord, which serves as a gateway to the central nervous system. The assumption is that the insertion and manipulation of the acupuncture needle stimulates the larger A fibers and in so doing blocks the transmission of pain signals from the C fibers through the substantia gelatinosa. This counter irritant effect is utilized in other forms of pain relief, such as transcutaneous stimulation. However, counter irritation does not explain the reported pain-reducing effects in areas remote from the stimulated site. More recent work suggests that the acupuncture effect may be mediated through the endorphin system, the internally produced opiate-like substances.[34] This second theory would account for the effects of stimulating acupuncture points on remote sites. A third explanation, suggested by other investigators, is that the acupuncture ceremony is merely a formula for inducing a hypnotic response.[35] The literature in this regard is contradictory: some papers suggest that sham points are not as effective as true points; some studies suggest otherwise.[36]

For whom is acupuncture indicated? Which kinds of chronic pain can be expected to respond? The answers are not in. Successful use has been reported for a wide variety of chronic pain. However, no criteria have been established to predict which patients will respond or for how long. Even for responsive patients, the results are only temporary, lasting from weeks to months and therefore, requiring repeated treatments.

Is it harmless? Probably. Disposable needles and sterile technique are used by legitimate operators. Battery-powered electrical stimulation is also safe, although more powerful sources of current can be quite dangerous.

HYPNOSIS IN PAIN CONTROL[35,37]

Spiegel has described hypnosis as the capacity for a certain style of concentration.[35] It is not a form of sleep. The EEG during a trance may show increased alpha but never sleep spindles. The hypnotist is, therefore, viewed as a teacher who helps the subject become aware of his or her capacity, if any, to achieve this state.

A variety of methods have been devised to measure hypnotizability. However, the issue is clouded by the observation that patients presenting for hypnosis to meet a clinical need may react differently from normal volunteers in a laboratory setting. It is likely that the motivation of patients with clinical problems enhances hypnotic responsivity.

The technique used to relieve pain will depend on the patient's capacity for hypnotizability. The most hypnotizable may be able to achieve a true sense of dissociation and numbness. The mid-range hypnotic subject will respond best to instructions that the pain sensation be altered, for example, from pain to a sense of tingling; least hypnotizable subjects will respond best to a distraction technique, in which they are instructed to direct attention to some other sensation and, by inference, to ignore their pain.

Hypnosis has been used as the sole form of anesthesia for surgical procedures. However, we are concerned here with its use in the management of chronic pain. For hypnosis to be useful for chronic pain, the patient must be taught a technique of altered perception using self-hypnosis. Patients are instructed to restructure their perception of chronic pain at those times when it becomes less tolerable. For example, many patients find they can tolerate the pain when distracted by work or social activities but not when trying to fall asleep in the quiet of their bedrooms. The self-hypnosis exercise can thus be used to diminish pain awareness and help the patient fall asleep. Other patients may find their pain intensified during the stresses of the day and can use the self-hypnosis strategy much as others use a coffee break. Some more hypnotizable patients, through the process of posthypnotic compliance can provide on-going pain relief for two hours or more after a brief self-induced trance.

It is interesting to speculate on the possible common mechanism of self-hypnosis and relaxation response therapy (Chapter 5), two techniques that can relieve physical symptoms related to stress. They are different ceremonies but they may be tapping the same natural capacity in a given patient.

TRANSCUTANEOUS NERVE STIMULATION

Transcutaneous nerve stimulation[38] probably works through the counter irritation principle, which has been used for years in various liniments. The gate theory of Melzack and Wall [33] best explains this phenomenon. Approximately 25 percent of patients with unselected chronic benign pain report some improvement. This technique is best used for shoulder, back and leg pain.

The device consists of a battery operated pack the size of a deck of cards and electrodes that are placed along the course of the nerve involved in the pain process or over the affected muscles. The patient controls the current and learns to deliver only enough to stimulate the larger nerves. Some patients keep the current on for hours while others use it only for a few minutes each day. The stimulator can be rented so that the patient can learn whether it will be effective before purchasing it.

OPERANT CONDITIONING FOR PAIN

The past ten years have seen the establishment of a number of interdisciplinary pain clinics that utilize the concepts of behavioral psychology and the early work of Fordyce.[39,40] They are dedicated to modifying "pain behavior," for example, the use of medication, excessive complaints of pain, or reduced activity. The treatment is based on the assumption that patients have learned to use pain in a specific way because of reinforcing responses (reinforcers) in their environment. Therefore, the treatment is designed to modify the environment and, in that way, to change the patient's behavior.

Treatment requires four or more weeks of hospitalization. The approach is most likely to succeed with chronic pain patients who have no clear indication for alternative treatment; the capacity to walk; a family relationship with positive reinforcers for pain behavior; a likelihood of responding to hospital reinforcers; a history of activities to which they can reasonably be expected to return; and a willingness to participate in the following program in a hospital:

1. Reinforcers are withdrawn, e.g., medication is not made contingent on pain behavior but is given at fixed time intervals. Narcotic doses are gradually reduced as other forms of treatment are introduced.
2. Favorable consequences, such as praise and rest, are associated with behaviors incompatible with pain behavior. Demands for performance are based on a careful assessment of the patient's capacities. Pain is no longer the threshold for discontinuation of a task.
3. The family are trained to modify their behavior so that pain reinforcers are withdrawn and well behavior is reinforced.

These pain units report significantly increased activity and reduced use of narcotics at the time of discharge for most patients.[41] However, there are not enough follow-up studies to ascertain how long lasting these effects will be. In one study at one year follow-up, 25 percent of admitted patients maintained the improvement achieved in the hospital, that is, pain was still present but at a lower reported level, and there was less need for analgesia and more activity.[42]

It is important to note that this approach requires a well-motivated patient. These inpatient units therefore treat a self-selected population. More long range follow-up studies with larger numbers are needed before their effectiveness can be accurately assessed. Using these behavioral techniques may therefore not have universal application. However, the multidisciplinary approach to diagnosis that most pain clinics employ is of great potential value and certain elements of the treatment approach can probably be helpful to some patients.

THE TREATMENT OF CHRONIC PAIN: WHAT CRITERIA FOR SUCCESS?

Chronic pain patients will often report that although their pain has not been completely relieved by a particular remedy they are better able to tolerate their pain. This may be the optimal goal to be realized in many patients with chronic pain. The patient and the doctor must both learn to tolerate the fact that some pain does continue to exist. We must resist the call of more radical forms of treatment to deal with a problem that may not be totally resolvable. As Aring has said, "The problem in the treatment of chronic pain is that we persist in ignoring the patient to fix our attention on his symptoms." As a result, he says, "The patient reaches the technically proficient physician where the temptation is unresisted to employ this proficiency quickly toward a hoped for relief."[1] Most patients expect us to be omniscient and omnipotent. For the physician who accepts that as his personal standard of performance these patients will elicit anxiety, guilt, or anger at what is perceived as a personal failure. Such feelings underly the decision to do one more procedure with the hope that this will produce that elusive cure.

The English neurologist Penman's experience with the removal of pain from a series of patients with tic doloreux prompted him to write a paper in 1954 entitled "Pain as an Old Friend."[43] Penman reported that a significant percentage of patients continued to complain vigorously of discomfort from the paresthesias produced by their operations or developed other psychiatric symptoms. He became aware that for some of these patients the pain had become integrated into their lives and, therefore, could not be given up easily. Its removal demanded a significant reorganization of their lives for which they had not been well prepared. He, therefore, recommended that every patient being considered for radical treatment of chronic pain have his personality and social circumstances assessed by the treating doctor or someone working closely with him. This is a time-consuming process, since we must know about the emotional make-up of the patient prior to the onset of pain, and a good deal about the setting in which the pain began, but it is essential if we are to save both the patient and physician from considerable grief. After all, the pain may play an important role in the patient's relationships with his or her family and it certainly plays a role in the dependent relationship on his or her physician.

Good results can similarly be destroyed when the treating physician discharges an improved patient too quickly from his care or makes office visits too far apart or strictly "as needed." Some of these patients will then experience more pain as a means of reestablishing the relationship. They are the ones who need the opportunity to share some knowledge of their lives with you. However, if you establish a regular, reasonably frequent, appointment schedule they will realize that your interest in them is not totally dependent upon the existence of excruciating pain. You should then find a reduction in urgent calls for appointments and in the need for hospitalizations.

With chronic pain patients, the treating physician should keep in mind the level at which the patient is functioning, and not the fact that the patient is still complaining of pain. As Szasz puts it, "What is our goal, to relieve pain or to stop the patient's complaint of pain?"[44] It is when we focus on the complaint alone and not on what the patient is able to do in spite of the pain that we are most readily deceived. It is therefore often necessary to allow patients to continue to complain of their pain and to maintain their dependence upon you. An important motivation for their continued activity may be your expression of respect for their ability to function despite the pain. We can always hold out the possibility of additional pain relief without doing our patients harm with radical procedures. Keep in mind that if the individual is functioning adequately, you have effected a very good therapeutic result.

REFERENCES

1. Aring CD: The nature and significance of chronic pain, in Medical Clinics of North America. Philadelphia, WB Saunders, 1958, pp 1467–1479
2. Levine JD, Gordon NC, Fields HL: The mechanism of placebo analgesia. Lancet, September 23, 1978, pp 654–657
3. Beecher HK: the powerful placebo. JAMA 159: 1602–1606, 1955
4. Shapiro A: Factors contributing to the placebo effect. Am J Psychother 18 (suppl 1:73–88, 1964
5. Chapman CR, Feather BW: Effect of diazepam on human pain tolerance and pain sensitivity. Psychosom Med 35:330–340, 1973

6. Beecher HK: Anxiety and pain. JAMA 209:1080, 1969
7. Egbert LD, Battit GE, Welch CE, et al: Reduction of postoperative pain by encouragement and instruction of patients. N Engl J Med 270:825–827, 1964
8. Jaffe J: Drug addiction and drug abuse, in Goodman LS, Gilman A (eds): The Pharmacological Basis of Therapeutics. New York, Macmillan, 1975, pp. 284–324
9. Marks RW, Sachar EJ: Undertreatment of medical inpatients with narcotic analgesia. Ann Intern Med 78: 173–181, 1973
10. Cassem NH, Hackett TP: Psychiatric consultation in a coronary care unit. Ann Intern Med 75:9–14, 1979
11. Saunders C: The treatment of intractable pain in terminal cancer. Royal Soc Med Sect Surg 56:195–198, 1963
12. Twycross RG, Wald SJ: Long-term use of diamorphine in advanced cancer, in Bonica JJ, Albe-Fessaro D (eds): Advances in Pain Research and Therapy, vol 1 New York, Raven Press, 1976, pp. 653–656
13. Forrest Jr. WH, Brown BW, Brown CR, et al: Dextroamphetamine with morphine for the treatment of postoperative pain. N Engl J Med 296:712–715, 1977
14. Maltbie A, Cavengar J: Haloperidol and analgesia. Milit Med 142:946–948, 1977
15. Loeser JB: The family doctor vs. chronic pain. Patient Care 12:35–37, August 15, 1978
16. Chodoff P, Lyons H: Hysteria, the hysterical personality and hysterical conversion. Amer J Psychiatry 114: 734–740, 1958
17. Engel GL: "Psychogenic" pain and the pain prone patient. Am J Med 26:899–918, 1959
18. Raskin M, Talbott JA, Meyerson AT: Diagnosis of conversion reactions. JAMA 197:102–106, 1966
19. Bradley JJ: Severe localized pain associated with the depressive syndrome. Br J Psychiatry 109:741–745, 1963
20. Mandel MR: Electroconvulsive therapy for chronic pain associated with depression. Am J Psychiatry 132:632–636, 1975
21. Lascelles RG: Atypical facial pain and depression. Br J Psychiatry 112:651–659, 1966
22. Taub A: Relief of post-herpetic neuralgia with psychotropic drugs. J Neurosurg 39:235–239, 1973
23. Davis SL, Lewis SB, Gerich JE, et al: Peripheral diabetic neuropathy treated with amitryptiline and fluphenazine. JAMA 238:2291–2292, 1977
24. Hart FD: The use of psychotropic drugs in rheumatology. J Int Med Res 4 (suppl 2): 15–19, 1976
25. Merskey H, Hester RA: The treatment of chronic pain with psychotropic drugs. Postgrad Med J 48:594–598, 1972
26. Theobald W, Wilhelm G, Krupp W: Analgesic and anticonvulsant activity of derivative of dibenzapine, in Souclairac A, Cahn J, Charpentier J (eds): Pain: Proceedings of International Conference London/New York, Academic Press, 1968
27. Lee R, Spencer PSJ: Anti-depressants and pain: A review of the pharmacological data supporting the use of certain tricyclics in organic pain. J Int Med Res 5 (suppl 1): 146–156, 1977
28. Hirschfeld AH, Behan RC: The accident process 1. Etiological considerations of industrial injuries. JAMA 186:193–199, 1963
29. Behan RC, Hirschfeld AH: The accident process II. Toward a more rational treatment of industrial injuries. JAMA 186:300–306, 1963
30. Hirschfeld AH, Behan RC: The accident process III. Disability: acceptable and unacceptable. JAMA 197:85–89, 1966
31. Fordyce WE: Stress and behavioral medicine: New frontiers in pain control. Read before the International Conference on Stress Research, Lugano, Switzerland, 1979

32. Chu LSW, Yeu SDJ, Wood DB: Acupuncture Manual: A Western Approach. New York, Marcel Dekker, 1979, pp. 150–153
33. Melzak R, Wall R, Wall PD: Pain mechanisms: A new theory. Science 150:971–978, 1965
34. Pomeranz B, Chiu D: Naloxone blockade of acupuncture analgesia: Endorphin implicated. Life Sci 19:1757–1762, 1976
35. Spiegel H, Spiegel D: Trance and Treatment: Clinical Uses of Hypnosis. New York, Basic Books, 1979
36. Frost EAM: Acupuncture and hypnosis. NY State J Med 78:1768–1772, 1978
37. Hilgard ER, Hilgard JR: Hypnosis in Relief of Pain. Los Altos, Calif, W Kaufman, 1975
38. Shealy CN, Maurer D: Transcutaneous nerve stimulation for control of pain. Surg Neurol 2:45–47, 1974
39. Fordyce WE, Fowler RS, Lehmann SF, et al: Operant conditioning in the treatment of chronic pain. Arch Phys Med Rehabil 54:399–408, 1973
40. Fordyce WE: Behavioral Methods for Chronic Pain and Illness. St. Louis, CV Mosby, 1976
41. Fordyce WE: Operant conditioning in the treatment of chronic pain. Arch Phys Med Rehabil 54:399–408, 1973
42. Swanson DW, Maruta T, Swenson WM: Results of behavior modification in the treatment of pain. Psychosom Med 41:55–61, 1979
43. Penman J: Pain as an old freind. Lancet, March 27, 1954, pp. 633–636
44. Szasz T: Pain and Pleasure. New York, Basic Books, 1957

Irene B. Seeland, M.D.

17

The Management of Cancer Patients and Their Families

Cancer has been the second most frequent cause of death in nearly all age groups during recent decades in this country. Up to 25 percent of the population in the United States will eventually develop some form of a malignant disease and up to 17 percent will die from cancer.

Much has been accomplished in recent years in dealing with cancer. Early detection and treatment, improved techniques in surgery, radiation, and chemotherapy all have resulted in increased cure rates for some patients and in longer survival rates and improved ability to function during the progression of the illness for others. However, the diagnosis of cancer is still one that most physicians and all patients dread.

DIAGNOSIS: THE ROLE OF THE PRACTITIONER

Public education has made the public increasingly aware of and knowledgeable about early signs and symptoms of different cancers, the importance of early treatment, and the different treatment modalities. Often, therefore, when a patient presents a particular symptom to the physician, the fear of a possible malignancy is already on his or her mind, even if the question is not directly asked. A lump in the breast, a bloody discharge, a rapidly growing mole, consistent pain and unusual weight loss bring the possibility of cancer to the mind of the patient. Even before any statement is made or a suspicion directly voiced by the physician, this possible diagnosis is apparent from the obvious concern of the doctor, through his request for specific and often extensive laboratory tests, x rays or biopsies.

The early interviews provide an opportunity to gather data on how the patient will respond to a diagnosis of cancer. The word "cancer" can be introduced into your discussion of the differential diagnosis. The patient has undoubtedly had it in mind, so your mentioning it should not come as a surprise; however, the response to it will provide you with useful information.

You can say, for example, to the patient with rectal bleeding, "We do have to get more tests to make the diagnosis. This may be a polyp, or diverticulitis, or possibly a tumor or cancer." Should the patient appear to be upset at your mention of the word, it provides you with an opportunity to reassure him or her that, even if it were a cancer, modern treatment methods have improved the prognosis greatly, thus setting the stage for future discussions should they become necessary. Your use of the word *cancer* also shows the patient that you can use it comfortably and makes it easier for the patient to do so.

In their response to the word, your patients may tell you a great deal about themselves and their attitudes toward this illness. Their responses may provide you with an early opportunity to dispel myths and diminish unrealistic fears. Using the word *cancer* at this point certainly will begin the process by which you gather data to help you construct your approach to a particular patient and his or her illness.

The practitioner will usually refer his or her cancer patient to a specialist for a final diagnosis and treatment recommendations. The need for mutual consultation and open communication between the primary physician and the oncological specialist or surgeon is vital. Primary care practitioners know about their patients' abilities to deal with stress and they know what information patients have already been given. Practitioners should inform the specialist of any psychological, social, or family problems that may have an important impact on the treatment and future disposition of the patient.

Should Patients Know the Truth?

One of the difficult questions that both general practitioner and specialist must confront is: What should the patient be told? This question has been explored and at times agonized over by many generations of physicians. The more recent growing concern with "patient's rights" and informed consent and the increasing attitude that a patient can be considered an active participant in the treatment process have encouraged more physicians to present the diagnosis of cancer openly to the patient. Euphemisms such as *premalignancy, tumor, mass,* or *rapidly growing tissue* may still be used by doctor and patient alike in order to at least, temporarily delay the full impact of the work *cancer,* which usually evokes the image of a progressive and destructive process and a fatal outcome. Yet it appears that many patients fare better, provided they are given adequate emotional support, when they are allowed to deal with known factors. This allows them to discuss their questions, fears, and often unrealistic fantasies openly. This is often preferable to surrounding them with a wall of silence, and then forcing them to cope with procedures, treatments, and progressive deterioration that stands in gross contrast with the promise, "Everything is going just fine."

At the same time, the ability of a patient to deal with the full burden of the diagnosis and prognosis needs to be carefully assessed by the physician. Discussions regarding "truth telling" often fail to make a distinction between providing accurate information regarding diagnosis and providing "the truth" about prognosis. They also fail to acknowledge the clinical observation that most patients provide us with clues as to what they want to know and when. Many patients want to know and are able to deal with a truthful answer about the diagnosis of their illness, provided it is given with a hopeful attitude regarding prognosis. For them the really important question is "What does this diagnosis mean to me, to my life, to my ability to function and to be with those people I care about?" Most patients need to know that even the most catastrophic illness has a chance of treatment, of cure, of extended and tolerable living. They need to know that something can and will be done for them. An element of constructive action and realistic hope is, therefore, a vital factor in discussing the diagnosis of a malignant illness with patient and family.

Patients usually will react in the way that they have coped with other difficult situations in their life—they will quietly withdraw, have violent emotional outbursts, turn for support to another person, or deny the whole situation. In the very best circumstances, facing serious illness, extensive treatment, and possibly pain and death still takes getting used to for most people. Your hopeful attitude and support for patient and family is, therefore, essential.

The prognostic statement is more problematic. Much has been written recently about the patient's "right to know the truth." Unfortunately, the most vociferous spokesmen have been laymen with inadequate understanding of the complexities of medical "truth." To know the outcome statistics for a sample of 100 patients does not tell us "the truth" for an individual patient. Even where this "truth" is known it is dangerous to assume that all patients want that kind of truth or would benefit from it. We have all known patients who have been told "the truth" and have chosen to deny it. Others have been told "the truth" and become depressed or anxious, living in fear of death. There were also those who heard "the truth" and benefited from this knowledge, living out their days the better for having known it. The question is, what truth, for which patient, at what time?[1]

The knowledge of an unfavorable or catastrophic prognosis therefore constitutes an awesome burden for the physician. He must decide in each instance what is the appropriate message and when it should be given. The knowledge that death may be impending leaves the physician with the responsibility to let a patient know that time may be short to finish up specific tasks, to deal with unresolved issues in human relationships, to take time to contemplate one's life. On the other hand, there are patients who cannot deal with this knowledge. It is a disservice to them to confront them with a reality that they have chosen to deny. We should not allow the practice of medicine, a very individualistic art, to be governed by rigid, doctrinaire positions. The patient's very real right to the truth must be balanced by his or her right to a physician who will treat him as an individual.

As Reiser has written, "Those who argue that disclosure of threatening news should be the rule instead of the exception bear weighty burdens. They must have prepared themselves to learn spoken and silent cues patients telegraph about facts they know or crave about their illnesses; to communicate effectively with patients and sustain them emotionally once the news is out; to understand psychological difficulties that can accompany disclosure and to allocate time for the often lengthy period over which disclosure can take place. They must also recognize that the harm created by inadequate mastery of the techniques and skills of communicating bad news may outweigh the benefits to the individual of learning the truth."[2]

The thoughtless dispensation of "the truth" is no more helpful than an arbitrary policy of providing only falsehood. The one overriding consideration should be to do what is necessary to maintain your patient's trust in you.

Protecting the Patient

At times the physician who "protects" a patient from a diagnosis may do so on the specific request of the patient's family or friends. Often out of respect for the "better" judgment and more intimate knowledge that the family may have of the patient's ability to cope, the physician will follow the request of the family and communicate only with one or several designated members of the family about all the important aspects of diagnosis, treatment, and prognosis. This "conspiracy of silence" often creates a social and emotional isolation of the patient who finds himself or herself surrounded by people who show obvious signs of serious concern, depression, overprotection, or withdrawal yet do not give any explanations for their behavior to the patient.

A 78-year-old Cuban woman, mother of 5 daughters, grandmother of 12 grandchildren, and a well-loved and respected matriarch in her family, was kept in the dark by her well-meaning and very concerned daughters about the fact that she had an inoperable cancer of the colon. Bloody stools, occasional partial obstructions and increasing weight loss were explained to her with a variety of "diagnoses." Although the treating physician had questioned the wisdom of leaving this intelligent and reasonable older woman completely in the dark, he respected the wishes of her daughters, and their explanation that "mother could not face a diagnosis of cancer and impending death, she would just become severely depressed and give up." The constant presence of one or the other daughters during clinic visits and a language barrier allowed no direct communication with the patient until one day the accompanying daughter had to leave the examination room temporarily and the patient indicated an urgent wish to speak to the physician herself. A Spanish nursing aide translated the patient's strong distress with her present situation, her awareness that she was seriously ill, her suspicion that she had cancer, and her sadness about the secretiveness and resulting dishonesty and emotional isolation that she had experienced in her relationship with her daughters.

The physician decided to confirm her suspicions. The subsequent conversations with her daughters provided a coming together and sharing of the concerns, the sadness, and aloneness they all had experienced. This allowed finally a much closer and richer time for the family together.

Does the Patient Want to Know

At times, the physician may feel that his or her patient may not want to know the diagnosis or may not be able to cope with it. Some patients indicate their initial inability to cope with bad news by not asking any questions that may result in difficult answers. Often these patients will direct their questions toward treatment and other functional issues and clearly avoid any discussion involving an open exploration of the nature of their illness or their prognosis.

Other patients will not "hear" the clearly spelled out diagnosis of "cancer" or "malignancy," and approach their illness and the treatment with an apparent lack of understanding that stands in clear contrast to the actual information already given to them. Often these patients need some time to prepare themselves emotionally to deal more directly with the somber news they are asked to face. Given time and support, they may eventually be able to ask more specific questions and to tolerate more direct answers. There are other patients who directly refuse to know what their medical situation is and who prefer to relinquish all responsibility of decision making to the physician: "Doctor, you know what is best for me, you just take care of everything." Yet even these patients sooner or later are faced with the realities of their illness, with treatment side-effects, and with progressive symptoms that require the treating physician to come up with a complicated and ever expanding network of explanations that often conflict with reality. The naive trust that both patient and doctor had tried to maintain begins to be undermined. The anxiety level of the patient often becomes high, and he or she requires increasing "reassurance." Titrated doses of truth are often a better method of dealing with such patients than promises of improvement or cure that have to be continuously retracted or reexplained with a new "diagnosis."

Informed Consent

The trend toward requiring "informed" consent for treatment of all patients, especially for surgery or chemotherapy, has led to an increasing number of more or less well-informed patients. Once again, some physicians have allowed what they believe to be the requirement of the law to govern their practice of medicine. Such physicians read their patients a detailed list of every possible side-effect, often creating considerable unnecessary anxiety. Most state laws do not require such disclosure. They ask only that we share with the patient that knowledge which is reasonable. Often "informed" patients show evidence of a disconcerting lack of real information regarding the illness, the required treatment, treatment side-effects, their own future functioning, and expectations for cure or long-term survival. This should not surprise us when we realize that anxious patients with little or no medical background or sophistication have been given perfunctory or highly technical explanations, leaving the patients not only poorly informed but at times more confused, anxious, and bewildered than before, as well as embarrased about their apparent inability to understand what has been explained to them.

This communication gap between the medical profession and the layperson can be bridged by simple, nontechnical explanations and simple drawings, by describing tests and procedures and giving a rationale for them. Time should be allowed for digesting the information and asking questions. At times one must repeat information that has already been given once or even several times. The anxiety level in most patients who suspect that they have cancer, and then are told that they do, is very high. Much information that is presented during that initial time is lost, because the patient is trying to cope with the overwhelming news, the prospect of radical surgery or other treatments, and the possibility of a considerable shortening of his life expectancy.

The value of thoughtful and caring early communication will emerge at a later point when the patient realizes that he has been well prepared for the experiences that confront him. This will assure him that he can maintain an honest and trusting relationship with his physician.

Societal Attitudes Toward Cancer

The question of honest communication about the diagnosis of cancer becomes considerably more complex when it involves people other than the patient or people closest to him. At present, though it is slowly changing, society still considers cancer a repugnant, disgraceful process, thus eliminating and isolating the "incurable" cancer patient as a relevant member of society. Patients with cancer often (and usually for good reason) fear discrimination in employment and severe restriction in obtaining health and other insurance policies and see their already burdened financial situation further complicated through such discrimination. Many patients also hesitate to share their diagnosis of cancer with fellow workers and friends for fear of social isolation and rejection. They may fear pity or unnecessary overprotection at a time when they feel quite capable of coping normally or adequately with their work or social tasks.

> A 57-year-old surgeon with malignant lymphoma responded well to chemotherapy and was able to maintain a busy professional practice and hospital appointment for 3 years. He didn't inform any of his colleagues or friends, except his wife and one very close friend, of his illness, for fear that their response to the knowledge of his illness would restrict his work responsibilities or that they would "pity" him, a thought he could not tolerate. When his illness began to progress more rapidly he sent his wife and two children abroad under an excuse of better schools for his children but really to "spare them the pain and the misery of my dying." He continued to work until he collapsed with sepsis in the hospital and died in complete human isolation. His fear of being rejected for an illness that still carries such ominous connotations for many people made it impossible for him to ask for some help and human support during the most difficult time in his life.

The physician should be aware of the particular social or work situation of his or her patient and of possible implications that a "public" diagnosis may have for both patient and family.

It is becoming very evident, as our understanding of the psychological and social stresses that affect cancer patients and their families grows, that an adequate emotional support system is vital in order to help all involved in an often prolonged process to cope with their difficult life situation. Primary practitioners, even if they are not directly involved in the actual treatment of the disease, can play an important role in assessing whether adequate support systems exist for their patients and their families. They can make recommendations to the treating physician regarding the utilization of social service, mental health professionals, or other agencies that provide assistance to cancer patients.

THE TREATMENT

Preparing the patient

Most patients as well as their families will respond to the initial diagnosis of a malignant disease with shock, some with initial denial, and many with fear and worry about the chances of real cure, progression of the disease, and eventual, premature death. During the initial explorations it is often necessary to give considerable time to exploring with the patient the relevant treatment modalities currently in use. Presentation of treatment in highly technical terms will add little to the patient's real understanding of what is actually going to happen to him or her. Simple explanations that leave time for questions, concerns, and fears are of great importance in the preparation of the patient. Even so, the physician must realize that the real impact of a treatment procedure, such as radical surgery, will not affect patients until after the surgery, when they must face the actual destructive results on their bodies, the serious changes of their body image, and possible impairment of function.

John, a 19-year-old, tall, well-built college student, who had never been ill in his life and received medical treatment only for some injuries sustained in playing football, was admitted to the hospital for a below-the-elbow amputation of his left arm for a synovial sarcoma. Considerable time was spent on exploring with John the need for the amputation, the chances for cure, and the possible need for further chemotherapy. John took all of this in stride and showed little evidence of fear or concern. He had quick and, on the surface, adequate explanations for how he might cope with the impact of the amputation or side-effects such as hair loss that might occur after chemotherapy. It became obvious that John, at this point, needed to deal with these issues on a safe, intellectual level only, and could not allow himself to respond emotionally to the radical disruption of his up to now very "normal" life.

The impact of what was happening to John did not hit home until the surgical dressing was changed on the second day after surgery. Then John had to face the reality that his left hand was no longer there. On returning home, and being confronted with many "normal" tasks requiring the use of two hands, John, who had coped well with the restricted range of activities in the hospital, became severely depressed, withdrawn, and avoided all contact with friends and peers. He felt he could no longer participate in their usual activities. The loss of his thick, blond hair, which when anticipated he had joked away with comparisons to the TV character Kojak, led to further social isolation. These reactions had been anticipated in view of John's initial inability to prepare himself for the expected changes in his life situation. Clinic visits had been scheduled to ensure follow-up contacts. It took John several months and several explorations with a mental health professional to come to deal with these painful and radical changes of his life.

Cancer treatment is often painful and at times destructive, and it often begins before the illness has created any major discomfort. The discrepancy between the initial complaint and the extensive treatment is hard to understand and at times hard to tolerate, especially for the younger patient. The physician needs to be aware of this to help the patient understand the need for specific treatment. Simple explanations outlining the rationale for treatment and the expected results may help the patient to deal in a more rational manner with his or her anxiety about the proposed treatment and its aftermath. However, even with such preparation such patients may vent their anger, resentment, and despair over their new fate on the physician, who has executed his or her medical responsibility in carrying out the required treatment. Understanding the basis for this anger should help us to deal with it.

Emotional Reactions to Treatment

It is important for physicians to realize that procedures that the medical profession has come to consider routine and necessary for the appropriate treatment of cancer, may have a considerably stronger effect on the patients and their families. Family members may respond with fear, disgust, or withdrawal after radical surgery, radiation, or chemotherapy have made their impact on the appearance of the patient. The effect of such reactions on the patient, who is in particular need of help and emotional support at that time, can be very destructive, if not disastrous.

A very attractive 30-year-old nurse had to undergo a radical mastectomy for breast cancer. Her medical background appeared to help her understand the procedure and its consequences better than other young women in similar circumstances. She appeared to cope as well as could be expected with her situation while in the hospital. During a 3-month post-operative check-up it became obvious that she was severely depressed. It was clear that she was functioning only minimally in spite of little physical impairment. It was only in response to a direct question about her sexual relationship with her husband, who had always adored his very beautiful young wife, that the reason for her depression became clear. Her husband had been unable to touch her physically since she returned from the hos-

> pital. Several meetings with the husband helped him to reach a better understanding of his own fears and exaggerated fantasies of the effects of the surgery as well as of the great need that his wife had for his support. The reestablishment of a closer interpersonal relationship was slow but was possible because the husband felt a strong enough commitment to his wife and their marriage to cope with his own fears and needs. He helped her by his acceptance of her despite her illness and the loss of her previously "perfect" body.

Meetings with the patient's husband before and after surgery to explore the expected physical results and the psychological implications for himself as well as for his wife would have been helpful in preventing the increased isolation that this young couple experienced in their still fairly new relationship.

The range of available treatments, some still in the research stage, can be overwhelming even to many physicians. How much more so for the nonmedical person who is to be subjected to them. It is important that the practitioner who is referring his or her patient to a specialist for treatment of cancer be sensitive to the impact that some of the treatment complications can have on the physical and emotional state of the patient. Treatment effects such as repeated nausea, vomiting, mouthsores, or hair loss—though not "life threatening" and therefore, not "serious"—often have deep, emotionally debilitating effects on patients and their families and can require as much medical and psychological supportive treatment as the primary disease.

Treatment "Drop-Out"

The cancer patient, who is already struggling to cope with the stresses that the diagnosis of a potentially fatal disease, repeated hospitalizations or ongoing clinic visits have on his emotional status, now finds his already diminished sense of well being further disrupted by the effects of treatment meant to "make him well," or at least "better." Many patients, especially after extended courses of treatment, find it increasingly difficult to tolerate the side-effects of a treatment that they experience at times as "being worse than the illness." The unwillingness of some patients to continue with treatment protocols is often related to the fact that they find little available time for normal living.

This is especially true with treatment in the face of progressive disease. It can be experienced by the patient as a futile exercise, robbing him or her of precious time free of painful, disabling complications. Therefore, the spacing of therapeutic regimens, allowing for "time out" for physical as well as emotional recuperation, can be an important factor in helping a patient deal with the burden of modern treatment modalities.

Frequent hospitalizations, with their onslaught of tests and procedures administered by a well-trained but at times overworked or impersonal hospital staff, can leave patients overwhelmed, helpless, frustrated, and often angry and resentful. Primary physicians may not see themselves as having any specific medical function during that time, especially if a patient has been admitted to a hospital with which the practitioner is not affiliated. However, the physician's willingness to continue contact with the patient through brief visits or telephone calls—whether for clarification, emotional support, or as a communication bridge between patient and specialist—can be a vital factor in the patient's ability to continue in a difficult treatment process.

THE "CURED" PATIENT

Modern medicine has produced an increase in cure rates and long-term survival rates for certain malignant diseases. The practitioner will find himself increasingly dealing with patients who have undergone treatment for cancer and are, at present, not showing any further evidence of malignant disease.

Fear of Recurrent Disease

For many patients it will take months and years before the fear of recurrent disease begins to subside. Some patients will observe the slightest change in body function, minor illness, or pain as ominous signs of the feared recurrence. It is not always easy to help a patient to establish a healthy balance between caution and resuming life in a normal manner. Many patients will need the security of physician contacts between-regular check-ups for a period of time until the normal demands of life and the progression of improvement give the patient a clear message that things are all right again.

The overanxious patient who shows evidence of a constant preoccupation with signs or symptoms of recurrent cancer or new disease may be struggling with other emotional issues. These may be directly related to the previous illness, such as difficulties in interpersonal or social relationships resulting from the disease. However, the behavior may reflect earlier psychological problems that did not emerge until the stress of the disease and treatment weakened the patient's usual coping mechanisms. Persistence and intensity of the fear of recurrence as well as an unusually slow resumption of normal activities or a marked discrepancy between the level of physical recovery and the level of functioning will give the practitioner clues to the existence of underlying emotional problems that need exploration. Often some questions about the patient's sense of recovery, ability to work, social activities, and family relationships may bring to the surface existing emotional, social, and interpersonal problems. Many of these issues can be dealt with in the practitioner's office using techniques outlined in other chapters. If the emerging issues appear to be of a more serious or longstanding nature, intervention by mental health professionals can be useful to clarify and help resolve existing problems. What is essential is the effort by the practitioner to explore these areas.

The Denying Patient

Some patients will assume an attitude of denial as means of coping with their underlying fear of recurrent disease. These patients will find it difficult to return for routine checkups; they will not follow through with adjunct chemotherapy and may even delay returning to their physician when symptoms of recurrences appear. The primary practitioner, who does not present the same association with the dreaded disease, can often follow their future progress, provoking less anxiety than a return to the "cancer specialist" or "cancer hospital."

> Jimmy, a 19-year-old college student, had been referred to an oncology clinic for evaluation of adjunct chemotherapy after amputation of his right leg for osteosarcoma. There had been no evidence of local lymph node involvement. Jimmy had a very difficult time adjusting to the loss of his leg as well as to loss of mobility and employability. He was, at this time, not willing to enter into a treatment process that would bind him to the clinic for a period of many months and possibly debilitate him further. After many discussions with the clinical physician who understood Jimmy's reasons but also felt strongly about the need for adjunct chemotherapy, Jimmy refused to return to the clinic. The clinic physician then contacted the physician in a small local clinic who had initially referred Jimmy and asked him to keep an eye on Jimmy. Jimmy has been followed in this way for the past 2 years without having to deal directly with the dreaded "cancer institution" and as no recurrence of disease has occurred, treatment has not been necessary.

THE PROGRESSIVELY ILL PATIENT

The diagnosis of cancer still allows hope of a cure for some patients. Yet there are a greater number who, after an initial expectation of cure or long remission will have to deal with the fact that the illness has recurred and requires further treatment. Implied, though rarely directly expressed by physician and patient alike, is the understanding that the first recurrence usually also eliminates the hope for real cure for most patients. However, the development of new treatment techniques permits, at times, considerable extension of the patient's life expectancy, at the cost of having to subject himself or herself continuously to modern medical procedures. The recurrence may come about in a variety of ways and have varying implications. For example, the leukemia patient with a recurrent infiltration of his or her bone marrow can still hope for another "good" remission; the breast cancer patient with metastasis to the liver or bone may have to face slowly progressive disease and increasing debilitation.

Refusal of Treatment

There will be the occasional patient who finds the thought of continuing life in an increasing state of debilitation, dependency, and possible pain intolerable and who may refuse any further treatment. Such patients often have few meaningful activities or relevant human relationships left in their lives, and the prospect of death may be experienced more as a relief than a dreaded interference with a full life. A treatable depression may also be present. This must be distinguished from unhappiness, since the depression can respond to specific treatment. Chapter 6 deals with this important differential diagnosis.

Some patients may also refuse treatment at this point because they prefer to use their remaining time free of the interruptions or side-effects of continuous treatment. The primary physician may be particularly helpful in exploring with the patient the pros and cons of such a decision, pointing out the potential benefits of active treatment. The physician should also try to understand and alleviate the fears and fantasies that some patients have of the final stages of their disease. These concerns are often related to past experiences with terminally ill relatives. Often specific reassurance can be given that their illness and its treatment need not have such dire consequences. A continuous dialogue and an established trusting relationship will be the best remedy to counteract a patient's feeling so helpless that he or she wants to "give up." The physician may, however, also have to face the fact that discontinuation of treatment may, at times, be in the overall interest of the patient and thus allow him or her that freedom of choice.

Anticipation of Death

Although patients will occasionally ask a physician about the exact progression of their disease and the "common" form of problems that will ultimately lead to their death, most patients are not really interested in the explicit details of terminal disease. They want to be reassured that they will not suffer intolerable distress or pain that might render them helpless or make them lose their dignity and control. Although no physician will be able to guarantee any patient an easy death, we can reassure most of our patients that intolerable suffering can be avoided. The most important factor for most patients remains, however, again and again the promise that they will not be abandoned during the final stages of their life.

Peter K, a 28-year-old married accountant, was found to have malignant lymphoma. His parents—divorced, both remarried, and wealthy—were convinced that the best medical treatment their money could buy would cure their son. The illness progressed rapidly, and within 3 months Peter K, was obviously approaching a terminal stage of his disease. His 20-year-old wife, who was taking care of their first child, then 14 months old, was becoming increasingly overwhelmed, both physically and psychologically, by the constant demands her very frightened husband was making on her. He demanded her presence with him day and night and would not allow for any substitutes. Further deterioration of his illness led to his rehospitalization. At this point, the disease had made a marked impact on his physical appearance: cervical lymph node enlargement, petechiae, and marked weight loss had changed Peter's appearance to that of an obviously, terminally ill person.

During the last 2 weeks of his life in the hospital, both his parents and stepparents could no longer face the failure of their "power over illness through money" nor could they face the physical deterioration of their son. His wife continued her visits until 3 days before his death. Then she stopped her visits and only called the ward daily to inquire about her husband's status. Several attempts were made to contact the family by telephone to explain to them Peter's urgent need for their support and physical presence. The family responded with a variety of excuses and was clearly unable to deal with the situation. Peter remained conscious until the last 3 hours before his death and was painfully aware of being deserted by all of his close family. He was extremely frightened and restless, but finally calmed down when the social worker and his primary nurse stayed with him and promised that either they or some other member of the staff team would remain with him at all times. He died the next day with both young women at his bedside holding his hand.

The Patient Who Cannot Give Up

In contrast to the patient who will question the relevance of further treatment is the patient who cannot accept the fact that further treatment will be of little or no benefit to him or her. For some patients the discontinuation of a protocol or any other active form of treatment means being abandoned and arouses great anxiety. These patients are often unable to accept the fact that their illness is no longer responding to treatment and that their death is approaching. Some patients respond to this situation with a request for further treatment, offer themselves as subjects for "any experimental drug," or resort to treatments and "healers" outside the medical establishment. They become easy prey to psychological and financial misuse and often find themselves and their families emotionally and financially depleted. These patients also may place a particular burden on their physicians, because they will continue to ask for additional consultations, hoping to find some physician who will again take on their "hopeless" case and promise them a cure or at least more time. Primary practitioners, if they have previous trusting relationships with such patients or their families, may be able to use these relationships in dealing with the anxiety and pain involved in facing the inevitable fact of impending death.

These patients may respond to a firm but supportive physician who will offer palliative care but is also willing to take a stand against useless experimentation. Most important, again, is the clear message that the physician will not abandon the patient and the family now that things have become "hopeless," but that he or she is more than ever available to them. Often this may require more of the physician's physical presence at the patient's bedside. It also requires that the practitioner himself or herself come to some resolution about the ultimate inevitability of death so that they can stand by the patient at this time.

Progressive Physical Decline

The progressive physical decline that cancer imposes on most patients presents a serious and challenging problem to the patients and their families as well as to the physician who is available for continuous care to patients. Most patients, especially those whom old age has not yet taught its lessons of infirmity and diminishing functioning, find it hard to adjust to an increasingly limited range of physical and social activities. Some patients tend to withdraw from all social contact; some abandon activities or hobbies from which they have derived much pleasure because they cannot any longer perform at their expected previous level or cannot compete with others. The inability to continue work, which becomes a reality for most patients at some point in the progression of the disease, usually has serious social, psychological, and financial implications for both patient and family. Patients begin to feel useless, unworthy, and a burden to others. The strain on the family or other supportive people in their environment becomes increasingly great as the illness progresses. The hope of cure no longer provides any light at the horizon, and a downhill course with increasing problems seems to be the only reality of life. It is of great importance during this time that the patient be helped to find meaningful and joyful experiences in life. Involvement in normal family activities, celebrations, social interactions with friends and peers give the patient a sense of the continuity of life and can be a source of encouragement and hope. Small excursions and trips into beautiful environments, tailored to the physical capacity of the patient, can lift the sense of being closed in and surrounded by illness and death. The practitioner can often be of great help by encouraging the patient and alleviating the family's anxiety about taking some "risks" in allowing the patient to continue to live as fully and actively as his or her physical and emotional stamina will allow.

The Resentful Family

As the illness process continues patients cannot help but be aware of the occasional resentment that their families experience at the continuous stress that the illness is imposing on everybody. Family members usually feel considerable guilt for being resentful, and either withdraw further or become overprotective and unreal in their extreme concern for the patient. During this period of progressing disease, intervention by a third party can be of vital importance in achieving a constructive resolution of existing expressed or unexpressed conflict.

> Mrs. B, a 57-year-old recent widow, had been undergoing treatment for multiple myeloma for 6 months, with only moderately successful results. During her recent readmission for further chemotherapy she expressed a wish to stop treatment and "get it over with." There were clear indications that Mrs. B felt her continuing illness was becoming an overwhelming burden to her two children, both young adults in graduate training. Although her 21-year-old daughter paid her only perfunctory visits on weekends, her 23-year-old son visited his mother daily for hours, had taken a leave of absence from school, and had postponed his impending graduation. During several meetings with the son it became evident that he greatly resented his mother's continued illness, which had disrupted his last year of graduate school. But he felt guilty for not having given more time to his dying father two years ago, and therefore felt guilty and obliged to be available to his mother. Mrs. B was obviously well aware of her son's ambivalent feelings as well as the more openly expressed resentment of her daughter. Mrs. B's physician involved other relatives in the care and visiting schedule of the mother. He had open discussions with the son and daughter about their resentment and explained that this was a common reaction of people in their situation. This led to a considerable lessening of tension in the family. The relationship between mother and daughter improved, and Mrs. B decided to resume her treatment.

Such meetings with members of the family to review the overall emotional, social, and financial status of the patient and the family can be quite helpful. The physician and family members can explore problems in interrelationships within the family, as well as practical problems such as the patient's need for home care, nursing care, financial support, or social service intervention or the need for mental health intervention for either the patient or for one or more family members. Sometimes simple solutions can greatly improve a difficult situation.

> Mrs. P. was a 32-year-old, married Greek woman, the mother of two small children. She and her husband, both immigrants, had found life in the United States difficult, and they had had to work very hard to make ends meet. Mrs. P's leukemia had completely exhausted their small savings, and because of her freqent hospitalizations, Mr. P was in danger of losing his job because he often had to stay home to care for their children. Both parents were becoming increasingly despondent, and Mrs. P felt particularly hopeless about the future of her husband and her two children. During several meetings with a mental health consultant and a social worker, several resources in the local community and the availability of volunteer and cancer organizations were discussed. Within 2 weeks one cancer organization had provided a full-time homemaker for Mrs. P, a local nursery school consented to have the older child attend its classes, and a volunteer organization was beginning to raise funds to have Mrs. P's widowed mother come to the United States to be available for the future care of her children. These arrangements eased the stress and despondency of Mrs. P and her husband, and her remaining time became more meaningful to the whole family.

The Spouse

The physician must, in particular, keep in mind the stressful situation of the patient's spouse and children. The spouse of any cancer patient may find himself or herself confronted with some of the following life issues: loss of a very important person; loss of a sexual partner; loss of one part of a parental team, leaving the other with the full burden of financial, emotional, and educational responsibilities for the children; responsibility to care for an ill and increasingly debilitated partner who can no longer provide his or her full share in the overall tasks of a family; responsibility to make or help make decisions concerning treatment, disposition, and plans for the future following the patient's death. Some spouses will try to deal with these tasks by themselves, trying to protect the patient from the added burden. Some will ask and perhaps receive help from friends, other family members, or outside agencies. Some spouses will be unwilling or unable to ask for or receive help, and finding themselves increasingly overwhelmed, seek inappropriate or destructive answers to their stress.

The incidence of extramarital relationships in marriages where one of the partners has cancer is not a public statistic. Clinical impression, however, seems to indicate that it is significant, especially in younger couples. The healthy partner who feels incapable of maintaining a sexual relationship with a spouse who suffers from cancer or who, because of the poor health of the other, is prevented from continuing a sexual relationship, has to decide whether to express and receive care and love on a nonsexual basis, or resort to extramarital gratification. The latter solution usually increases conflict, guilt, isolation, and breakdown of communication when support and closeness is most needed. It is a difficult subject to raise for most physicians, and not always gratefully received by a spouse of a cancer patient. However, it can be a relief for a partner in such a situation to find an opportunity for an open and nonjudgmental discussion and to be reassured that he or she is not a callous and uncaring human being but a person who is struggling with a difficult human situation. The final solution still will have to be found by each individual, but the physician can be of much help in being available for clarification and support.

The Children

Children of cancer patients have to deal with their own specific problems and, according to their age and the degree that the parents are willing to include them in the process of dealing with the illness, may cope well or poorly with a parent's disease and death.

Very young children, up to the age of three or four, usually do not yet have a clear concept of an illness leading toward death. They will respond most strongly to the absence of a parent, to the impact that illness may have on the physical appearance of the parent as well as the impact that decreased availability or changed mood and behavior of important family members has on their own lives. At this age children need much warmth, closeness, and support and some simple explanation of an illness that requires a parent to be in the hospital or receive medicines, both concepts with which they are familiar.

School age children are usually more exposed—through television, peer contact, and education—to the concept of cancer and terminal disease. Death is an idea they understand and have begun to deal with. At this point, it is nearly impossible to "hide" all the facts from a child without completely isolating him or her from the family or leaving the child unprepared in the case of the parent's death. An appropriate amount of information should be given, indicating that there is a serious illness requiring the parent's hospitalization and treatment. Children should be prepared for some of the more visible physical side-effects such as hair or weight loss. Such problems as pain or increased irritability, which may have a direct impact on the parent–child relationship, should be discussed. These efforts can help to alleviate fears and exaggerated fantasies. Continued communication and availability of both parents as much as the demands of the illness and treatment allow are important factors in avoiding the isolation of children during this stressful time. Availability of other close relatives to spend time with children and provide some continuity of normal family life can also help to lighten the anxiety and loneliness of a child whose parents are preoccupied with illness, hospitalization, and their own despair.

Direct questions from a child about the nature of the illness or the possibility of the death of a parent are usually better dealt with by giving an open-ended answer such as "Yes, this is a really serious illness, but the doctors are working very hard to make things better," or, "Yes, sometimes people can die of such an illness, but we sure hope that it won't happen to us." Complete denial of a serious situation often stands in direct contrast to the behavior and mood of the family and leaves the child confused and vulnerable to the fears aroused by his or her own fantasies and interpretations.

Children may exhibit a certain amount of anxiety, depression, and resentment at the fact that "normal life" is so radically interfered with by the parent's illness. They may suffer from insomnia, loss of appetite, and preoccupation with physical symptoms. The primary physician or pediatrician called to deal with such symptoms can be of much help by giving reassurance, after an appropriate examination, that everything is all right with their bodies, as well as by asking some questions about how things are going at home and how the ill parent is doing. This may provide an opportunity for these children to share some of their concerns, fears, and anxieties or to ask questions that they may find difficult to bring to either of their parents.

The Adolescent

Adolescents often have a particularly hard time with an ill or dying parent. Being in a process of separating emotionally from the parent, at times being in rebellion or "distancing" themselves as part of the normal adolescent process, they are suddenly confronted with the possibility of the premature loss of the person whose importance they are busy denying yet on whom they still depend for emotional, social, and financial support and guidance. Some adolescents react with complete withdrawal from the family during this period of time, keeping busy with school and social life, holding themselves basically unavailable to the needs of the family or being resentful if demands are made upon them. Other adolescents temporarily give up the adolescent growth process and return to a preadolescent closeness and dependency on the family, thus avoiding the guilt of abandoning the ill parent.Some adolescents have to take on major responsibilities in caring for the household, younger siblings, or even the ill parent, if the other parent is working. This may be rewarding, but it can also be an overwhelming experience for an adolescent, exceeding his or her physical and emotional resources. Emotional or somatic symptoms may then appear and should be taken seriously as a response to a stressful situation, requiring intervention, understanding, and support. At times a minor rearrangement of circumstances may make a major impact on the problem with which the adolescent is dealing.

Mary, the attractive, 16-year-old stepdaughter of a terminal lung cancer patient came to visit her stepfather daily in the hospital and stayed during and beyond all visiting hours. It became clear that she was also the main caretaker of the father when he was at home, doing all the shopping, cleaning, cooking, and physical care. She had dropped out of high school, and had at this point no social life. Her mother worked as a bar waitress, and slept during the day. Mary suffered from insomnia, had lost 10 pounds over the past 3 months, and had occasional attacks of migraine headaches. Her relationship to her stepfather was "very close," and concerned the nursing staff who felt uncomfortable with the extreme amount of time and care Mary lavished on him.

During a few brief meetings with Mary it became evident that several things concerned her greatly; her stepfather had been the first man in a long time who had been able to stop her mother from drinking too much and had brought some stability to a very disrupted family during the 2 years of his marriage to her mother. Mary would stay awake at night until her mother would come home, hoping that she would be sober. Mary also apparently felt that giving her stepfather the kind of care he needed to survive as long as possible would maintain the recent stable family structure, the first that Mary had ever experienced. Caring for the father had assumed high priority in Mary's mind to the exclusion of all else.

During the discussion with Mary the physician explored the need for her own schooling as a means of providing herself with a more stable life and regular income in the future; her need for more rest to avoid becoming so weakened that she could not care for her father, and the fact that she had not in the past, and would not now, be able to control her mother's actions. A homemaker was provided to take on some of the responsibilities of cooking and cleaning and caring for her father after his discharge. This allowed Mary to return to school and to spend some time with her peers. All of these changes made the remaining time for Mary and her father more worthwhile. After her father's death she was less isolated, with other human relationships to turn to and better prepared to take on the responsibilities of her own life.

The "Depleted" Family

The physical and psychological stress that family members of cancer patients are subject to, especially if the patient suffers from a long-drawn-out and slowly progressing illness, leaves the family often depleted, increasingly unable to give emotionally to the patient and at times reacting with withdrawal, resentment, and abandonment. "I wish it were over," is not an uncommon thought in the mind of a family member of a cancer patient, yet it is nearly always accompanied by feelings of guilt and shame. It is important that the professional staff remain aware of this fact and, when appropriate, point out to the family that feelings of depletion, resentment, and guilt are common, understandable, and normal human responses to an extremely painful experience. The need for physical and emotional respite has to be communicated to the family. Where possible, help from relatives, social agencies, or other support systems such as church organizations or private groups should be called on to assist the family in maintaining their own level of energy and equilibrium so that they can remain available to the patient. As in the case of Peter K, described previously, the terminal patient's fear of being abandoned may be intense, demanding constant attention and attendance and allowing little space for the family to take time to recover. The physician may, at times, have to strongly encourage family members to limit their visiting hours and to "take time out" in order to restore their own ability to cope and to relate constructively to the patient rather than to allow a debilitating bedside watch to continue. The acceptance of outside help needs to be explored with a resistent patient in the light of the needs and long-term availability of those close to him. Once a patient understands that a part-time nursing aide has not been called into the house or to the bedside as a substitute for the wife's or husband's participation in the care, but rather to free up energy, time, and greater availability for more relevant human interaction, he or she may react with less fear and resistence to such a change.

THE DYING PATIENT

The final stage of progressive disease usually brings the patient again back into a medically oriented setting—a general hospital, the cancer center, or, if the illness has progressed rapidly and with critical symptoms, into a more intensive treatment setting.

The General and Teaching Hospital

In spite of much recent public and professional discussion about death and dying and increased education and consciousness-raising of professionals and public alike, most hospitals and research institutions are not physically and pyschologically equipped to deal in a humane and supportive manner with the actual dying process. Professionals working exclusively with cancer patients, understandably, cannot allow themselves to get too emotionally close to their patients. Aggressive medical treatment makes quiet and peaceful periods difficult if not impossible for both patient and family. The professional staff will often respond to their own sense of helplessness or feelings of uselessness by withdrawing completing from the dying patient. Hospital regulations, space limitations and staff attitudes often allow little opportunity for families or friends to come and stay with a patient during his or her last days or hours. Intensive care units especially make any supportive human contact impossible and are probably the most isolating place for a terminal patient to die.

The primary physician may be able to fill some of this emotional void. He or she can contribute to the decision regarding the need to admit a patient to the ICU. Although no longer involved in making daily decisions regarding the patient's care, he or she can still play an important role in providing emotional support to the patient and family. Regular visits by a familiar physician in these frightening hospital settings can have a powerful therapeutic effect. The patient will feel freer to discuss his or her needs and fears with his or her own doctor than with the hospital staff.

Alternatives to Hospital Care

The primary physician can be of much help to a patient and his or her family in exploring alternative settings for the care of the terminal patient. Depending on the local community, any of the following alternatives should be considered and explored, and the problems and advantages of the specific situation for each particular patient considered.

Dying at Home

Many patients express a wish, when facing impending death, to be able to stay at home in their own environments and among their families. This is becoming again an increasing possibility. It may place much stress on the family, however, so it is important that the problems and possible complications be discussed well in advance. Many families find themselves quite overwhelmed with the idea of being confronted at home with sudden medical complications with which they are unprepared to deal. Some would feel uncomfortable in rendering simple medical or nursing care that the patient may require. However, if there is a real willingness on the part of both family and professional staff to take on this task, it can become a meaningful and enriching experience for all involved. Medical and nursing staff can assist family members in acquiring some specific skills, such as giving injections for pain, handling oxygen masks or suction pumps, and changing dressings, thereby increasing their confidence and sense of security. Arrangements for back-up services, home visits, and rehospitalization in case of a crisis can also alleviate much anxiety and allow a family to take on such a task.

Mrs. B, a 47-year-old divorced secretary was, after 3 years of valiant struggle with metastatic colon cancer, finally no longer able to take care of herself and her two preadolescent children. Her previously divorced husband had no contact with her or her children, and her only remaining support was a younger married sister who had adolescent children herself. Mrs. B's relationship with her sister had not been very close and not always very peaceful. She expected little help from her sister, other than to take her children and care for them after her death. During an extended hospitalization the nursing staff met with Mrs. B's sister and explored with her the medical stituation—the poor prognosis as well as the futility of any active treatment for Mrs. B. The sister had apparently not known of the terminal nature of Mrs. B's illness and began to reassess her relationship, as well as her own availability in this situation.

During the remaining weeks of hospitilization, the nurses, physicians, and Mrs. B's sister began to develop a plan for Mrs. B's discharge to her sister's home where she hoped to remain until her impending death. The sister and her oldest adolescent daughter came for instructions by the nursing staff and began to feel more confident and competent with the task that would confront them. Mrs. B remained in her sister's home for the remaining time of her life, except for a brief readmission for treatment of convulsions due to brain metastasis, which were controlled by medication. After Mrs. B's death at home, the sister expressed her gratitude for having been helped in taking on this task which allowed her to spend an intense and meaningful time of sharing and giving to her only sister. It allowed an easier transition and closer bondage for Mrs. B's two children who, during this time, participated in the care of their mother and came to appreciate the concern and care of their aunt.

The Hospice

In response to similar situations, the *ambulatory hospice* has been developed. Usually a group of professionals and volunteers are available to provide professional care, emotional support, and training of families in certain aspects of patient care and to act as consultants to staff in hospital settings. These ambulatory hospices, or similar support groups, exist in increasing number in many communities in the United States. They have proven to be of much help in those situations where patients and family would like to let the patient remain at home but need help to deal with the situation.

For those patients whose families cannot keep the patients at home, or for the patient who is alone and has no other human support, the inpatient hospice, if well run, can be a better place for a patient to die than a general hospital. Recent years have proven the value of such hospices, and the educational work of places such as St. Christopher's in London, have done much to eliminate from the public image the fear of "terminal" institutions. Hospices usually provide not just for their patients' physical welfare but also for their emotional well-being and peace of mind. A pleasant physical environment; liberal visiting policies for spouses, children, and friends, which allow for extended visits or even a continuous presence; and a willingness to accept death as a real and nonthreatening part of life allow for a more positive experience of the dying process for all involved. Some hospices attempt to maintain contact and give support to a patient's family after the patient's death.

Physicians and nurses in general hospitals or cancer treatment centers often are inadequately informed about the nature and functioning of existing hospices in their environment. Most hospices welcome and encourage visits from interested professionals, and such visits can do much to change one's image of such institutions, enabling physicians to make more appropriate referrals and easing their concern and anxiety about "sending patients away."

The Death of a Cancer Patient

The death of a cancer patient usually is expected and at times is welcomed by the patient as well as his or her family. The actual loss of a close person, however, no matter how long anticipated, will always remain an intense, and at times shattering experience to those involved. The survivors, depending on their closeness to the deceased, their own fears of death, and their specific life situations, will respond in a variety of ways to the death of the patient. Some family members will experience a sense of numbness or shock and will be unable for a period of hours or days to experience or express their grief. Often immediate practical demands surrounding a death, such as funeral arrangements, notification of other family members, payments of hospital bills, or arrangements of insurance claims, will leave little time to face and deal with the immediate loss. Widowed parents are not only left to face their own grief but are expected to be available to ease the pain of their children.

After the turmoil that often follows the death of a patient, a period of loneliness and depression sets in. Yet overwhelming new tasks, responsibilities, and demands may face the surviving members of a family or the widowed spouse. Several studies over the past decade have shown that the recently widowed population has a significantly increased health risk and mortality rate as compared with a "normal" population.[3] The primary physician should, therefore, be on the alert for physical and psychological symptoms that may indicate that the recent loss is taking a serious toll on the physical and emotional well being of the surviving family members. Occasional follow-up visits and phone calls inquiring about the physical and emotional well being of the family can provide this information and be highly supportive. Specific interventions may be indicated to deal with these problems.

The role of the practitioner in the diagnosis and treatment of malignant disease is clearly important and manifold: he or she is a provider of human and professional support to patient and family alike; a liaison between specialist and layman; a provider of continuity and consistency of care against the backdrop of large impersonal institutions. These are some of the vital functions that the practitioner can perform in a process that subjects patients and their families to serious and continuous physical, emotional, and social stress.

REFERENCES

1. Kornfeld DS: What Truth for Which Patient, at What Time. Guest editorial. CA, A Cancer Journal for Clinicians 28:256, 1978
2. Reiser SJ: Words as scapels: Transmitting evidence in the clinical dialogue. Ann Intern Med 92:837–842, 1980
3. Jacobs S, Ostfeld A: An epidemiological review of the mortality of bereavement. Psychosom Med 39:344–357, 1977

BIBLIOGRAPHY

Kavanaugh R: Facing Death. Baltimore, Penguin Books, 1974

Explores the meaning of death in the life of the individual and society; deals with attitudes toward death and dying within specific interpersonal, societal, and professional frameworks.

Kübler-Ross, E: On Death and Dying. New York, Macmillan, 1970

Kübler-Ross, E: Questions and Answers on Death and Dying. New York, Collier-Macmillan, 1974

Based on rich clinical experience; provides an elementary, step-by-step understanding of the psychological process related to dying and mourning.

Schoenberg B, Carr, Peretz, Kutcher: Loss and Grief—Psychological Management in Medical Practice. New York, Columbia University Press, 1970

Compendia of articles on psychosocial issues in terminal illness; provides useful material on practical patient-management issues; sections on "The Dying Patient" and "Reaction to Partial Loss" are particularly useful.

Weisman A: On Dying and Denying. New York, Human Sciences Press, 1972

Section on "Dying from a Fatal Illness—Cancer," gives rich psychological dynamics of "fatal illness."

Rollin, B: First You Cry. New York, New American Library, 1977

A well-known reporter describes her own experience of the diagnosis and treatment of breast cancer; gives a good sense of the subjective experience of illness and treatment.

Samuel C. Klagsbrun, M.D.

18

The Management of the Dying Patient and Death

Most readers of this chapter will have had ample experience in treating the dying patient. What have I, a psychiatrist, to offer to those of you who may have seen more death, experienced more responsibility for the dying, and suffered alone with this burden more than I have? You have all found your own ways of coping with death in your practices. You have developed techniques to help patients and families go through a very difficult period of time and you will not—and, probably should not—alter successful patterns that have grown out of your own experience. Yet it is my hope that you will find some of the following suggestions useful.

Know Thyself

To begin with, the biblical injunction "Know thyself" applies to all of us in medicine in a highly significant way. There is no point in having any one of us learn and attempt to use techniques that do not suit our personalities. For those of us who are reserved, who show little emotion, and who prefer to treat our patients from a distance, it is perfectly all right for us to continue in this style as long as we allow our patients to let us know of their suffering and worries. Those of us who are more effusive or emotional can use approaches that allow for that outgoing part of our personalities to function but within constraints that protect and safeguard our patients. We must guard against getting overinvolved and interfering excessively in their lives.

"Know thyself" also refers to being responsible for ourselves and setting limits on the amount of stress that we can tolerate. We must take into consideration the high suicide rate among physicians. That statistic suggests that we do not take care of ourselves adequately. Certainly for those of us who have had a great deal of exposure to dying patients, that statistic ought to serve as a significant warning. "Know thyself," therefore, means taking stock of our own inclinations to behave in a predictable fashion toward patients and to know ahead of time which situation, which patient, which kind of problem we have dealt with well in the past and which are the ones where our track record is not as good.

A person skilled in the area of mental health or supportive care should be available to any physician whose practice includes taking care of chronically sick and dying patients. That person—whether psychiatrist, social worker, or other professional—by virtue of knowing the physician's practice can serve as a consultant to both the physician and his or her patients. This arrangement ought to be one in which you feel comfortable getting advice over the phone or in making a referral of patients and families for supportive care. No physician ought to handle the entire burden alone, endlessly.

Know the Situation

Know the situation you are getting into. To the extent possible, know the total potential problems of the patient and the family ahead of time. For example, are you responsible for a patient who is quite independent and whose family members take their cues from the patient, or are you dealing with a patient whose family is the dominant force in his life? Ought you to speak to the family through the patient or should you spend more time in direct contact with the family?

Let me illustrate this issue with a clinical example:

> Mr. B, a 56-year-old man, was dying of a rapidly spreading carcinoma of the prostate. He was the founder and president of a bakery chain. He was a self-made man whose two daughters had married men who then became vice-presidents of his corporation. Mr. B's wife was a warm, adoring, and self-effacing woman who had desperately tried to keep her husband comfortable over the last year of illness and pain.
>
> Mr. B's physician was given explicit orders by Mr. B at the time of the original diagnosis not to discuss any aspect of his illness, and especially his prognosis, with his wife or family. "I will take care of this in my own way and in my own time," he told his physician. His doctor's admiration turned to confusion as time passed. He noticed that Mr. B was not preparing to transfer his business affairs to his sons-in-law. He was also aware that after a time Mr. B avoided all visitors and phone calls. Most of all, he noted that Mr. B had stopped asking him any questions. Mr. B was depressed. The physician, by following Mr. B's request not to discuss anything with Mrs. B or the family, had found himself at a loss as to how to proceed. When Mr. B died, his business was left in chaos. Mrs. B went into a profound depression and lived out her life in isolation and despair.

Both the physical and the emotional course of a patient's illness are fairly predictable if we pay attention to the clues presented to us. It was easy to predict Mr. B's behavior in the future when he gave the order to keep his illness a secret. His need to control his family right to the end was a paramount motivating force. His physician could have pointed out that Mr. B could have actually maintained far better control over the future of his wife, his business, and their family were he to have given his wife intensive training in business skills. He could have suggested how others could be of help to her in complex business matters. The recognition that Mr. B was using denial in an attempt to maintain control could have led his physician to find a way of helping him by actively insisting that he share the details of his illness with the family in order to help them prepare adequately for the future.

Stoic dying patients may thus present more severe problems to us and to their families than patients who demand endless help and support. The dependent patient prepares his family by constant reminders of the presence of illness and the nearness of death. The essential lesson is that most communications, even painful and irritating ones, are usually more helpful than the conspiracy of silence that surrounds so many dying patients.

The Use of Technical Skills

We physicians have had very little training either in medical school or in subsequent years in the nontechnical parameters of medicine. And yet, at the terminal stages of life, it is precisely those nontechnical aspects of medical care that increasingly matter as the disease takes its toll. At that time, technical medical expertise, though valid and important, will take second place to other values and issues in the life of the physician and his or her patient. We do not need to disparage technical expertise but to acknowledge that there is a need for other clinical skills in the terminal phase of life.

There are most certainly basic technical skills that a physician must utilize in managing the terminal phase of life. The old adage, "First of all, do not harm," applies here possibly more than at any other time in a patient's life, since this is the point when the patient has little strength, little stamina, and probably little hope. Doing no harm means decreasing the assaults on the body and on the spirit of the patient as much as possible. Therefore, research, academic interests, and fears of malpractice suits should all be laid aside in favor of focusing on the real needs of the patients. Tests seeking information that will not alter treatment plans—for example, identifying metastases in a patient for whom any further manipulation, chemotherapy, surgery, or radiation therapy would be fruitless—makes no sense. And what of the patient, near death, who develops an intercurrent infection? The decision regarding the use of an antibiotic then becomes as much a philosophical question as it is a technical medical question. Here we have an example of the possible conflict between the values of the patient and the family and the values of the physician.

In any treatment situation that has been based on reasonably open discussion from the beginning, such issues, ones hopes, would have been anticipated and discussed by the physician, the patient, and the family prior to entering expected moments of crisis. Clear guidelines ought to have been established before facing the terminal phase of life. For example, it seems reasonable to suggest that most families would agree that aggressive life support measures, such as the use of antibiotics in the situation just described, are not indicated. *The availability of medical skills does not necessarily mean the obligation to use them.*

Unfortunately, some physicians cannot accept their inability to control illness and as a consequence avoid patients in the final stages of disease. It is precisely when the more technical aspects of treatment become less important that the physician becomes more important as a person. Again, this does not mean having to spend a great deal of time at the bedside or becoming sentimental and maudlin. What it does mean is that by paying attention to patients' specific physical symptoms and using our clinical knowledge to relieve each one, we are paying attention to the entire person. After all, as physicians, our obligation is not only to cure but also to provide relief of suffering. For many patients in the late stages of illness, that is their only expectation of us. A physician who inquires daily at rounds about sleep patterns, constipation, nausea, skin breakdown, fatigue, mouth care, and so on is a physician who will be able to use his or her medical knowledge to provide total care. The skillful use of pain medication, tranquilizers, antidepressants, and steroids as palliative measures become of crucial importance to the patient in the latter stages of illness. We still have to "deliver the goods," treating the patient so as to make him or her more comfortable, even though we may have lost the battle for arresting the process of disease.

Communication

A physician who keeps the patient and his or her family realistically well informed of the patient's condition has a chance to help each person deal optimally with changing situations. The worst aspect of a progressive and fatal disease is often the lack of communication that obtains between family members, the patient and the medical staff. Hopes need to be kept within reasonably realistic boundaries for all. By helping each person anticipate the next phase that a patient faces, the physician is both preventing excessive grief and self-recrimination and allowing an opportunity for the healthy mourning that is so necessary for the health of the survivors.

An essential ingredient in treating a patient's terminal illness is honesty in the relationship between you and your patient. The trust the patient has in you as a physician is your most important tool. Your medical skills obviously also influence the extent to which the patient places his trust in you. But that is probably of secondary importance. That is why it is so important for physicians to pay very careful attention to the first meeting between themselves and their patients. It sets the tone for all future meetings. For example, if you, as the treating physician, have dealt with the patient in an honest and forthright manner from the initial moment of the diagnosis of a malignancy all the way through to the terminal phase of the illness—if you have been consistent, have predicted most of the turning points, and have described the side-effects and potential complications of all treatments accurately, you will have laid down a foundation of trust and reliablility. Therefore, any subsequent difficult aspect of your continuing work with the patient, will be accepted with little unnecessary difficulty. On the other hand, if you had been falsely hopeful and had sidestepped important issues in the course of the disease, if, in order to protect the patient from unnecessary mental pain, you had grossly misled the patient and the family (granted for the highest motives), you would have precious little to rely on in the terminal phases of the illness. It is at the end when you need the trust and faith of the patient the most.

There has been considerable discussion in recent years regarding the patient's right, or need, to discuss his or her impending death. In the final phases of illness there are patients who wish to delve philosophically into the questions of dying and the meaning, or lack of meaning, of life. There are patients who wish to express their fears of death. These patients should be able to have such talks as a matter of choice. However we should not force such discussions on patients in the name of truth or patient's rights. Certainly we should provide our patients with the opportunity to discuss these matters. This is done by allowing some time at the bedside for talk. Those patients who wish to have such a discussion will grasp the opportunity. Those who choose not to enter into such talks, won't.

Maintaining Hope

It is essential to maintain hope, but hope has to be based on a realistic acknowledgement of the patient's current situation and on reasonable expectations. Hope based on fabrications that are soon revealed as such can lead to a much greater loss of hope and more profound depression and bitterness. Such a situation often leads patients to seek false hopes elsewhere, and we may witness the sad spectacle of patients traveling to distant countries in search of miracle cures. In discussing the course of a disease in a positive fashion within realistic parameters, you can help the patient develop a sense of trust and faith in your ongoing efforts to find ways of being helpful.

We have learned a great deal from St. Christopher's Hospice in London—a facility that specializes in the care of the dying—about the roles of hope, comfort, and pain control. Patients who come to St. Christopher's know full well that they are most likely going to end their lives in that setting and yet, the atmosphere that permeates the hospice is filled with a sense of peace and comfort. Because of the magnificent pain control skills of the staff, the patients appear to have no anxiety and very little depression. There are often discussions at St. Christopher's about the possibility of living longer and even on occasion, beating the disease. Those discussions are not based on fantasies but on serious recognition that excellent care may mean being around long enough to benefit from new and ongoing research in the treatment of disease.

The patients, for the most part, are quite clear about the reality of their lives but they also seek, in a very active fashion, pleasure, joy, and control over their lives. Their energies are not channeled into chasing false dreams but rather into utilizing whatever is available to them in their environment that can make them feel special. Having your bed in the garden and watching the goldfish in the pond, taking part in services in the chapel from your bed on wheels, being able to listen to music from a small band in the garden—these things can all be part of feeling full of life in spite of major disease. This is what the finest care can offer to a patient and his or her family.

It is important to stress that it is not up to the physician alone to undertake this entire, complicated, time-consuming and trying task. A physician who has an ally in the form of a skilled interviewer, such as a social worker, a psychiatrist, a psychologist, or a skilled nurse, can delegate some of the responsibility for maintaining contact with everyone to that person. Physicians who practice with colleagues and are open to the idea of mutual help and support are clearly able to remain more involved, supportive, and attentive to dying patients and their families than are physicians who practice alone.

The Role of Denial

There is a great deal of discussion, in the terminal illness literature, of the role of what psychiatrists call *denial.* Denial seems like something heavy and negative, something one ought not to do. Denial actually is a terribly important and healthy phenomenon in all of our lives. As children we used it daily in our recess periods: playing ball in the schoolyard for a few minutes allowed us to forget the math quiz that awaited us as soon as we walked back into the classroom. Denial was very important for us then and it certainly continues to be important for us as adults. Vacations are a kind of denial. Reading an exciting novel, listening to music, playing golf—all of these things can be normal, healthy, and essential ways of using denial. Denial becomes unhealthy only if we spend our entire time in recess and never go back to take that math quiz, or never return to work from vacation.

Denial for a patient who faces death means running away mentally or even physically. What harm is done when the patient who has been told he has cancer chooses to talk about his "tumor" or his "ulcer"? What harm is done when a patient interrupts hospital routine for a family gathering or puts off a very important x-ray for a day in order to be present at an affair set up by a local church? Denial can allow for a moment of intimacy with people who are close and loving, ignoring the paraphernalia of the sick room.

Although, as the reader can see, denial is extremely useful, it can be self-destructive in those instances where symptoms of treatable illness are ignored. It can lead to the search for quack cures. It can prevent families from taking the proper financial steps to avoid unnecessary estate tax problems for survivors. Denial also can lead to profound psychological consequences. For example, families that remain unprepared for death can suffer from profound pathological mourning reactions, leaving them unable to reattach to life. Denial prevents proper mourning for the loss, and incomplete mourning prevents new relationships from forming. Impoverished relationships can lead to isolation, loneliness, and depression and, finally, to illness, where the cycle begins again.

Dealing With Family and Friends

The way you handle your relationship with the family and friends of the patient takes on added significance during the terminal phase of an illness. It is often helpful for the physician to suggest specific tasks family and friends can carry out; for example, minor nursing responsibilities, running errands, sitting with the patient (by assignment, to share the responsibility), and reading to the patient. These constructive tasks become meaningful as part of the ongoing process of bereavement, which begins before death actually occurs. As in every other situation discussed here, a balance must be maintained between inviting the family to participate in the care of the patient and taking care to prevent them from overdoing it. You may have to "order" family members to limit their help and their visits in order to prevent them from abusing themselves and neglecting other responsibilities. Their feelings of guilt may not permit them to limit their time at the bedside unless you take responsibility for their doing so.

After the death of a patient, it is extremely important for the physician to set up follow-up appointments in subsequent months for close family members and make sure that they do not fall prey to pathological mourning. Since it is often not possible for practicing physicians to assume all of these responsibilities, it is important for them to acquaint themselves with community resources that may be available to carry on the tasks required in these situations. For example, the clergy can be encouraged to maintain scheduled contact with the bereaved for a year and trained to detect the signs and symptoms of major depressive disorders. A referral to a physician can then be made.

A clinical example that combines a number of suggestions expressed in this chapter follows.

Mr. W, a man of considerable talent and success developed prostatic carcinoma at the age of 62. His family consisted of his wife, two daughters and one grandson. Mr. W. spent a year having elaborate and absolutely first-rate treatment for his cancer. Unfortunately, he developed metastases to his spinal cord with the suggestion of metastases to the brain. At the end of the year he was quite sick, confined to bed, and getting increasingly weaker and more dependent on everyone around him. His family, physician, and community hospital did a superb job in treating him.

When it became increasingly clear that his disease was getting the best of him, Mr. W became despondent and, in the hope of cheering him up, everyone who loved him increased the tempo of their encouragement. Promises for cures that earlier were dealt with in a much more rational fashion became more strident. Plans for the future, which earlier were circumspect, now were portrayed as definite plans. Mr. W, a realistic man, smiled and became less communicative. He stopped reporting symptoms though he was noticed by the nurses to groan and wince periodically, indicating pain and discomfort. The physician and his consultants offered more experimental chemotherapy and other increasingly drastic measures. Mr. W refused to accept the treatment offered and explained that he was well aware, by virtue of his past experience, of the side-effects and did not wish to die (as he put it), "while vomiting." His family despaired.

Finally, at Mr. W's insistence, the family began exploring the possibility of having him moved from the hospital to a local hospice. One of Mr. W's daughters visited the hospice and made the arrangements for his transfer. The first question that the admitting physician asked him at the moment when he was transferred to his bed was, "Where is your pain?" Adequate doses of oral morphine were given around the clock on a four-hour basis, with additional prn doses in between. Mr. W was awakened during the night and given the pain medication since it was predictable that were he to be allowed to sleep through the fourth hour, he would awaken with pain shortly thereafter. In this way he was guaranteed freedom from pain for the price of occasionally interrupted sleep. He began to experience severe headaches, probably related to his metastases. No CT scan or skull x-rays were ordered, but he was given steroids to decrease intracranial pressure and, within a short time he had relief from his headaches.

It was essential during Mr. W's short stay at the hospice to treat his discomfort sufficiently so that he could spend a little time with his grandson, something he so desperately wanted to do prior to his death. The little boy, who was five years old, was prepared carefully for the changes in his grandfather, since he had not been allowed to see him for the past two months because of the rules of the previous hospital forbidding children under 13 from visiting. The boy spent time in the room, chatted with his grandpa, drew pictures, touched him and commented quite openly on how grandpa had changed. During the visit, which turned out to be the last one, Mr. W was able to compliment his grandson on his lovely pictures, and with everyone weeping, said goodbye, for him, his most important remaining task. The hospice physician spent time with the child and his parents afterward to be sure that there was no fear, just sadness, and a sense of completion and thankfulness for having been able to experience this moment. Mr. W died a few hours later.

This, in the author's view, is a fine example of good medical care; that is, care focused on relief of symptoms that allowed the patient to go on with the business of his life, whatever was left of it, to take control and do what he wanted to do most of all, to say goodbye to his grandson. It is also good preventive medicine because it allowed this family to grieve, free of many of the unresolved issues that can interfere with the mourning process.

Death in the Young

The management of fatal illness in the young can be an overwhelming experience for medical staff as well as families. A physician who has responsibility for the care of young children, adolescents, or even young adults has to face these situations periodically. There is no better way to help everyone, including the patient, the family, and the rest of the staff, face the impending death of that young person than to prepare the families, from the beginning, for the likelihood of the death of the patient. Here, introducing reality becomes an essential, though most difficult, ingredient in the care of the family and the patient. And yet, in these situations, because of the age of the patient, our tendency is to be most hopeful. Of course it is important to maintain hope and, most certainly, it is important to keep as positive an attitude as possible, but almost never at the cost of distorting reality. A family that is able to grieve before the death of the youngster is a family that will be better able to come to terms with that death, pay attention to the other children, and plan for its own future than the family for whom denial has been the way of dealing with the illness.

Harry, a 10-year-old dying of leukemia, had been protected repeatedly by his parents from knowing the terribly grim prognosis of his disease. After his fourth admission in about two years of treatment, Harry became uncooperative, fighting the staff, the treatment, and, most painfully, his parents. The ward suggested a psychiatric consultation.

The psychiatrist described his first few moments with Harry as among the most important learning experiences in his life. Harry, he said, had looked at him with the darkest, saddest, and wisest eyes he had ever seen, and said, "Are you also selling hope today?"

To his credit, the psychiatrist said, "No, not today—the sale ended yesterday." Harry smiled and said, "OK, we can talk."

This conversation could undoubtedly only take place with a 10-year-old who had seen and experienced enough for a 30-year-old—but that too is the reality of these children. Their experiences call for a different level of relating—a more honest level, if they ask for it, and a more realistic level, if they sound doubtful about your overenthusiastic assurances.

The words to use ought to be words validating their feelings, such as, "You are right, this stinks," "I don't blame you for being angry," "Let's cry first and then take the shot," "Let's think of a reward that will make this miserable day that's coming up worthwhile." Encouragement, bribing, special treats—all the techniques of childrearing are stretched to the fullest—but at the core is the desperate need to maintain a relationship of trust and integrity along with hope. Those who can manage it well are to be praised as true healers. The demands are enormous, and all of us falter.

The physician, in his relationship with a young patient, must thus use concepts, language, and images commensurate with the patient's level of sophistication. Avoid technical language such as the names of organs that may be unfamiliar. Use simple drawings to show areas affected. Though most physicians are totally aghast at the notion of carrying dolls around on rounds, it is a useful way of being more graphic with a child and also of entering their normal world rather than forcing them to try to understand our world and ways of talking. Allowing the patient to maintain as much control as possible over his or her activities, especially at this time of life, is part of the proper treatment approach. Having patients go home periodically, handle their own medication, continue their education with a tutor is a statement that their life is still to be lived.

A pediatric oncologist in Cleveland has each one of his adolescent patients take his home phone number with the full expectation that from time to time his patients will want to call him. One wonders how that man manages to balance the needs of his own family with the needs of his patients. He and his family are most remarkable for offering themselves in that way. However, it is interesting to note that he reports that patients rarely call. Just knowing that he is available is usually enough. Offering such help before it is demanded often results in its never being required excessively. That same oncologist also offers his patients and their families an open-ended invitation to visit his laboratory to see the nature and extent of his research as an expression of hope in the constant work going on in the lab which may be of help to the visitors. This is an example of excellent support within the bounds of reality.

Young and old often fear abandonment and isolation more than death itself. Therefore, a child, as well as an adolescent, must be informed in suitable language about the state of his disease. This places a tremendous burden on the physician, who often has to overcome the reluctant parents' hesitation in facing this ordeal as well as his own natural feelings of wanting to spare the child undue psychological pain. Frequent meetings with family and friends, keeping them posted and helping them by gradually using reality-bound words will encourage a realistic approach to the patient and prepare them for the inevitability of their loss. It is far better to work through the depression and the difficulties while going through the process of working with the patient and the family than to deal with the complications that follow the death of a patient whose family has not been adequately prepared.

Having presented the above in as positive and helpful a fashion as I know, I must, for the sake of truth and in the service of reality, add a comment about the effect of death in the young on those involved. I know of no parent, physician, or other involved health professional who has experienced the death of a young person without being affected in a damaging way. The death of a young patient can never be rationalized. There is no "acceptance" of young death—only a "coming to terms", an absorption of the blow, which always leaves a mark.

Parents who have experienced the loss of their child, therefore, require long term follow-up treatment as part of proper medical management. Marriages fail, depression takes its toll, acting-out behavior takes place for months, and even years after the death of the child. This is not to say that psychopathological reactions are universal occurrences, but certain kinds of suffering are beyond our ability to endure without the development of scar tissue. The more serious disruptions are more likely to occur in families where relationships are already tenuous, although all families are at risk. The appropriate prophylactic intervention is referral to an experienced psychotherapist. Should the family reject this suggestion, the situation should be monitored with follow-up visits and phone calls. They will appreciate your support and may become motivated for a referral at a later date.

Health care professionals must also be conscious of their own needs. The experience of loss is a constant accompaniment of this area of health care. The loss of young patients is an especially difficult burden to bear. For the physician facing continuing losses of young patients, frequent vacations, a supportive environment, and active interests in matters beyond medicine are essential. Having taken all the possible precautions, the scars will still be there. Those who continue in this field, therefore, deserve a special level of recognition and respect.

The Unexpected Death

Unexpected deaths are always enormously difficult for medical staff to handle, and they are certainly traumatic for families. The physician has a unique responsibility in these situations to pay careful attention to the survivors. There has long been a tradition surrounding unexpected death of having sedation available for the survivor who is overcome with grief, shock, and fear. Whether the untimely death is due to an unexpected physical disease, to an accident, or to suicide, the need for the physician on the spot to help the family find a way of coping with the death is great. The job of the physician at that time is to urge the family, at the risk of seeming to ignore their pain, to verbalize their feelings over and over again in order to gain control over a tragedy. The physician, who may already know the course of events that took place, should still have the family describe the details of these events—repeatedly. The tendency on the part of many people surrounding a family at such moments is to shield them from the event and to expect and hope that the physician will sedate them. Unless there are terribly unusual circumstances, sedation is probably the worst treatment a physician might offer at such a time.

The desperate need is to push the family to find a vocabulary through which they can express their feelings—whether they are rage, anger, shock, grief, or even embarrassment—about what has occurred. A family that can find a way to describe what has happened is a family that is in the process of regaining control both over themselves and over the event. A family that is too overcome to describe what happened may live with a sense of dread and fear, crippled in the future by virtue of never having been able to overcome the overwhelming experience. That family is also more prone to handle future pain and stress in a much more anxiety-laden manner.

A most terrible event that I can share with you—and one that I hated at that time and still dread ever to face again—involves the circumstances surrounding the death of an 8 year-old girl who was standing behind her father's car as he backed out of the driveway. The father brought his dead girl into the emergency room. We were all horrified at this terrible accident. My treatment of the father consisted of insisting that this poor man talk about the accident in great detail. Only after I helped him put words to his experience did I allow him to go home. He came back to the hospital the next day and talked some more. Many months later this grief and guilt-ridden man told me that he would never get over his carelessness but that he would have to live with it. He had a sense of responsibility and of unalterable loss, but because he could also talk about it he could go on living—although he would never be the same man. I think facing the horror of that moment at the time helped him come to grips with a reality from which he might otherwise have continued to flee. Words of comfort and solace are extremely important but only after the fact and experience of death has been mastered. Mastery means putting impossible situations into words, which can then be dealt with. The theme, therefore, that has run through this entire chapter is that of the need to master events, not be crippled by them.

A physician is often called upon to respond to a person who is dying not from illness or accident but because the person chooses to die at his or her own hand. More often than not, in spite of many warning signals, the family may be totally surprised by the event they face. The wish to deny the reality serves two purposes: one is to undo the guilt that may be felt if the suicide is aimed as an accusing finger at the family. The second is to avoid the embarrassment the family may feel over such an event. It was not that long ago in the history of civilization that people who had committed suicide were forbidden burial in cemeteries as an expression of disapproval of the deed. The family's apparent embarrassment and guilt often put pressure on the physician to camouflage the events. But to do this can have tragic consequences.

Most certainly, if the patient has attempted suicide but has not died, clearly identifying the event as a suicide attempt may be a life-saving move. For example, a patient who is seen as having "accidentally" fallen onto the subway tracks rather than having jumped in front of a train and who is discharged from the hospital after a negative physical examination is a patient who has been misdiagnosed and inadequately treated. Such a patient, without proper care, will most likely try to kill himself or herself again. Similarly, the patient who has attempted suicide by ingesting pills but who has recovered and now appears quite cheerful is a patient who may have released a certain amount of tension by the behavior but who remains in desperate need of psychiatric treatment. Such a patient, left alone in a hospital room, may again attempt suicide in that very setting if not watched by the staff. Even more likely is the repetition of the suicide attempt after discharge from the hospital if this desperate act of communication is ignored. Psychiatric consultation should therefore be mandatory with any suicide gesture or attempt. The psychiatrist should be called immediately even if the patient is unconscious. In this early stage, the family or friends may provide important information that they may later choose to withhold when the patient is clearly out of danger.

What of the family that has been left behind when a suicide has taken place? Here the sad fact is that every suicide I have ever worked with or discussed with a colleague had a finger-pointing aspect to it. In every circumstance, that finger is pointed at another individual, often a family member, sometimes a particular friend. It is not that the patient is saying, "You did this to me"; it is more that he or she is saying, "You could have stopped this," or, "Had you done something, this might have been prevented." And because it is true that this often is the case, many times someone is left with a dreadful burden of guilt.

Do not be misled by the foregoing statement, however. Often the person who commits suicide has been in psychiatric treatment and the family has done a great deal to offset the patient's pain and depression but to no avail. With such families, the physician who appears on the scene can point out all the efforts that had been made to help the patient and that the family has done all it could. When the death is a surprise or when a family feels it might have prevented the suicide, it is important for the physician not to placate and soothe the family's feelings by denying that possibility but to try to find a way to help the family live with it. It is extremely important to help such individuals learn to forgive themselves—to acknowledge their errors of omission or commission but at the same time to recognize that none among us is infallible. Families who choose to ignore or deny that reality will usually find some way to punish themselves in the future.

What are some of the comments that a physician may make at such a time? You must always acknowledge the loss involved. "Yes, this is a terrible experience." Or, "Sometimes I wonder how it is possible to tolerate such pain." Or, "We would all feel terrible in such circumstances." Or, "It's impossible to avoid feeling some responsibility and guilt when faced with such a tragedy." These words invite recognition of the loss and the responsibility and underline your sharing of that feeling with the family. These are accepting, not judgmental, statements. They encourage the family to express their conflicted feelings. It is important to find a language that helps the family realize that they are not alone, and that you, as a representative of society, can understand and forgive. This, in turn, will make it easier for them to forgive themselves.

Summary

The management of the dying patient and death are among our most difficult tasks. Here are some basic principles that can guide you in their management:

- Help the people involved, patients and families, to verbalize the fact that something terrible, frightening, and unfair is happening. Use simple words to help them identify and express these feelings.
- Spend time with the patient and the family without feeling called upon to be falsely encouraging. Your presence is what counts, not your false promises or empty encouragement.
- Offer continuity of care, both for the patient and the family. Provide appointments even when you feel you have nothing to offer except your presence. Use your community resources as an extension of your office. You will ward off isolation, depression, and future morbidity by offering such continuity of care.
- And finally, take care yourself. Make sure that you build in ample opportunities to share with colleagues or friends the weariness of doing this kind of work. Build into your practice plenty of time off for pleasure so that you can be a more open and more caring physician. If you take good care of yourself, you will take better care of others.

Donald S. Kornfeld, M.D.

19

The Management of the Psychiatric Referral

So many of the chapters in this book come with the recommendation that if all else fails, refer your patient to a psychiatrist. The referral itself, however, requires skill in order for it to be effective. If not done properly, the physician will have made a recommendation that will not be followed. Some of the author's colleagues have patients who universally seem to follow their advice and call for appointments. Patients of other colleagues, however, just never do follow through on the advice that has been given. Later in this chapter, we will review some reasons for such differential success in making this kind of referral. Let us begin, however, by reviewing the circumstances in which we feel a psychiatric referral should be made.

The first type of patient who needs psychiatric referral is the person who manifests severe psychopathology. We have spent considerable time reassuring practicing physicians that they have the skills and knowledge, and more importantly, a relationship that can be used as the basis for the treatment of considerable psychopathology in their own offices. However, we must be realistic and acknowledge that there are certain situations in which they must refer a patient for more specialized help. Certainly, the suicidal patient must be referred. This patient will probably require hospitalization and treatment by a psychiatrist. Detailed management of that situation is outlined in Chapter 6. Acutely psychotic schizophrenic patients also require referral. Some can be managed in the office with the use of phenothiazines or haloperidol. However, when patients are very agitated and seriously delusional and a potential threat to themselves or others, hospitalization under psychiatric care is usually indicated (Chapter 7).

Certain serious family difficulties must also be referred for specialized help. Milano has reviewed a number of techniques that can be used by the family practitioner. However, certain complex family interactions will require a psychiatric referral (Chapter 8).

Perhaps the most subtle indication for referral is the presence in a patient of serious character pathology. Such individuals exhibit behavior patterns that have a significant detrimental effect on themselves and/or those around them. For example, individuals with extreme obsessive compulsive character traits, passive-aggressive character styles, or overly dependent behavior will require a psychoanalytic form of psychotherapy which is beyond the training of the average physician.

Certain diagnostic problems will also require psychiatric consultation. Although family practitioners, with their considerable knowledge of their patients, are in a position to make many diagnostic decisions regarding the role of psychological factors in illness, there will be certain situations in which they will require a psychiatrist to confirm their impressions. Often, however, the psychiatrist may be asked to go beyond the confirmation of the diagnosis and determine if some form of psychiatric treatment is indicated. The consultant can also be used when referring physicians are not sure that they have adequate psychiatric knowledge to treat particular cases. The physician and the consultant together can then make a decision regarding who can best treat the patient.

Why do some referrals fail? If improperly handled, referrals can make some patients very angry or frightened based on the following common misconceptions: (1) The doctor thinks they are imagining their complaints. (2) The doctor thinks they are crazy. (3) The doctor is trying to get rid of them as patients.

The physician must be alert to nonverbal cues in the patient's reaction to the suggestion of a referral. The patient may not state openly that he or she is offended, frightened, angered, or embarrassed at the suggestion of a psychiatric referral. However, the failure to pick up nonverbal cues will make the referral a meaningless exercise. The patient's chart may indicate that a referral has been made, but, in reality, nothing may come of it. Dealing with the patient's feelings in an open, direct way can neutralize them and allow the patient to get the help you think he or she needs.

How can these three misconceptions be dealt with? Let us assume that we are dealing with the common situation of a patient with a physical complaint that has been thoroughly evaluated with no organic findings. Perhaps the family doctor has evaluated the psychological factors and wants another opinion confirming his or her own, or perhaps the physician is convinced that emotional problems are contributing to the patient's difficulty and is now interested in having the patient consider some form of psychiatric treatment. In these situations, it is best to have the referring doctor make it clear to the patient that he or she is being referred to the psychiatrist only for a consultation. The doctor should point out that he retains the patient as his patient and that they both have the option of reviewing the psychiatrist's advice prior to moving ahead with any kind of plan.

The patient must be reassured that we do not think his or her complaints are imaginary. The patient should be told that the absence of positive findings on x ray or other diagnostic tests is good news. However, this does not mean that the patient is not suffering. Most patients, these days, have some understanding of the concept of psychosomatic illness. For example, many patients are willing to accept that illnesses such as peptic ulcer or coronary disease may be related to stress; that stress can reduce the body's resistance to illness; and that stress can produce pain through muscle spasm or hyperacidity, etc. Therefore, once reassured that *psychosomatic* does not mean "imaginary," the average patient will usually accept the psychiatric referral for consultation.

When patients fear that seeing a psychiatrist means that they are "crazy," their fear must be dealt with directly, in the referring doctor's office. It cannot be left to the psychiatrist to deal with this issue, since most such patients will never get to his or her office. It will also be a great deal more effective if the referring doctor makes this point. If patients express this concern, a flat statement should be made that you do not consider them "crazy" but, since doctors do not usually use that term, you would like to know what they mean by it. This may allow patients to share with you some previously unspoken information or fear. For example, a patient may reveal that a family member has a history of depression that required hospitalization back in the era before antidepressants and office management. The patient can be reassured that you do not anticipate the psychiatrist would recommend hospitalization. Or a patient may reveal some specific symptom not previously mentioned, such as a suicidal idea, a paranoid thought, or a phobia. The patient can be relieved by your accepting the information in a matter of fact manner and reassuring him or her that these are treatable problems. In most situations, however, you need only to reassure them that psychiatrists are not just for "crazy" people, but can also be of help to people with their kind of problem.

Some depressed patients can interpret the psychiatric referral as further evidence of their personal inadequacy. This self-derogation is part of the depression syndrome. Such patients should be told that we now understand that depression has a biological component that is beyond their control. They should know that their mood is probably the result of a defect in the neurotransmitter system in the central nervous system, that their depressed mood and thoughts cannot be changed by strength of will, and that the psychiatrist with his special knowledge of medication can do much to reverse the condition.

A referral for psychotherapy usually reflects your feeling that the patient needs help with intrapersonal or interpersonal conflict. Most patients will respond well to your acknowledgement of the problem and recommendation for professional help. The chronically anxious woman can be told that the answer to her problem cannot be the lifelong use of tranquilizers, and that the underlying sources of tension must be sought and dealt with. The depressed middle-aged man in a "mid-life crisis" should accept quite readily the concept that the resolution of this problem requires more than antidepressant medication. The patient with marital difficulty usually will accept, with great relief, your recommendation for marriage counseling.

Some patients assume that going to a psychiatrist means that somebody else is going to have to solve their problems. They can feel demeaned by the implication that they can't do it themselves. The referring doctor can point out that psychiatrists do not solve peoples' problems for them. However, as specialists who have worked with many people with similar difficulties, psychiatrists can often help patients to think about themselves and their situations from a different point of view. In this way patients may be better able to solve their problem themselves.

Patients have also derived their ideas about what psychiatrists are like from television and movies where the representation is not always flattering. It is helpful to point out that the psychiatrist to whom you are referring the patient is someone whom you know personally and someone you respect as a colleague. Patients should be told that the psychiatrist is going to want to know about their lives in order to help understand the stresses they may be experiencing; that the psychiatrist is interested in many more things than patients' sex lives; that the psychiatrist is not going to solve their problems with a brilliant interpretation in the first hour they meet. Above all, patients must sense that the psychiatrist is someone the referring doctor respects and a person to whom the doctor has referred other patients in the past. Patients must be assured that the psychiatrist is to be a consultant and not a substitute for the family physician.

The referring physician should call the psychiatrist and inform him or her of the referral and of the nature of the problem. Your knowledge of the patient and his family will be helpful to the psychiatrist. Be sure to tell the patient you are going to discuss him or her with the consultant. Most patients find it a lot easier to know that the psychiatrist is expecting their call and knows something about them. It also places a little more pressure on them to follow through on your recommendation.

One way of assuring that the referral is successful and of simultaneously communicating that the relationship with you continues is to suggest that the patient call you after the visit to the psychiatrist to discuss the patient's reaction. Tell the patient that you will also expect to confer with the psychiatrist regarding his or her recommendations. This will give you a chance to discuss any questions that the patient may have. It is advisable not to refer your patient to any psychiatrist who is unwilling to get back to you with a reasonable summary of what has transpired. There is nothing in the doctor–patient relationship between a psychiatrist and a patient that precludes a discussion of the patient's history between the referring physician and the psychiatrist as long as the patient understands that this is going to be done. It is a rare patient, indeed, who will not want his or her family physician to be apprised of the consultant's opinion and the data on which it is based. The psychiatrist need not go into great detail. Neither of you have that kind of time available. But a summary of the findings, formulations, and recommendations should be made. It may be difficult for some psychiatrists to supply this in writing as many of them do not have secretaries. However, a telephone call is a reasonable expectation, and you should have a consultant who is willing to do that.

In some cases where, despite your best efforts, the patient cannot accept your advice regarding the need for psychiatric treatment you may have to manage the case yourself. Such a patient may be persuaded to go for a consultation with the psychiatrist with the understanding that this will allow you to get expert advice regarding an appropriate treatment regimen. The psychiatrist can then be used for additional advice as needed.

There will also be those infrequent situations where, despite your best efforts, the patient refuses to accept your recommendation for either psychiatric consultation or treatment. With the suicidal or homicidal patient you may have to elicit the help of the local police and the patient's family in arranging for hospitalization. If you suspect that the patient will not go voluntarily, it is best not to tell the patient of your plan to call the police until after they have arrived in your outer office. This will prevent the patient's bolting out of the office once you have made your plan clear. Your receptionist can place the necessary calls while you engage the patient in conversation. Although we all hesitate to use coercion, it is obviously indicated in such a situation and in most cases, the patient is ultimately grateful.

What about the more common situations in which patients refuse to go for consultation and there are no indications for enforced treatment? In some cases, especially where you believe drugs can be helpful, you should try to get some advice from a psychiatric colleague. Such supervised treatment can be quite effective. After all, that is the way most psychiatrists are trained.

Where drugs are not indicated and the patient resists a referral for psychotherapy, you must learn to be patient and hope that at a future date the patient will be motivated. You might suggest that the patient give the idea more thought and return for another appointment to discuss it further with you. Patients who pride themselves on their independence may need to decide for themselves when treatment should begin. Above all, patients must not be made to feel rejected for failing to take your advice.

What do you do if the patient calls to tell you the psychiatric visit was so upsetting that he or she is not going back? First, call the psychiatrist and get his or her perception of what transpired during the hour. It is possible that the patient misunderstood something that was said or not said. You are in the best position to clarify this. Try to determine what the misperception may have been, and then encourage your patient to return to the psychiatrist to discuss it with him or her directly. All this may be difficult at first for the patient. However, if the relationship with the psychiatrist is to continue, it will help the patient to understand that the basis for that relationship has to be one of complete openness and honesty. If, however, the "chemistry" between the patient and your first consultant was not right, it may be necessary to make another referral. Your first psychiatric consultant may be the best person to suggest another psychiatrist who may have different personality characteristics and thus provide a better fit for this particular patient.

A word about the psychiatric referral in the general hospital is pertinent here. House officers are sometimes reluctant to tell their patients that they have requested a psychiatric consultation, fearing that the patient will get upset and angry with them. They may forget to tell the patient, or use a euphemism in telling the patient a psychiatric consultation has been requested. Unfortunately, these techniques invariably backfire because the patient is quick to learn that the consultant is a psychiatrist. The patient will then surely get angry at the house officer, not for requesting the consultation, but for not telling them of the plan. This difficulty can be avoided if the house officer uses the principles outlined above in dealing with his or her own projected concerns.

In summary, the referring doctor must take the process of referral seriously. This will require attention to what you say, how you say it, and how you deal with your patient's reaction to it. If you fail to do these things, the patient's chart may show a referral for a form of treatment that the patient clearly needs but may never receive because of the manner in which the referral process was handled.

Index

a
b
c
d
e
f
g
h
i
8 2 j